Allen & Hanburys®
DIVISION OF GLAXO INC.

D0075299

Dear Doctor:

Allen & Hanburys, developer of VENTOLIN® (albuterol, USP/albuterol sulfate, USP) and BECLOVENT® (beclomethasone dipropionate, USP), is pleased to present you with this complimentary copy of the 1992 edition of <u>Current Pulmonology</u>. This new book demonstrates Allen & Hanburys' dedication to the medical profession and effort to be an indispensable partner in health care.

For information about Allen & Hanburys products, please contact your Allen & Hanburys sales representative.

Sincerely,

Charles A. Sanders, MD
Chairman & Chief Executive Officer
Glaxo Inc.

Please consult complete prescribing information for VENTOLIN and BECLOVENT on last pages. VIN836

Five Moore Drive, Research Triangle Park, NC 27709 • Telex 802813 • Telephone (919) 248-2500

CURRENT

PULMONOLOGY®

VOLUME 13

Edited by

Daniel H. Simmons, M.D., Ph.D.

Professor of Medicine, Emeritus
Department of Medicine
Division of Pulmonary and Critical Care Medicine
UCLA School of Medicine
Los Angeles, California

Donald F. Tierney, M.D.

Professor of Medicine
Department of Medicine
Division of Pulmonary and Critical Care Medicine
UCLA School of Medicine
Los Angeles, California

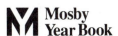

**Mosby
Year Book**

St. Louis Baltimore Boston Chicago London Philadelphia Sydney Toronto

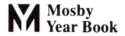
Mosby
Year Book

Dedicated to Publishing Excellence

Sponsoring Editor: Amy L. Reynaldo
Associate Managing Editor, Manuscript Services: Denise Dungey
Assistant Director, Manuscript Services: Frances M. Perveiler
Production Supervisor: Timothy A. Phillips
Proofroom Manager: Barbara M. Kelly

Produced in association with Clinical Communications,
Inc. Greenwich, CT 06830

Editorial Office:
Mosby–Year Book, Inc.
200 North LaSalle St.
Chicago, IL 60601

International Standard Serial Number: 0163-7800
International Standard Book Number: 0-8151-7743-7

Contributors

Deborah J. Cook, M.D., F.R.C.P., M.Sc.
Assistant Professor
Department of Medicine
Division of Critical Care and Department of Clinical Epidemiology and
 Biostatistics
McMaster University School of Medicine
McMaster University Medical Center
Hamilton, Ontario, Canada

Diana S. Dark, M.D.
Associate Professor of Medicine
Division of Pulmonary Disease and Critical Care Medicine
University of Kansas Medical Center School of Medicine
Kansas City, Kansas

Scott F. Davies, M.D.
Associate Professor of Medicine
University of Minnesota Medical School—Minneapolis
Director, Pulmonary Division
Hennepin County Medical Center
Minneapolis, Minnesota

Lisa L. Dever, M.D.
Fellow, Infectious Diseases Division
Department of Medicine
University of Texas Health Science Center at San Antonio
San Antonio, Texas

v

J. Bernard L. Gee, M.D.
Professor of Medicine
Pulmonary and Critical Care Section
Department of Internal Medicine
Yale University School of Medicine
New Haven, Connecticut

W.G. Johanson, Jr., M.D.
Professor and Chairman
Department of Medicine
UMDNJ New Jersey Medical School
Newark, New Jersey

Theodore W. Marcy, M.D.
Assistant Professor of Medicine
University of Minnesota
Pulmonary and Critical Care Section
St. Paul–Ramsey Medical Center
St. Paul, Minnesota

John J. Marini, M.D.
Professor of Medicine
University of Minnesota
Pulmonary and Critical Care Section
St. Paul–Ramsey Medical Center
St. Paul, Minnesota

Nestor L. Müller, M.D., Ph.D.
Associate Professor
Department of Radiology
University of British Columbia
Vancouver General Hospital
Vancouver, British Columbia, Canada

Susan K. Pingleton, M.D.
Professor of Medicine
Division of Pulmonary Disease and Critical Care Medicine
University of Kansas Medical Center School of Medicine
Kansas City, Kansas

Richard J. Pisani, M.D.
Assistant Professor of Thoracic Disease and Critical Care Medicine
Mayo Medical School
Mayo Clinic
Rochester, Minnesota

Jonathan D. Plitman, M.D.
Senior Fellow
The Center for Lung Research
Vanderbilt University School of Medicine
Nashville, Tennessee

Thomas A. Raffin, M.D.
Chief, Division of Pulmonary and Critical Care Medicine
Co-Director, Stanford University Center for Biomedical Ethics
Stanford University School of Medicine
Stanford University Medical Center
Stanford, California

Edward C. Rosenow, III, M.D.
Arthur M. and Gladys D. Gray Professor of Medicine
Thoracic Disease and Internal Medicine
Mayo Medical School
Mayo Clinic
Rochester, Minnesota

Frederick L. Ruben, M.D.
Professor of Medicine
University of Pittsburgh School of Medicine
Montefiore University Hospital
Pittsburgh, Pennsylvania

George A. Sarosi, M.D.
Clinical Professor of Medicine
University of Arizona College of Medicine
Chairman, Department of Internal Medicine
Maricopa Medical Center
Phoenix, Arizona

James R. Snapper, M.D.
Professor of Medicine
The Center for Lung Research
Vanderbilt University School of Medicine
Nashville, Tennessee

Stephen R. Thom, M.D., Ph.D.
Assistant Professor of Medicine
Chief, Hyperbaric Medicine
Institute for Environmental Medicine
University of Pennsylvania School of Medicine
Philadelphia, Pennsylvania

Charles V. Zwirewich, M.D.
Clinical Instructor
Department of Radiology
University of British Columbia
Vancouver General Hospital
Vancouver, British Columbia, Canada

Publisher's Preface

Publication of *Current Pulmonology*®, volume 13, marks the end of an outstanding era of editorship by Daniel H. Simmons, M.D., Ph.D. During each of Dr. Simmons' 13 years as editor of the series, the volume's readers have been treated to a wealth of information about the most important topics in pulmonology. Dr. Simmons' leadership and vision inspired the series and fostered its tradition of quality and success. We extend to him our deepest appreciation for the services he has provided and for his unending support and enthusiasm for *Current Pulmonology*®.

Donald F. Tierney, M.D. joins Dr. Simmons in editing volume 13. Beginning with volume 14, Dr. Tierney will edit *Current Pulmonology*® alone, carrying on the tradition of distinguished editorial direction. We welcome Dr. Tierney as we extend our heartfelt thanks and appreciation to Dr. Simmons for his years of excellent contribution.

Preface

Since 1979, I have edited 12 annual volumes of *Current Pulmonology*®. This year, I am happy to announce that there are two coeditors, Dr. Donald F. Tierney and myself. And next year there will be another change: Dr. Tierney will be the sole editor.

My twelve years as sole editor and my one year as coeditor were both enjoyable and fruitful, but I feel it is time to hand over the entire job to someone else to avoid my arranging new volumes to reflect the past rather than the present and the future.

I cannot imagine a new editor more appropriate and qualified than Dr. Tierney. He has been a prominent investigator, teacher, and clinician for many years. But he has also been very active in pulmonary organizations—a few years ago he was president of the American Thoracic Society—and therefore he knows well which other investigators, teachers, and clinicians are most appropriate authors for *Current Pulmonology*.®

Over the years, I have worked with four publishing houses and with numerous editors to whom I owe gratitude for allowing the series to continue with its initial bent toward both the basic science of pulmonary disease and its clinical aspects. To my knowledge, this format is still unique to *Current Pulmonology*® and it justifies the series continuation even at a time when there are so many publications in the pulmonary field.

But of those connected with *Current Pulmonology*,® I must thank its authors the most. They have given a great deal of their time and expertise—with little reward—to keep others current in the many old and new areas of pulmonary disease.

To all these people, another thank you. And to Dr. Tierney, my best wishes.

Daniel H. Simmons, M.D., Ph.D.

Contents

Publisher's Preface ix
Preface xi

1 / Nosocomial Pneumonia
by Lisa L. Dever and W.G. Johanson, Jr. 1

2 / Ethics in Cardiopulmonary Medicine
by Deborah J. Cook and Thomas A. Raffin 29

3 / Modes of Mechanical Ventilation
by Theodore W. Marcy and John J. Marini 43

4 / Nutritional Support of the Critically Ill
by Diana S. Dark and Susan K. Pingleton 91

5 / Viral Infections of the Respiratory Tract
by Frederick L. Ruben 119

6 / Nonspecific Airway Hyperresponsiveness: Mechanisms and Meaning
by Jonathan D. Plitman and James R. Snapper 143

7 / Conventional and High-Resolution Computed Tomography of Chronic Infiltrative Lung Disease
by Charles V. Zwirewich and Nestor L. Müller 193

8 / Occupational Lung Disease
by J. Bernard L. Gee 221

9 / Fungal Diseases
by George A. Sarosi and Scott F. Davies 257

10 / Carbon Monoxide Poisoning
by Stephen R. Thom 289

11 / Drug-Induced Pulmonary Disease
by Richard J. Pisani and Edward C. Rosenow, III 311

Index 313

CHAPTER 1

Nosocomial Pneumonia

Lisa L. Dever, M.D.

Fellow, Infectious Diseases Division, Department of Medicine, University of Texas Health Science Center at San Antonio, San Antonio, Texas

W.G. Johanson, Jr., M.D.

Professor and Chairman, Department of Medicine, UMDNJ New Jersey Medical School, Newark, New Jersey

Hospital-acquired pneumonia is not a new problem, nor is it solely a product of advancing medical technology. Seriously ill patients with either acute or chronic illnesses have always been susceptible to the development of pneumonia, usually with disastrous consequences. These pneumonias, often referred to as "terminal bronchopneumonias," were caused by a variety of organisms.[1] Although aerobic gram-negative bacilli (GNB) were isolated from the secretions and lung tissue of patients dying of pneumonia well before the advent of antibiotics, their significance often was overlooked in favor of the far more virulent organisms that did, and still do, cause community-acquired pneumonias.[2, 3] Over the past 40 years or so, medical progress has created large new groups of patients at risk and the organisms responsible for respiratory infections acquired in the hospital have shifted in response to several factors, including antibiotic pressure, environmental hazards, and remarkable changes in host resistance. In recent years, significant progress has been made in understanding the pathogenesis of these infections and in defining the organisms responsible. In addition, more effective antimicrobial agents hold the promise of improved patient outcomes. We will review advances in each of these areas.

PATHOGENESIS

Pneumonia for our purposes here can be defined as an inflammatory condition in the distal lung caused by the presence of microorganisms. Requirements include an organism, a route of inoculation into the lungs, and an inadequate response by the host's defenses. The latter must always exist regardless of the causative organism, but the impaired elements of defenses may differ widely for infections caused by bacteria, viruses, fungi, or protozoa.

Most nosocomial pneumonias are caused by bacteria. The causative organisms usually are not found in samples of hospital air and transmission to the patient is by direct contact, either on the hands of hospital personnel or by fomites.[4] Alternatively, the patient's own bacterial flora, usually resident in the gastrointestinal tract, may be translocated to the oropharynx.[5] Colonization of the oropharynx allows the organisms to persist and multiply. Successful colonization of this region requires that the newly implanted organism be able to avoid removal by host defenses, and this usually is accomplished by adherence of the bacterial cell to host epithelial cells. A variety of adherence mechanisms have been described and it appears that this is a general phenomenon that mediates many, if not all, bacterial interactions with mucosal surfaces.[6] One of the features of serious illness is an increase in the binding of GNB by buccal epithelial cells in vitro, an alteration in host defense that appears to correlate well with susceptibility to colonization and pneumonia caused by these agents.[7] Certain organisms, notably *Pseudomonas aeruginosa,* appear better able to bind to tracheobronchial cells than to buccal cells, a feature that may explain the occasional presence of this organism in tracheal secretions while it apparently is not in the oropharynx.[8]

Some evidence suggests that colonization of the stomach may be an important step in the pathogenesis of some nosocomial pneumonias.[5] Serious illness often is accompanied by a decrease in gastrointestinal motility, with a resultant proliferation of the indigenous gut flora. It has been proposed that this flora may propagate retrograde to colonize the small intestine and stomach.[9] Alternatively, bacteria entering the oropharynx are swallowed and may colonize the stomach by that route.[5] Under normal circumstances, the acid milieu of the stomach provides an effective barrier to colonization and bacterial counts in the normal stomach are low, if present at all.[10] Diminishing gastric acid by either neutralization or inhibition of secretion is associated with an increased bacterial burden, especially when the pH rises above 3.0. Clinically, acid inhibition for prophylaxis of stress bleeding has been associated with an increased risk of nosocomial pneumonia in several studies.[9, 11] Prophylaxis with sucralfate does not raise pH and does not appear to increase the risk of pneumonia, although the number of patients in each of these trials is small. In addition, there is some evidence that sucralfate has direct antibacterial activity that may contribute to its effectiveness.[12] Studies done with sequential cultures at various sites have yielded somewhat inconclusive results as to the order of these events.[5] It seems clear that colonization of the oropharynx occurs first in some patients, followed by colonization of the stomach and tracheobronchial tree. In other patients, organisms are detected first in the stomach, followed by colonization of the oropharynx. It should be kept in mind when considering these studies that cultures of the oropharynx, in particular, may miss organisms that are present in one or another area but are not uniform in distribution, or may be present only in low concentrations. The important concept is that the oropharynx and stomach are contiguous with the tracheobronchial tree and, at least in seriously ill patients, in virtual direct contact, so that changes in the bacterial flora of one region are reflected quickly in the others.

Colonizing organisms, whether newly acquired or long-term residents of the oropharynx, are aspirated into the tracheobronchial tree regularly in small volumes of secretions.[13] Nocturnal aspiration has been documented in both patients with impaired levels of consciousness and normal people and is probably a common occurrence. The volume inoculated by this mechanism may be very small, but since bacterial concentrations in oral secretions may achieve 10^8 mL or more, only minute volumes are required to cause inoculation of large numbers of bacteria. However, the tracheobronchial tree is sterile in normal subjects, whereas it regularly contains the oropharyngeal flora in seriously ill patients. This difference is explained by two factors; (1) it is likely that seriously ill patients aspirate more often and greater amounts, and (2) antibacterial defenses of the tracheobronchial tree and distal lung of seriously ill patients are less effective, leading to persistence and multiplication of aspirated organisms.

Antibacterial defenses of the normal lung can inactivate rapidly enormous numbers of viable bacteria. This process is somewhat more effective for organisms presented as a widely distributed small-particle aerosol than for those presented in a liquid bolus, as is the case with aspiration.[14] This difference probably is explained by a greater local concentration of organisms in a bolus and by the antiphagocytic function of secretions. Mucociliary removal mechanisms contribute only a small fraction of the lung's antibacterial function, as long as they are operational.[15] The great majority of organisms that are "inactivated" are phagocytosed and killed in situ, not transported out of the lung.[16] Circulating neutrophils or specific antibody are not required for the clearance of many organisms. However, for others, notably the GNB often associated with nosocomial pneumonia, prompt mobilization of neutrophils into alveolar spaces appears to be a critical aspect of host defense.[17, 18] Organisms that escape phagocytosis and killing may multiply, depending on local conditions within the lung. Factors that decrease bacterial killing include pulmonary edema, alveolar hypoxia, preceding viral infection, and systemic acidosis, among many others. The nature of the defects in host defenses leading to decreased killing are widely varied, including, for example, impaired phagocyte mobility, phagocyte membrane abnormalities, and impaired intracellular killing. On the other hand, severe acidosis, hypoxia, or the lack of essential nutrients in areas of consolidation each may impair bacterial multiplication. The outcome of these interactions, inactivation or clearance on the one hand and bacterial multiplication on the other, has been referred to as "net clearance" in experimental studies. If removal/killing functions predominate, the bacterial population progressively diminishes; if bacterial multiplication predominates, the bacterial population increases and progressive pneumonia results.[19, 20]

In critically ill patients, these processes of microaspiration, mucociliary clearance, phagocytosis and killing, and bacterial multiplication are repeated many times each day if not operating continuously. Thus, foci may be present in different areas of the lungs representing various stages of these interactions. The concentration of bacteria in these regions may vary, depending principally on the effectiveness of defense mechanisms locally. The species of bacteria present in a given region reflects the bacterial population of the more proximal regions of the respiratory tract, especially the oropharynx and trachea. Samples collected simultaneously from several sites within the lung usually show similar bacterial populations, although quantitative relationships may vary among regions. In general, when samples from the trachea or oropharynx are compared with samples from the distal lung, fewer bacterial species are present in the distal lung.[21] This shift represents a selection phenomenon in which those organisms most capable of evading the host's defenses survive in greatest numbers. It is a manifestation of "virulence," a concept that is defined best in terms of both the organism and the host. These considerations underlie many of the difficulties in the diagnosis of pneumonia in seriously ill patients, especially intubated, mechanically ventilated patients.

Whereas the aforementioned mechanisms account for the great majority of nosocomial pneumonias, other pathogenetic mechanisms may be important on occasion. Transmission of organisms in hospital air might be one such possibility. However, the requirements for airborne transmission of an organism are such that most bacterial agents are precluded. These conditions include the capacity to withstand extremes of environmental conditions, especially drying and ultraviolet irradiation, and the capacity to produce disease with a very small inoculum. A few bacterial agents are well-suited for this type of transmission. *Legionella* species, for example, have produced several hospital outbreaks, both through contaminated water and through airborne transmission from contaminated air-handling units.[22-26] Hospital outbreaks of influenza and respiratory syncytial virus (RSV) are well known and may occur following hospitalization of infected persons. *Mycobacterium tuberculosis* has caused numerous instances of infection among both patients and staff, usually due to failure to recognize the disease promptly in the index case.[27] However, the onset of pulmonary infiltrates following infection with *M. tuberculosis* requires several weeks at least and the nosocomial acquisition of this infection may be overlooked. Fungal agents, notably *Aspergillus* species, may be spread through the air of hospitals, as well as elsewhere, since these are ubiquitous organisms. They are recognized as potential problems in hospitals because markedly neutropenic patients are most susceptible to infection with them, and such patients tend to be hospitalized. Housing such patients in laminar flow rooms has been shown to be effective in reducing the incidence of *Aspergillus* infections, good evidence for the airborne route of transmission. For the most part, airborne transmission is unusual and not a major factor in nosocomial pneumonias.

Early experience with inhalation therapy demonstrated very clearly how hazardous medical advances can be. Over 70% of therapy devices incorporating reservoir nebulizers were shown to contain high concentrations of bacteria, often *P. aeruginosa*, and to produce contaminated aerosols.[28] The incidence of gram-negative necrotizing pneumonia at one hospital was 12% in a consecutive autopsy case series; this was reduced to less than 3% by the institution of effective decontamination procedures.[29] Respiratory medications can become contaminated, usually through faulty technique.[30] Even resuscitation equipment and spirometers used to monitor lung function in ventilated patients may become contaminated and transmit organisms that cause infections. Currently, contamination of respiratory therapy equipment is uncommon and such devices are not important factors in the pathogenesis of nosocomial pneumonia, largely because of the use of disposable equipment.[31]

DIAGNOSIS

The distinction between community-acquired and hospital-acquired infections usually has been set as the onset of pneumonia 48 or 72 hours after admission. Various combinations of clinical signs and symptoms have been used as diagnostic criteria for nosocomial pneumonia. Virtually all investigators have required the presence of "new or progressing" radiographic infiltrates for a diagnosis of pneumonia, along with fever and leukocytosis or leukopenia.[32] Most have required the presence of purulent tracheobronchial secretions. Some have required a positive Gram stain and/or culture of secretions; others have not. Conventional clinical wisdom would predict that, among previously healthy nonhospitalized individuals, the onset of fever, purulent sputum, leukocytosis, and a new infiltrate in the lungs usually indicates the presence of pneumonia. It is somewhat perplexing that a definite etiologic agent can be identified in only about 50% of patients with community-acquired pneumonias when rigorous diagnostic criteria are used.[33] That finding suggests that as-yet-unidentified organisms may be responsible for a significant proportion of pneumonias, or that noninfectious processes may mimic lung infection among nonhospitalized patients.

The problems of diagnosis are compounded in hospitalized patients because of two central problems: the high rate of colonization of the respiratory tract by pathogenic bacteria and the frequent presence of processes other than pneumonia that may cause fever, leukocytosis, and radiographic infiltrates. Since bacteremia appears to complicate nosocomial pneumonia in fewer than 10% of cases,[34] a suitable "gold standard" on which to base the diagnosis of pneumonia has been elusive.

Andrews et al.[35] used the histologic presence of pneumonia at autopsy as definitive evidence of pneumonia. By this technique, over 70% of patients dying with the adult respiratory distress syndrome (ARDS) were shown to have had pneumonia at the time of death. Clinicians who were blinded to the autopsy findings attempted to determine whether or not pneumonias had been present at the time of death, based on clinical criteria. Approximately 30% of patients with histologic pneumonia and 30% of those with no histologic evidence of pneumonia were misclassified by clinical criteria. Findings such as fever, leukocytosis, and the presence of bacteria in secretions were present in the great majority of patients, whether or not histologic pneumonia was found at autopsy. The major shortcoming of the histologic approach is obvious; it has little clinical utility. It is important to note in addition that pneumonias identified by the pathologist at necropsy are of uncertain clinical significance. There can be little doubt that widespread necrotizing pneumonia is a highly significant finding, but many of the pneumonias identified in the aforementioned study were focal bronchopneumonias and the significance of these is open to some question. Histologic pneumonias have been found by this group in similar percentages of patients dying of ARDS in other studies as well, so it seems that focal bronchopneumonia of varying degrees is present in most patients who die after a period of ventilatory support for ARDS.[36, 37] Whether this is true of other types of patients is not known.

Histologically recognizable pneumonia requires a bacterial population of at least 10^4/g of lung tissue in both humans and experimental animals.[38, 39] It would seem that quantitative cultures of respiratory secretions would provide a clear differentiation between infected and colonized patients. This is an intuitively attractive hypothesis that has been investigated for many years.[40–42] It seems only reasonable that organisms that are merely colonizing the mucosal surface would be present in lower concentrations than those that are causing infections. Unfortunately, analysis of sputum or tracheal aspirates in intensive care unit (ICU) patients generally has failed to show conclusive differences between infected and apparently uninfected patients due to several confounding factors, including the presence of multiple organisms and overlap of values.[32]

The use of invasive techniques to collect specimens may avoid some of these problems by sampling closer to the actual site of infection. One study in experimental animals compared quantitative cultures of tracheal aspirates, bronchoalveolar lavage (BAL), protected specimen brush (PSB), and needle aspiration of the lung parenchyma. The results from each of these were compared to quantitative cultures of homogenates of the same portion of lung[43] (Table 1). Bacterial species present in lung tissue were more likely to be identified by BAL than by PSB or aspiration. However, bacterial species present in concentrations greater than 10^5/g in lung tissue were detected equally well by PSB or BAL; aspiration was inferior to either of these. Transthoracic needle aspiration had the highest sensitivity and specificity of these techniques in another study of experimental pneumonia, but was associated with a 20% to 30% risk of pneumothorax.[44] That risk has prevented transthoracic aspiration from becoming a useful technique for the evaluation of ICU patients.

In a very interesting study, Chastre et al.[38] obtained PSB samples and matching lung tissue from patients who died while receiving mechanical ventilation. Histo-

TABLE 1.
Bacterial Species Recovered by Different Sampling Techniques*†

Bacterial Concentration in Lung Tissue	Number of Species in Lung Homogenate	PSB	BAL	ASP	TA
$<10^4$/g	18	4	11	8	12
$\geq 10^4$/g	9	7	9	7	9
Total (%)	27	11 (41)	20 (74)	15 (56)	21 (78)
False-positive results		4	3	3	14

*Data from Johanson WG Jr, Seidenfeld JJ, Gomez P, et al: *Am Rev Respir Dis* 1988; 137:259–264.
†PSB = protected specimen brush; BAL = bronchoalveolar lavage; ASP = needle aspiration; TA = tracheal aspirate.

logic evidence of pneumonia was associated with bacterial colony counts of at least 10^4/g in homogenized lung tissue. PSB sampling of these lungs recovered at least one species in a concentration of 10^3/mL or greater. The specificity provided by PSB cultures, using a cutoff value of 10^3 colony-forming units per milliliter is due to the characteristics of these samples. The PSB device collects a sample volume of about 0.001 mL and customarily is diluted in 1.0 mL of sterile saline. The presence of 10^3 colony-forming units per milliliter in that dilution would require that the concentration of organisms at the sampling site in the lungs be at least 10^6 colony-forming units per milliliter. It is not surprising to learn that most patients with that finding have significant infections. It would be expected that some patients with significant infections would have lesser bacterial concentrations, depending on several factors. Thus, the PSB is likely to err on the side of false-negative results, but in the few well-validated studies to date, this appears to be a small error.

It is important to understand the limitations of quantitative bacteriology in discriminating between infection and colonization in the setting of serious illness. The *presence* of the organisms in airway secretions is not in doubt, so the term "false-positive" to describe a culture containing few organism seems inappropriate. The question, then, is why does the bacterial population remain low in some patients whereas it increases to high levels in others? The answer is to be found in the lung defense mechanisms described previously, with perhaps an additional contribution from antimicrobial therapy in some patients. If lung defenses are relatively intact, the bacterial population will remain low, and perhaps even disappear; recovery without specific antimicrobial therapy does not seem out of the question, at least for some patients. On the other hand, if lung defenses are impaired seriously, the bacterial population will increase and a spreading, invasive infection will result. Thus, it is not surprising that a bacterial concentration might be identified that would predict a clinically important infection accurately, particularly if sampling is performed at a site near the possible infection. However, the virtually 100% accuracy of a concentration of 10^3/mL in distinguishing pneumonia from "nonpneumonia" cannot and will not hold as further experience is gained with this approach, for the simple reason that there is not a static equilibrium between the bacteria present and lung defenses.

A second approach toward a "gold standard" for the diagnosis of nosocomial pneumonia has been to withhold antimicrobial therapy from certain groups of patients who are suspected of having nosocomial pneumonia, if invasive sampling with the PSB technique did not indicate a high bacterial population in the distal lung. It seems resonable to believe that, if a seriously ill patient with clinical signs of pneumonia improves without antimicrobial therapy, pneumonia was not present. This approach can be used only in clinical circumstances in which a few days' delay in treatment would not be expected to lead to marked worsening of the patient's status and it has been employed in few studies. It should be added parenthetically that the usual practice has been to treat all patients and to include those whose "clinical course was consistent with pneumonia" or for whom another diagnosis was not established as having pneumonia. This presumes that the investigators know the expected course of pneumonia in that particular patient or that pneumonia and other processes do not coexist. Both assumptions are likely to be wrong, especialy in seriously ill patients.

Fagon et al.[45] studied 147 intubated, mechanically ventilated patients during episodes of suspected nosocomial respiratory infections; over 50% of patients met all four of the criteria commonly used by other investigators (fever, infiltrates, leukocytosis, purulent secretions) and 90% had at least three of these findings. Despite this clinical evidence of pneumonia, PSB samples revealed bacterial growth of 10^3/mL or less in 102 (69%) patients. Patients whose cultures were "negative" by this definition received either no antimicrobial agents or no change in antibiotics, or, if treatment had been started pending culture results, it was discontinued. The bases for excluding pneumonia in these 102 patients are shown in Table 2. These data emphasize the fact that clinical signs of infection are poor predictors of pneumonia in this patient group, at least by the standard that "pneumonia is not present if the patient improves without therapy."

There are several shortcomings in this study. The patients studied were predominantly postoperative patients who had suffered one or another complication; only 12 (8%) had ARDS. Thus, they differ significantly from the patients present in most medical ICUs. Only 26 of 102 (26%) of patients with "negative" PSB samples in fact recovered without treatment and the exclusion of pneumonia might have been less certain in the others.

The technique of BAL is not as well standardized as that of PSB, especially when used in ICU patients, and widely disparate findings have been reported. BAL should be used in immunocompromised hosts undergoing diagnostic bronchoscopy because of the larger area of the lung that is sampled and the availability of specimens for a variety of techniques. Stover et al.[46] reported an overall diagnostic yield of 66% in immunocompromised patients with new infiltrates with greater than 80% accuracy for diagnosing infections. Similar findings have been reported by others.[47–50] BAL has been less successful in the ICU environment. Chastre et al.,[51] for example, found virtual total overlap in the BAL quantitative culture results in intubated patients with infection and without infection. In another study, multiple BALs were performed in 29 patients who were free of pul-

TABLE 2.
Patients With Protected Specimen Brush Cultures
of $<10^3$ Colony-Forming Units per Milliliter*

Number of Patients	Basis For Excluding a Diagnosis of Pneumonia
Pneumonia definitely excluded:	
34	No pneumonia at autopsy within 2 weeks
26	Recovered without antibiotics
12	Recovered with no change in therapy
Pneumonia probably excluded:	
5	Died quickly, no autopsy
21	Change in therapy for other reasons
4	Other

*Data from Fagon JY, Chastre J, Hance AJ, et al: *Am Rev Respir Dis* 1988; 138:110–116.

monary disease but receiving mechanical ventilation for other reasons[52]; BAL cultures were positive in 34%. BAL was performed in 30 patients who subsequently died and had pneumonia at autopsy; BAL cultures were negative in 20% of these patients. Further, only 74% of the organisms recovered from lung homogenates were found in BAL. Torres et al.[53] compared PSB and BAL in 34 mechanically ventilated patients with suspected pneumonias. They found close agreement between these two techniques, with cultures disagreeing in only one case (3%). These investigators used a bacterial concentration of 10^3/mL in BAL to define a "positive" result for bacteria other than *Legionella* species. All patients received antibiotics, so the accuracy of diagnosis is difficult to determine. Somewhat surprising, the sensitivity of BAL was only 22% for patients with community-acquired pneumonia and 72% for those with nosocomial pneumonia. These low sensitivity values appear to be due to the 10^3/mL cutoff, since many patients had positive cultures at lower concentrations. On balance, BAL remains a useful technique because of the samples obtained and its lack of complications. It is particularly useful when unusual organisms or those difficult to culture are suspected. Although BAL culture results best reflect the spectrum of organisms present in the lung, quantitation of BAL specimens is of uncertain significance.

Awaiting the results of quantitative cultures of a PSB sample has obvious drawbacks in the care of seriously ill patients. Several approaches have been proposed to circumvent this problem. Examination of serial smears of tracheal aspirates has been used by some.[54] Results were compared for patients who developed lower respiratory infections according to clinical criteria and those who did not. Clinically infected patients demonstrated greater numbers of polymorphonuclear cells and bacteria in smears when mean values for apparently infected and apparently uninfected patients were compared. However, the overlap between groups was extensive and no one value would have identified an infected patient satisfactorily.

Staining of samples obtained by BAL has been suggested as another means of providing a prompt diagnosis of lung infection. The empiric observation has been that infected patients' lavagates contain a number of cells that have phagocytosed bacteria; in fact, finding that more than 7% of lavaged cells contained bacteria identified 86% of infected patients with a specificity of 96%.[55] This should not be surprising in concept, given the previous discussion of lung defenses, although the exact percentage of phagocytosing cells found to be predictive of infection is likely to vary under differing clinical circumstances. This approach does offer a quick initial appraisal of whether infection is likely or not and additional information on the likely causative organisms. By sampling at the alveolar level, much of the contamination of the proximal airways is avoided. BAL samples can be processed in various ways and subjected to a variety of special stains and cultural techniques. These may be of great value in determining the etiology of pulmonary processes, particularly in immunocompromised hosts. However, for the diagnosis of bacterial nosocomial pneumonia, only the PSB technique has been validated against a reasonably rigorous standard.

One interesting and as-yet-unconfirmed approach is to search for elastin fibers in sputum or tracheal aspirates. The rationale is that gram-negative infections are often necrotizing and that tissue destruction liberates elastin fibers into the airways[56]; since elastin is extremely resistant to degradation, these fibers remain intact for detection while being removed from the lungs. In fact, using a simple potassium hydroxide wet mount, one group found that the presence of elastin fibers accurately identified all patients with clinically suspected gram-negative infections.[54] The two patients with "false-positive" results each had entered the hospital with gram-negative pneumonias several days before a new infection was suspected and probably were still positive from the initial infection. The source of these fibers is not known, but they could arise from either bronchial walls or alveolar septa. The overall usefulness of this technique remains uncertain.

ETIOLOGIC AGENTS

The microbiology of nosocomial pneumonia differs from that of community-acquired pneumonia. The reported frequency of pathogens isolated varies significantly depending on populations studied, specimen collection and processing, and diagnostic methods. Perhaps the best source of information regarding the etiologies of nosocomial pneumonia, even though it is based on clinical criteria, is the National Nosocomial Surveillance System (NNIS), which has collected and analyzed data on the frequency of nosocomial infections in U.S. hospitals since 1970.[57] The ten most frequently isolated pathogens from lower respiratory infections in 1984 according to NNIS data are shown in Table 3.

Aerobic GNB account for 50% to 60% of all nosocomial pneumonias, with *P. aeruginosa* and *Klebsiella pneumoniae* the most frequent GNB recovered.[57-59] *Staphylococcus aureus* is the most frequent gram-positive isolate. *Streptococcus pneumoniae*, the most common cause of community-acquired pneumonia, accounted for less than 3% of isolates in the NNIS data from 1984.[57] Although a single organism is identified most often, an estimated 10% to 20% of nosocomial pneumonias are polymicrobic, and anaerobes may be underrepresented due to the difficulties of isolation and identification.[58, 60] In a prospective study of nosocomial pneumonias in which bacteriologic studies were restricted to transtracheal aspirates, pleural fluid, and blood, Bartlett and colleagues found that nearly 50% of specimens yielded polymicrobic flora with more than one potential pathogen.[61] The predominant isolates recovered were aerobic GNB (47%), *S. aureus* (31%), *S. pneumoniae* (26%), and anaerobic bacteria (35%). The recovery of *S. aureus*, *S. pneumoniae*, and anaerobes was higher than had been reported previously.

Mechanically ventilated patients are at high risk for the development of nosocomial pneumonia. Recent studies utilizing the PSB technique have defined better the organisms involved.[62-64] Table 4 shows the data collected by Fagon and coworkers on the frequency of organisms recovered by PBS in 52 episodes of ventilator-associated pneumonia.[64] In this study, *P. aeruginosa*, *Acinetobacter* species, and *Proteus* species were the predominant GNB isolated. At least one gram-positive organism was isolated in 52% of episodes; approximately 40% of infections were polymicrobic. Prior antibiotic therapy increased the frequency of isolation of *P. aeruginosa* and *Acinetobacter* and the frequency of methicillin resistance among staphylococcal isolates in these patients. In a similar study of mechanically ventilated patients in which the diagnosis of nosocomial pneumonia was made by

TABLE 3.

Most Frequently Isolated Pathogens From Lower
Respiratory Infections in the United States, 1984*

Pathogen	Frequency (%)
Pseudomonas aeruginosa	16.9
Staphylococcus aureus	12.9
Klebsiella species	11.6
Enterobacter species	9.4
Escherichia coli	6.4
Serratia species	5.8
Proteus species	4.2
Candida species	4.0
Enterococci	1.5
Coagulase-negative staphylococci	1.5

*Data from Horan TC, White JW, Jarvis WR, et al:
MMWR 1986; 35:17SS–29SS.

TABLE 4.

Frequency of Organisms Recovered From
Protected Brush Specimens in Significant
Concentrations ($>10^3$ Colony-Forming Units per
Milliliter) in 52 Episodes of Ventilator-Associated
Pneumonia*

Organism	Frequency (%)
Gram-negative bacteria	75
Pseudomonas aeruginosa	31
Acinetobacter species	15
Proteus species	15
Moraxella (Branhamella)	10
catarrhalis	
Haemophilus species	10
Escherichia coli	8
Klebsiella species	4
Enterobacter cloacae	2
Citrobacter freundii	2
Legionella pneumophila	2
Gram-positive bacteria	52
Staphylococcus aureus	33
Streptococcus pneumoniae	6
Other streptococci	15
Corynebacterium species	8
Anaerobes	2

*Data from Rouby JJ, Rossignon MD, Nicolas MH, et al:
Anesthesiology 1989; 71:679–685.

PSB or by blood or pleural fluid culture, *Acinetobacter* species, *P. aeruginosa*, and polymicrobic infections were the most frequent causes of nosocomial pneumonia.[62]

Legionella species account for a number of nosocomial pneumonias, with cases occurring sporadically or in clusters. As the diagnosis of legionellosis requires special serologic and microbiologic techniques, the exact frequency of infection is unknown. Estimates of frequency range from 3% to as high as 47% in hospitals where legionellosis is endemic and potable water is contaminated.[22–24]

Viral etiologies of nosocomial pneumonia may be more common than previously recognized. Nosocomial viral illnesses may go unrecognized due to the difficulties of diagnosis and the traditional emphasis of infection control programs on bacterial pathogens. In one prospective study of hospital infections, viral agents were found to be responsible for 20% of nosocomial pneumonia, with the majority of patients hospitalized on the pediatric ward.[65] Herpes viruses, most notably cytomegalovirus, are important pathogens in nosocomial pneumonias of renal and bone marrow transplant recipients.[66] Nosocomial viral respiratory infections, unlike bacterial infections, generally parallel the activity of agents in the community. The respiratory tract viruses, primarily RSV, influenza viruses A and B, and parainfluenza virus are responsible for at least 70% of nosocomial viral diseases.[67] Although young children are the major target of nosocomial viral infection, outbreaks of viral disease among institutionalized elderly, and chronically ill and debilitated patients have been well described and may have serious or fatal consequences.

Virtually any organism can cause nosocomial pneumonia. Less frequently isolated bacterial pathogens include *Citrobacter* and *Aeromonas species, Moraxella (Branhamella) catarrhalis,* and nonfermentative GNB, including nonaeruginosa pseudomonads, *Xanthomonas (Pseudomonas) maltophilia,* and *Alcaligenes, Achromobacter,* and *Flavobacterium* species. *Aspergillus* species may be an important cause of nosocomial pneumonias in selected patient populations that are severely neutropenic. *M. tuberculosis* as well as atypical mycobacteria have been reported as causes of nosocomial pneumonias.[68, 69] *Chlamydia pneumoniae* also has been reported recently as a cause of hospital-acquired pneumonia in immunocompetent hosts.[70]

Immunosuppression and myelosuppression are predisposing factors for the development of nosocomial pneumonia with both common and uncommon pathogens. Patients with neutropenia are particularly susceptible to GNB pneumonias.[71] Table 5 provides a list of unusual pathogens responsible for nosocomial pneumonias in immunocompromised hosts.

TABLE 5.
Unusual Pathogens Responsible for Nosocomial
Pneumonias in Immunocompromised Hosts

  I. Bacteria.
    A. *Nocardia.*
    B. *Legionella.*
    C. *Mycobacterium tuberculosis.*
    D. Atypical mycobacteria.
 II. *Chlamydia.*
III. Fungi.
    A. *Aspergillus.*
    B. *Cryptococcus.*
    C. *Candida.*
    D. *Torulopsis.*
    E. Zygomycetes.
IV. Viruses.
    A. Cytomegalovirus.
    B. Herpes simplex.
    C. Varicella zoster.
    D. Influenza.
    E. Respiratory syncytial virus.
 V. Protozoa.
    A. *Pneumocystis carinii.*
    B. *Toxoplasma gondii.*
VI. Helminths.
    A. *Strongyloides.*

THERAPY

Empiric Antimicrobial Therapy

Due to difficulties in obtaining a rapid and definitive diagnosis of the etiologic agents responsible for nosocomial pneumonia in the majority of patients, and the significant morbidity and mortality associated with these infections, early empiric antimicrobial therapy frequently is warranted. It has not been demonstrated convincingly that utilization of aggressive diagnostic measures to guide antimicrobial therapy improves outcomes over empiric therapy alone. The decision whether to begin empiric antimicrobial therapy must be individualized and relies on clinical judgment.

Initial therapy of nosocomial pneumonia ideally would be based on examination of the Gram stain or other specialized stains of a cytocentrifuged BAL specimen. In the absence of such specimens, sputum or tracheal aspirates may be used, recognizing that both false-positive and false-negative results are common.[72] Factors that should be considered in the selection of antimicrobial agents include the patient's underlying disease and immune status, the severity of the patient's illness, length of hospitalization, intubation and mechanical ventilation, prior antibiotic therapy, and previous isolates from respiratory tract cultures. Additional factors to be considered include hospital or ICU experience with nosocomial pathogens, particularly multiantibiotic-resistant organisms, hospital incidence of legionellosis, and any recent outbreaks of viral respiratory infections in the hospital and community.[73]

Traditional therapy for nosocomial pneumonia has consisted of broad-spectrum combination antibiotic therapy with an aminoglycoside in conjunction with a β-lactam agent.[68, 73, 74] In most instances, empiric therapy should include coverage for aerobic GNB and *S. aureus,* including resistant organisms such as *P. aeruginosa, Acinetobacter* and *Serratia* species, as well as *S. aureus.* In light of recent studies suggesting an increased frequency of isolation of gram-positive organisms as pathogens in nosocomial pneumonia, the use of appropriate gram-positive coverage is advisable.

There is increasing evidence that monotherapy with a third-generation cephalosporin, imipenam, or ticarcillin/clavulanic acid, is as efficacious as combination therapy with an aminoglycoside in nonneutropenic patients.[68, 75-84] Because of the lack of activity against gram-positive organisms, aminoglycosides and aztreonam have no role as single agents in empiric therapy of nosocomial pneumonia.[85] The third-generation cephalosporins show a broad spectrum of activity against the Enterobacteriaceae, *Haemophilus influenzae,* many gram-positive isolates, and some anaerobes. Ceftriaxone, cefotaxime, and ceftizoxime have greater activity against streptococci and staphylococci than do the other third-generation cephalosporins, whereas cefoperazone and ceftazidime have superior activity against *P. aeruginosa.* Though ceftazidime has been shown to be effective therapy as a single agent in the treatment of nosocomial pneumonia,[76-78] if there is a high likelihood that gram-positive organisms are the major pathogens involved, an additional agent to cover these should be added, or an alternative third-generation cephalosporin providing better gram-positive coverage should be used.[86]

Imipenam, a carbepenem, has an exceptionally broad spectrum of activity that includes activity against the Enterobacteriaceae, *P. aeruginosa, Acinetobacter* species, *H. influenzae,* many gram-positive organisms, and anaerobes. It lacks activity against methicillin-resistant staphylococci and nonaeruginosa pseudomonads, and should not be relied on as a single agent for enterococci. A major concern with imipenam has been the emergence of resistant organisms during therapy, particularly with strains of *P. aeruginosa*. If imipenam is used for therapy directed at *P. aeruginosa,* the addition of an aminoglycoside is recommended.[87-89]

Ticarcillin/clavulanic acid shows significantly greater antibacterial activity than ticarcillin alone against clinically important β-lactamase, producing gram-positive and gram-negative organisms due to the inhibition of β-lactamase by clavulanic acid. Ticarcillin/clavulanic acid has activity against the Enterobacteriaceae, staphylococci, streptococci, anaerobes, and ticarcillin-susceptible strains of *P. aeruginosa*.[84] The extended spectrum β-lactams, including the third-generation cephalosporins, imipenam, and ticarcillin/clavulanic acid, all have a broad spectrum of activity, achieve high serum bactericidal levels, and have good tissue penetration and a low level of toxicity, which makes them attractive agents for the treatment of nosocomial pneumonias either alone or in combination with other antibiotics.

The usefulness of aminoglycosides in the therapy of nosocomial pneumonias has been questioned due to the small differences between therapeutic and toxic serum levels, their poor penetration into bronchopulmonary secretions and infected lung, and their relative inactivity at the pH level found in respiratory secretions.[73, 90, 91] Moore and colleagues found an association of aminoglycoside plasma levels with therapeutic outcome of gram-negative pneumonia.[92] Therapy was more likely to have a successful outcome if mean peak plasma aminoglycoside levels were 6 μg/mL or greater for gentamicin and tobramycin and 24 μg/mL or greater for amikacin.

Rationale for using aminoglycosides in the therapy of nosocomial pneumonias include greater activity against certain GNB such as *P. aeruginosa* or *Acinetobacter* species, potential synergism between aminoglycosides and β-lactam agents against GNB, and prevention of the emergence of resistance.[73, 89, 90, 93] Although there is increasing evidence to support the use of monotherapy in the empiric treatment of nosocomial pneumonia, particularly in an era of cost containment, aminoglycosides remain the mainstay of therapy in serious infection with resistant GNB, most notably *P. aeruginosa* and GNB pneumonias associated with bacteremia, and in neutropenic patients. Table 6 provides options for empiric antimicrobial therapy of nosocomial pneumonias.

TABLE 6.
Empiric Antimicrobial Therapy for Nosocomial Pneumonia

Suspected Pathogens	Therapeutic Options*
Aerobic gram-negative bacilli *Staphylococcus aureus* Polymicrobic flora High probability anaerobes	Nafcillin/cefazolin + aminoglycoside; third-generation cephalosporin ± aminoglycoside; antipseudomonal penicillin† + aminoglycoside; timentin ± aminoglycoside; imipenam Clindamycin/penicillin G/cefoxitin + aminoglycoside; ticarcillin/clavulanic acid ± aminoglycoside; imipenam
High probability *Pseudomonas* *aeruginosa*	Ceftazidime ± aminoglycoside; imipenam + aminoglycoside; antipseudomonal penicillin† + aminoglycoside; ticarcillin/clavulanic acid + aminoglycoside
Legionellosis endemic	Include erythromycin
High probability methicillin- resistant staphylococci	Use vancomycin for gram-positive coverage
Aminoglycoside resistance	Substitute amikacin for gentamicin or tobramycin

*Aztreonam may be substituted for gram-negative coverage in some instances.[94, 95]
†Ticarcillin, mezlocillin, piperacillin, azlocillin.

Definitive Antimicrobial Therapy

When the pathogenic organisms responsible for the antimicrobial susceptibility patterns are known, modifications can be made to optimize antibiotic therapy of nosocomial pneumonias. In neutropenic patients and in seriously ill patients with pneumonias caused by resistant GNB such as *P. aeruginosa, Serratia* and *Acinetobacter* species, continued combination therapy with an appropriate β-lactam agent and an aminoglycoside is recommended.

Single agents (usually β-lactams) can be selected based on antimicrobial susceptibilities for continued antibiotic therapy in patients in whom resistant organisms have not been identified and when the patient has shown a clinical response to therapy. Susceptibility testing utilizing minimal inhibitory concentrations and minimal bactericidal concentrations may be useful in the selection of antibiotics, particularly when resistant organisms are involved. Duration of therapy should be based on clinical response, but a minimum of 2 weeks and preferably 3 weeks for GNB pneumonias and legionellosis is recommended.[24, 96] In critically ill patients, neutropenic patients, and patients with pneumonias complicated by abscess, empyema, or atelectasis, extended therapy may be required. Table 7 provides antimicrobial options for the treatment of nosocomial pneumonias when the pathogen has been identified.

Aminoglycosides have different levels of activity against various GNB; however, there is no clinical evidence to suggest that one aminoglycoside is superior to another in infections with susceptible organisms.[90] Gentamicin is more active against *Enterobacter* species than tobramycin or amikacin. Gentamicin also is more active against *Serratia* species than tobramycin; however, due to the in-

TABLE 7.
Therapeutic Options for Nosocomial Pneumonia of Known Etiology

Pathogen	Options
Gram-negative bacilli	
Acinetobacter	Ticarcillin/piperacillin + tobramycin; ceftazidime + tobramycin; imipenam; trimethoprim-sulfamethoxazole
Enterobacter/Serratia	Third-generation cephalosporin ± gentamicin/amikacin; trimethoprim-sulfamethoxazole
Escherichia coli	Cephalosporin; aztreonam
Haemophilus influenzae	Cefotaxime; ceftriaxone
Klebsiella	Third-generation cephalosporin ± aminoglycoside; aztreonam; imipenam
Proteus mirabilis	Ampicillin; third-generation cephalosporin
Pseudomonas aeruginosa	Ceftazadime ± tobramycin/amikacin; imipenam/antipseudomonal penicillin/ticarcillin/clavulanic acid + tobramycin/amikacin
Gram-positive cocci	
Staphylococcus aureus	Nafcillin; vancomycin
Methicillin-resistant staphylococci	Vancomycin
Streptococci	Penicillin G; erythromycin; vancomycin
Legionella	Erythromycin ± rifampin
Anaerobes	Metronidazole; clindamycin; penicillin G

creased resistance of *Serratia* to gentamicin, amikacin is recommended until susceptibilities are known.[96] Amikacin also is recommended for strains of *Pseudomonas* that are tobramycin-resistant. When aminoglycoside therapy is used in the treatment of gram-negative pneumonias, plasma levels must be followed to ensure high therapeutic levels.[92]

Ciprofloxacin is a quinolone with broad-spectrum antibacterial activity, including activity against the Enterobacteriaceae and *P. aeruginosa,* but it has only moderate activity against streptococci. The quinolones have the advantages of enteral absorption, a long half-life, excellent tissue penetration, and a low incidence of adverse reactions. Ciprofloxacin appears to be a promising agent in the treatment of acute respiratory infections in patients with cystic fibrosis; however, its role in the treatment of nosocomial pneumonias has not been well defined yet.[97] A parenteral preparation of ciprofloxacin has been approved only recently, and experience with its use in the treatment of nosocomial pneumonias is limited.

As the majority of nosocomial pneumonias are bacterial in origin, any discussion of therapy focuses on antibacterial agents. There have been, however, some advances in the treatment of nonbacterial pneumonias. Trimethoprim/sulfamethoxazole has been the preferred therapy for patients with histologically proven *Pneumocystis* pneumonia with pentamidine as an alternative therapy. Newer options that have been successful in treating *Pneumocystis* pneumonia in patients with the acquired immunodeficiency syndrome (AIDS) include pyrimethamine with sulfadiazine, trimethoprim with dapsone, and clindamycin with primaquine.[98, 99, 100] Adjunctive corticosteroid therapy should be given to patients with human immunodeficiency virus (HIV) infection and documented or suspected *Pneumocystis* pneumonia if they have moderate or severe pulmonary dysfunction.[101]

Advances in antiviral therapy include the use of ribavirin, a synthetic triazole available in an aerosolized form, for the treatment of severe RSV infection in children and intravenous acyclovir for pneumonias caused by herpes simplex and varicella zoster viruses.[66] Acyclovir has activity against both herpes simplex virus and varicella zoster virus in vitro and in vivo. There are no controlled studies of the efficacy of acyclovir in the treatment of herpes simplex and varicella pneumonia; however, given the low toxicity profile of acyclovir, its use is justified in serious disease.[66, 102]

Ganciclovir is an antiviral agent with excellent in vitro activity against cytomegalovirus. Initial reports in renal transplant patients with cytomegalovirus pneumonia treated with ganciclovir were encouraging; however, little impact on overall survival was demonstrated subsequently in allogeneic marrow transplant patients.[103, 104] More recent studies of ganciclovir in combination with high-dose human immune globulin or cytomegalovirus immunoglobulin in the treatment of cytomegalovirus pneumonia have shown a significant improvement in survival (52% survival with ganciclovir and cytomegalovirus immunoglobulin vs. 15% survival with previous antiviral regimens[105, 106]). Although further studies are needed, the combination of ganciclovir with cytomegalovirus immunoglobulin or human globulin offers promise for therapy of a disease with a mortality of 85% in allogeneic marrow transplant recipients.

Foscarnet, trisodium phosphonoformate, is an investigational antiviral agent with in vitro activity against herpes-class viruses and HIV. The primary experience with foscarnet in this country has been in the treatment of cytomegalovirus retinitis in patients with AIDS.[107, 108] Investigations in Europe have shown favorable clinical responses with foscarnet in serious cytomegalovirus infections in allograft recipients, and further studies are in progress.[109, 110]

Despite recent advances in the development of new azole antifungal agents, amphotericin B remains the drug of choice for serious pulmonary infections caused by the majority of fungi, including *Aspergillus, Candida,* and *Cryptococcus* species.[111–113] Flucytosine is synergistic with amphotericin B against *Candida, Cryptococcus,* and *Aspergillus* species, but myelosuppressive toxicities frequently limit its use. Further clinical trials with the new azole antifungals may define their role in the treatment of serious pulmonary fungal infections.

PREVENTION

Topical antibiotics have been used to provide prophylaxis against nosocomial pneumonia for high-risk patients. Early experience during the polio epidemic of the 1950s indicated that instillation of antimicrobial agents into the tracheostomy stroma of ventilated patients had some effects on the bacterial flora, but did not eliminate it.[114] The one exception was that polymyxin B was remarkably effective in preventing colonization of the airways by *P. aeruginosa*. Polymyxin are not absorbed topically, but adsorb to cell surfaces, thus providing high concentrations on the mucosal surface. Since they are bactericidal for many gram-negative bacteria, they are a good choice for a preventive agent. Polymyxin B as a single agent was studied extensively in the early 1970s in a respiratory intensive care unit in Boston.[115-117] The key observations were that polymyxin B markedly reduced the incidence of colonization and infection with *P. aeruginosa* and reduced the incidence of pneumonias diagnosed by clinical criteria. However, pneumonias developing in patients receiving prophylaxis usually were caused by polymyxin B–resistant organisms and 60% of such patients died, a marked increase over previous experience. The net effect was that deaths from pneumonia were not reduced and the authors concluded that polymyxin B prophylaxis should not be used.[117]

Prophylaxis of nosocomial infections with antimicrobial agents has become standard practice for certain groups of patients, especially those who are rendered markedly neutropenic by malignant disease or chemotherapy.[118] Prevention of infections in immunocompetent patients by this means generally has been regarded as futile, with the prevailing thought being that one could alter the responsible bacterial species by such therapy but not reduce the incidence of infections. A much more aggressive approach to prophylaxis has been developed in Europe over the past few years.[119] This approach calls for the use of multiple agents applied to the oral mucosa in a sticky paste to promote retention, and instilled into the stomach via a nasogastric tube. The agents that have been utilized most often are tobramycin, polymyxin E (colistin), and amphotericin B, each in concentrations of 2% by weight. These agents are applied shortly after the patient's admission to intensive care and are continued for the duration of stay in the unit. An important addition was discovered in early trials of this approach. It was learned in Groningen, Holland, that the use of the regimen described did not reduce the incidence of pneumonia, the most common nosocomial infection among trauma patients in that unit.[120] These investigators found that the pneumonias that continued to occur were those that developed early (<4 days) in the patient's course; these pneumonias were caused principally by organisms that commonly cause community-acquired infections and commonly are present in the upper respiratory tracts of healthy people. Presumably, these organisms were deposited in the patient's lungs during injury or initial reuscitation. To prevent these early pneumonias, caused by "normal flora" types of organisms, the Groningen investigators added a parenteral agent to the prophylactic regimen. Previous experimental work from that center had suggested that "colonization resistance" of the gastrointestinal tract required the presence of anaerobic bacteria in the gut. Therefore, they chose an agent that was thought to have little effect on anaerobic bacteria, cefotaxime. It has been shown subsequently that metabolites of cefotaxime are active against anaerobes, but these metabolites may not be present in the intestinal lumen.[121]

Thus, the full regimen was developed (topical tobramycin, colistin, and amphotericin B), applied to the oral mucosa, and instilled into the stomach, supplemented by parenteral cefotaxime. Because of the perceived importance of the gastrointestinal tract, it was called "selective digestive decontamination." This approach has been used in a number of clinical trials in Europe,[122-132] but in only a few in the United States.[133, 134] In general, the incidence of pneumonia has been reduced significantly in patients receiving active drugs. The effect on other infections has been inconsistent, and most studies have found no impact on mortality. The one group of patients that has demonstrated reduced mortality most often is trauma patients, interestingly enough, the group for which the regimen initially was developed. Some of these studies are summarized in Table 8.

Compared to usual clinical trials, these studies have a number of flaws. None have employed placebo controls, with the argument being that the effect of the regimen on bacterial flora is so dramatic that blinding could not be maintained. However, it would seem that the major end points could be determined by individuals who were not involved in the care of the patients and did not have access to all of the cultural data. Few trials used concurrent controls. This is a legacy from the Beth Israel trials with polymyxin B in which the authors reasoned that exposure of untreated patients to small amounts of the drug in the unit would promote the emergence of drug resistance.[115] The concept that all or none of the patients in a unit at one time must be treated has been adhered to by virtually all investigators since, even though there are no data to support that view and it seriously compromises the credibility of the existing data. Some trials have used the presence of bacteria in respiratory secretions as a necessary criterion for the diagnosis of nosocomial pneumonia, along with other findings. However, repeated local instillation of these drugs results in very high drug concentrations in secretions, and sterile cultures of those secretions would be expected, even if distal infection were present.[135] Since the major effect of selective digestive decontamination is to reduce the incidence of apparent pneumonias, but mortality of treated patients is no less than that of untreated patients, one must consider the possibility that the re-

TABLE 8.
Nosocomial Pneumonia and Mortality in Trials of Selective Digestion Decontamination*

Controls			SDD			
Number	NP (%)	Died (%)	Number	NP (%)	Died (%)	Reference
47	85	32	49	12†	28	Kerver et al.[127]
161	11	24	163	1.2†	24	Lewdingham et al.[125]
52	56	54	48	14†	31†	Ulrich et al.[128]
101	45	45	99	10†	34	Hartenauer et al.[126]
20	45	30	19	5†	26	Unertl et al.[124]
59	59	—	63	8†	—	Stoutenbeek et al.[122]

*NP = nosocomial pneumonia; SDD = trials of selective digestion decontamination.
†P <.05, compared with controls.

duction of pneumonias is an artifact caused by the regimen's effect on the bacterial flora of secretions. Finally, the existing trials have been done with very different patient groups. It seems quite clear that prophylaxis is destined to be futile in certain groups of patients and is not needed in others for whom the prognosis is good in any case. Trauma patients can be stratified readily on admission on the basis of well-standardized indices.[136] Further, most trauma patients are free of underlying diseases that greatly complicate determining the severity of illness among other groups of patients, especially those admitted to medical ICUs. Whereas stratifying systems such as APACHE II[124] are useful instruments for comparing the outcomes of groups of patients, they are less useful when applied to individual patients with a range of underlying diseases. The major question about selective digestive decontamination at the present time is whether or not it should be used at all and, if so, in what groups of patients. These questions cannot be answered on the basis of existing data and will require well-designed trials for clarification. In the meantime, selective digestive decontamination is not a modality that should be implemented as a routine in any unit, in our opinion.

Prevention of nosocomial infections by active immunization with parenteral immunoglobulin has been attempted. As might be anticipated, such immunotherapy is relatively limited in scope, whereas the range of infecting bacteria has no such limitation. Immunization of patients against *P. aeruginosa* was quite effective in reducing the incidence of infections with that organism, but did not reduce the overall incidence of infection appreciably.[137] Human polyclonal antiserum directed against the endotoxin core determinants of gram-negative bacteria has been shown to be effective in reducing deaths from gram-negative sepsis.[138, 139] Ziegler and colleagues demonstrated that adjunctive HA-1A, a human monoclonal IgM antibody that binds to the lipid A domain of endotoxin, significantly reduced mortality in patients with sepsis and gram-negative bacteremia.[140] These agents have not been used prophylactically and appear to be of little benefit for patients with established gram-negative pneumonias.

REFERENCES

1. Kneeland Y Jr, Price KM: Antibiotics and terminal pneumonia: A postmortem microbiological study. *Am J Med* 1960; 29:967–979.
2. Ritchie WT: The bacteriology of bronchitis. *J Pathol Bact* 1901; 7:1–21.
3. Burn CG: Postmortem bacteriology. *J Infect Dis* 1934; 54:395–403.
4. Simmons BP, Wong ES: Guideline for prevention of nosocomial pneumonia. *Infect Control Hosp Epidemiol* 1982; 3:327–333.
5. du Moulin GC, Paterson DG, Hedley-Whyte J, et al: Aspiration of gastric bacteria in antacid-treated patients: A frequent cause of postoperative colonization of the airway. *Lancet* 1982; 1:242–245.
6. Beachey EH: Bacterial adherence: Adhesin-receptor interactions mediating the attachment of bacteria to mucosal surfaces. *J Infect Dis* 1981; 143:325–345.
7. Woods DE, Straus DC, Johanson WG Jr, et al: The role of salivary protease activity in adherence of gram-negative bacilli to mammalian buccal epithelial cells *in vivo*. *J Clin Invest* 1981; 68:1435–1440.

8. Niederman MS, Rafferty TD, Sasaki CT, et al: Comparison of bacterial adherence to ciliated and squamous epithelial cells obtained from the human respiratory tract. *Am Rev Respir Dis* 1983; 127:85–90.

9. Driks MR, Craven DE, Celli BR, et al: Nosocomial pneumonia in intubated patients given sucralfate as compared with antacids or histamine type 2 blockers. *N Engl J Med* 1987; 317:1376–1382.

10. Snepar R, Poporad GA, Romano JM, et al: Effect of cimetidine and antacid on gastric microbial flora. *Infect Immun* 1982; 36:518–524.

11. Tryba M: Risk of acute stress bleeding and nosocomial pneumonia in ventilated intensive care unit patients: Sucralfate versus antacids. *Am J Med* 1987; 83(suppl 3B):117–124.

12. Tryba M, Mantey-Stiers F: Antibacterial activity of sucralfate in human gastric juice. *Am J Med* 1987; 83:125–127.

13. Huxley EJ, Viroslav J, Gray WR, et al: Pharyngeal aspiration in normal adults and patients with depressed consciousness. *Am J Med* 1978; 64:564–568.

14. Harris GD, Woods DE, Fine R, et al: The effect of intra-alveolar fluid on lung bacterial clearance. *Lung* 1980; 158:91–100.

15. Green GM, Jakav GJ, Low RB, et al: Defense mechanisms of the respiratory membrane. *Am Rev Respir Dis* 1977; 115:479–514.

16. Goldstein E, Lippert W, Warshauer D: Pulmonary alveolar macrophage: Defender against bacterial infection of the lung. *J Clin Invest* 1974; 54:519–528.

17. Gross GN, Rehm SR, Pierce AK: The effect of complement depletion on lung clearance of bacteria. *J Clin Invest* 1978; 62:373–378.

18. Pierce AK, Reynolds RC, Harris GD: Leukocytic response to inhaled bacteria. *Am Rev Respir Dis* 1977; 116:679–684.

19. Jay SJ, Johanson WG Jr, Pierce AK, et al: Determinants of lung bacterial clearance in normal mice. *J Clin Invest* 1976; 57:811–817.

20. Johanson WG Jr, Jay SJ, Pierce AK: Bacterial growth *in vivo:* An important determinant of the pulmonary clearance of *Diplococcus pneumoniae* in rats. *J Clin Invest* 1974; 53:1320–1325.

21. Crouch TW, Higuchi JH, Coalson JJ, et al: Pathogenesis and prevention of nosocomial pneumonia in a nonhuman primate model of acute respiratory failure. *Am Rev Respir Dis* 1984; 130:502–504.

22. Muder RR, Yu VL, McClure JK, et al: Nosocomial Legionnaires' disease uncovered in a prospective pneumonia study. *JAMA* 1983; 249:3184–3188.

23. Rudin JE, Wing EJ: Prospective study of pneumonia: Unexpected incidence of legionellosis. *South Med J* 1986; 79:417–419.

24. Edelstein PH, Meyer RD: Legionella pneumonia, in Pennington JE (ed): *Respiratory Infections: Diagnosis and Management.* New York, Raven Press, 1989, pp 381–402.

25. Arnow PM, Chou T, Weil D, et al: Nosocomial Legionnaire's disease caused by aerosolized tap water from respiratory devices. *J Infect Dis* 1982; 146:460–467.

26. Zuravleff JJ, Yu VL, Shonnard JW, et al: *Legionella pneumophilia* contamination of a hospital humidifier. *Am Rev Respir Dis* 1983; 128:657–661.

27. Ehrenkranz NJ, Kicklighter JL: Tuberculosis outbreak in a general hospital: Evidence for airborne spread of infection. *Ann Intern Med* 1972; 77:377–382.

28. Reinarz JA, Pierce AK, Mays BB, et al: The potential role of inhalation therapy equipment in nosocomial pulmonary infection. *J Clin Invest* 1965; 44:831–839.

29. Pierce AK, Sanford JP, Thomas GD, et al: Long-term evaluation of decontamination of inhalation-therapy equipment and the occurrence of necrotizing pneumonia. *N Engl J Med* 1970; 282:528–531.

30. Sanders CV Jr, Luby JP, Johanson WG Jr, et al: *Serratia marcescens* infections from inhalation therapy medications: Nosocomial outbreak. *Ann Intern Med* 1970; 73:15–21.

31. Cross AS, Roup B: Role of respiratory assistance devices in endemic nosocomial pneumonia. *Am J Med* 1981; 70:681–685.

32. Johanson WG Jr, Pierce AK, Sanford JP, et al: Nosocomial respiratory infections with gram-negative bacilli. *Ann Intern Med* 1972; 77:701–706.

33. Bates JH: Microbial etiology of pneumonia. *Chest* 1989; 95:194S–197S.

34. *National Nosocomial Infections Study Report, Annual Summary*. Atlanta, Georgia, Centers for Disease Control, 1979, pp 1–13.

35. Andrews CP, Coalson JJ, Smith JD, et al: Diagnosis of nosocomial bacterial pneumonia in acute, diffuse lung injury. *Chest* 1981; 80:254–258.

36. Coalson JJ: Pathophysiologic features of respiratory distress in the infant and adult, in Shoemaker WC, Thompson WL (eds): *Critical Care. State of the Art*. Fullerton, California, The Society of Critical Care Medicine, 1982, pp 1–28.

37. Seidenfeld JJ, Pohl DP, Bell RC, et al: Incidence, site, and outcome of infections in patients with the adult respiratory distress syndrome. *Am Rev Respir Dis* 1986; 134:12–16.

38. Chastre J, Viau F, Brun P, et al: Prospective evaluation of the protected specimen brush for the diagnosis of pulmonary infections in ventilated patients. *Am Rev Respir Dis* 1984; 130:924–929.

39. Johanson WG Jr, Higuchi JH, Woods DE, et al: Dissemination of *Pseudomonas aeruginosa* during lung infection in hamsters. *Am Rev Respir Dis* 1985; 132:358–361.

40. Louria DB: Uses of quantitative analysis of bacterial populations in sputum. *JAMA* 1962; 182:1082–1086.

41. Monroe PW, Muchmore HG, Felton RG, et al: Diagnostic and therapeutic advantages of serial quantitative cultures of fresh sputum in acute bacterial pneumonia. *Am Rev Respir Dis* 1969; 100:831–838.

42. Guckian JC, Christiansen WD: Quantitative culture and gram stain of sputum in pneumonia. *Am Rev Respir Dis* 1978; 118:997–1005.

43. Johanson WG Jr, Seidenfeld JJ, Gomez P, et al: Bacteriologic diagnosis of nosocomial pneumonia following prolonged mechanical ventilation. *Am Rev Respir Dis* 1988; 137:259–264.

44. Moser KM, Maurer J, Jassy L, et al: Sensitivity, specificity, and risk of diagnostic procedures in a canine model of *Streptococcus pneumoniae* pneumonia. *Am Rev Respir Dis* 1982; 125:436–442.

45. Fagon JY, Chastre J, Hance AJ, et al: Detection of nosocomial lung infection in ventilated patients. *Am Rev Respir Dis* 1988; 138:110–116.

46. Stover DE, Zamanm MB, Hajdu SI, et al: Bronchoalveolar lavage in the diagnosis of diffuse pulmonary infiltrates in immunosuppressed host. *Ann Intern Med* 1984; 101:1–7.

47. Broaddus C, Dake MD, Stulbarg MS, et al: Bronchoalveolar lavage and transbronchial biopsy for the diagnosis of pulmonary infections in the acquired immunodeficiency syndrome. *Ann Intern Med* 1985; 102:747–752.

48. Martin WJ, Smith TF, Brutinel WM, et al: Role of bronchoalveolar lavage in the assessment of opportunistic pulmonary infections: Utility and complications. *Mayo Clin Proc* 1987; 62:549–557.

49. Springmeyer SC, Hackman RC, Holle R, et al: Use of bronchoalveolar lavage to diagnose acute diffuse pneumonia in the immunocompromised host. *J Infect Dis* 1986; 154:604–610.

50. Williams D, Yungbluth M, Adams G, et al: The role of fiberoptic bronchoscopy in the evaluation of immunocompromised hosts with diffuse pulmonary infiltrates. *Am Rev Respir Dis* 1985; 131:880–885.

51. Chastre J, Fagon JY, Soler P, et al: Diagnosis of nosocomial bacterial pneumonia in intubated patients undergoing ventilation: Comparison of the usefulness of bronchoalveolar lavage and the protected specimen brush technique. *Am J Med* 1988; 85:499–506.

52. Rouby JJ, Rossignon MD, Nicolas MH, et al: A prospective study of protected bronchoalveolar lavage in the diagnosis of nosocomial pneumonia. *Anesthesiology* 1989; 71:679–685.

53. Torres A, De La Bellacasa JP, Xaubet A, et al: Diagnostic value of quantitative cultures of bronchoalveolar lavage and telescoping plugged catheters in mechanically ventilated patients with bacterial pneumonia. *Am Rev Respir Dis* 1989; 140:306–310.

54. Salata RA, Lederman MM, Shlaes DM, et al: Diagnosis of nosocomial pneumonia in intubated intensive care unit patients. *Am Rev Respir Dis* 1987; 135:426–432.

55. Chastre J, Fagon JY, Soler P, et al: Quantification of BAL cells containing intracellular bacteria rapidly identifies ventilated patients with nosocomial pneumonia. *Chest* 1989; 95(suppl):190S–192S.

56. Schales DM, Lederman MM, Chmielewski R, et al: Sputum elastin fibers and the diagnosis of necrotizing pneumonia. *Chest* 1984; 85:763–766.

57. Horan TC, White JW, Jarvis WR, et al: Nosocomial infection surveillance, 1984. *MMWR* 1986; 35:17SS–29SS.

58. Bryan CS, Reynolds KL: Bacteremic nosocomial pneumonia–analysis of 172 episodes from a single metropolitan area. *Am Rev Respir Dis* 1984; 129:668–671.

59. Levison ME, Kaye D: Pneumonia caused by gram-negative bacilli: An overview. *Rev Infect Dis* 1985; 7(suppl 4):657–665.

60. Veazy JM: Hospital-acquired pneumonia, in Wenzel RE (ed): *CRC Handbook of Hospital Acquired Infections*. Boca Raton, Fla, CRC Press, 1981, pp 341–369.

61. Bartlett JG, O'Keefe P, Tally FP, et al: Bacteriology of hospital-acquired pneumonia. *Arch Intern Med* 1986; 146:868–871.

62. Jimenez P, Torres A, Rodriguez-Roisin R, et al: Incidence and etiology of pneumonia acquired during mechanical ventilation. *Crit Care Med* 1989; 17:882–885.

63. Torres A, Aznar R, Gatell JM, et al: Incidence, risk and prognosis factors of nosocomial pneumonia in mechanically ventilated patients. *Am Rev Respir Dis* 1990; 142:523–528.

64. Fagon JY, Chastre J, Domart Y, et al: Nosocomial pneumonia in patients receiving continuous mechanical ventilation. Prospective analysis of 52 episodes with use of a protected specimen brush and quantitative culture techniques. *Am Rev Respir Dis* 1989; 139:877–884.

65. Valenti WM, Hall CB, Douglas RG Jr, et al: Nosocomial viral infections. I. Epidemiology and significance. *Infect Control Hosp Epidemiol* 1981; 1:33.

66. Kauffman RS: Viral pneumonia, in Pennington JE (ed): *Respiratory Infections: Diagnosis and Management*. New York, Raven Press, 1989, pp 427–442.

67. Graman PS, Hall CB: Nosocomial viral respiratory infections. *Semin Respir Infect* 1989; 4:253–260.

68. Toews GB: Southwestern internal medicine conference: Nosocomial pneumonia. *Am J Med Sci* 1986; 291:355–367.

69. CDC: Nosocomial transmission of multi-drug resistant tuberculosis to health-care workers and HIV-infected patients in an urban hospital-Florida. *MMWR* 1990; 39:718–722.

70. Grayston JT, Diwan VK, Cooney M, et al: Community- and hospital-acquired pneumonia associated with Chlamydia TWAR infection demonstrated serologically. *Arch Intern Med* 1989; 149:169–173.

71. Valdivieso M, Gil-Extremera B, Zornoza J, et al: Gram-negative bacillary pneumonia in the compromised host. *Medicine (Baltimore)* 1977; 56:241–254.

72. Towes GB: Nosocomial pneumonia. *Clin Chest Med* 1987; 8:467–479.

73. Pennington JE: Hospital-acquired pneumonia, in Pennington JE (ed): *Respiratory Infections: Diagnosis and Management.* New York, Raven Press, 1989, pp 171–186.

74. Santoro J: Nosocomial respiratory tract infections, in Levison ME (ed): *The Pneumonias: Clinical Approaches to Infectious Diseases of the Lower Respiratory Tract.* Boston, Bristol London, 1984, pp 182–194.

75. Quenzer RW: A perspective of cephalosporins in pneumonia. *Chest* 1987; 92:531–535.

76. Mandell LA, Nicolle LE, Ronald AR, et al: A multicentre prospective randomized trial comparing ceftazidime with cefazolin/tobramycin in the treatment of hospitalized patients with nonpneumococcal pneumonia. *J Antimicrob Chemother* 1983; 12(suppl A):9–20.

77. Trenholme GM, Pottage JC Jr, Karakusis PH: Use of ceftazidime in the treatment of nosocomial lower respiratory infections. *Am J Med* 1985; 79(suppl 2A):32–36.

78. Mangi RJ, Ryan J, Berenson C, et al: Cefoperazone versus ceftazidime monotherapy of nosocomial pneumonia. *Am J Med* 1988; 85(suppl 1A):44–48.

79. Mangi RJ, Greco T, Ryan J, et al: Cefoperazone versus combination antibiotic therapy of hospital-acquired pneumonia. *Am J Med* 1988; 84:68–74.

80. Perkins RL: Clinical trials of cefotaxime for the treatment of bacterial infections of the lower respiratory tract. *Rev Infect Dis* 1982; 4(suppl):S421–5430.

81. Diaz-Mitoma F, Harding GKM, Louie TJ, et al: Prospective randomized comparison of imipenem/cilastatin and cefotaxime for treatment of lung, soft tissue, and renal infections. *Rev Infect Dis* 1985; 7(suppl 3):S452–456.

82. Acar JF: Therapy for lower respiratory tract infections with imipenem/cilastatin: A review of worldwide experience. *Rev Infect Dis* 1985; 7(suppl 3):S513–517.

83. Schwigon CD, Hulla FW, Schulze B, et al: Timentin in the treatment of nosocomial bronchopulmonary infections in intensive care units. *J Antimicrob Chemother* 1986; 17(suppl C):115–122.

84. Roselle GA: Nosocomial and nursing home-acquired pneumonia: Recent therapeutic advances. *Postgrad Med* 1987; 81:131–136.

85. Cook JL: Gram-negative bacillary pneumonia in the nosocomial setting: Role of aztreonam therapy. *Am J Med* 1990; 88(suppl 3C):345–375.

86. Goldberg DM: The cephalosporins. *Med Clin North Am* 1987; 71:1113–1133.

87. Lipman B, Neu HC: Imipenem: A new carbapenem antibiotic. *Med Clin North Am* 1988; 72:567–579.

88. Winston DJ, McGrattan MA, Busuttil RW: Imipenem therapy of Pseudomonas aeruginosa and other serious bacterial infections. *Antimicrob Agents Chemother* 1984; 26:673–677.

89. Rusnak MG, Drake TA, Hackbarth CJ, et al: Single versus combination antibiotic therapy for pneumonia due to Pseudomonas aeruginosa in neutropenic guinea pigs. *J Infect Dis* 1984; 149:980–985.

90. Pancoast SJ: Aminoglycoside antibiotics on clinical use. *Med Clin North Am* 1988; 72:567–579.

91. Pennington JE: Penetration of antibiotics into respiratory secretions. *Rev Infect Dis* 1981; 3:67–73.

92. Moore RD, Smith CR, Lietman PS: Association of aminoglycoside plasma levels with therapeutic outcome in gram-negative pneumonia. *Am J Med* 1984; 77:657–662.

93. Neu HC: Antimicrobial therapy of gram-negative bacillary pneumonia, in Sande MA, Hudson LD, Root RK (eds): *Respiratory Infections: Contemporary Issues in Infectious Diseases,* vol 5. New York, Churchill Livingstone, 1986, pp 235–251.

94. Swab EA, Cone CO, Muir JG: Summary of worldwide clinical trials of aztreonam in patients with lower respiratory tract infections. *Rev Infect Dis* 1985; 7(suppl 4):S675–678.

95. Nolen TM, Phillips HL, Hall HJ: Comparison of aztreonam and tobramycin in the treatment of lower respiratory tract infections caused by gram-negative bacilli. *Rev Infect Dis* 1985; 7(suppl 4):S666–668.

96. Crane LR, Komshian S: Gram-negative bacillary pneumonia, in Pennington JE (ed): *Respiratory Infections: Diagnosis and Management.* New York, Raven Press, 1989, pp 314–340.

97. Kemmerich B, Lode H: Rational use of new antibiotics in respiratory infections, in Pennington JE (ed): *Respiratory Infections: Diagnosis and Management.* New York, Raven Press, 1989, pp 648–657.

98. Toma E, Poisson M, Phaneuf D, et al: Clindamycin with primaquine for Pneumocystis carinii pneumonia. *Lancet* 1989; 1:1046–1048.

99. Kay R, Dubois RE: Clindamycin/primaquine therapy and secondary prophylaxis against Pneumocystis carinii pneumonia in patients with AIDS. *South Med J* 1990; 83:403–404.

100. Medina I, Mills J, Leoung G, et al: Oral therapy for Pneumocystis carinii pneumonia in the acquired immunodeficiency syndrome. A controlled trial of trimethoprim-sulfamethoxazole versus trimethoprim-dapsone. *N Engl J Med* 1990; 323:776–782.

101. Sattler FR, Allegra CJ, Verdegem TD, et al: Trimetrexate-leucovorin dosage evaluation study for treatment of Pneumocystis carinii pneumonia. *J Infect Dis* 1990; 161:91–96.

102. Schlossberg D, Littman M: Varicella pneumonia. *Arch Intern Med* 1988; 148:1630–1632.

103. Hecht DW, Snydman DR, Crumpacker CS, et al: Ganciclovir for treatment of renal transplant-associated primary cytomegalovirus pneumonia. *J Infect Dis* 1988; 157:187–190.

104. Shepp DH, Dandliker PS, de Miranda P, et al: Activity of 9-[2-Hydroxy-1-(hydroxymethyl) ethoxymethyl] guanine in the treatment of cytomegalovirus pneumonia. *Ann Intern Med* 1985; 103:368–373.

105. Reed EC, Bowden RA, Dandliker PS, et al: Treatment of cytomegalovirus pneumonia with ganciclovir and intravenous cytomegalovirus immunoglobulin in patients with bone marrow transplants. *Ann Intern Med* 1988; 109:783–788.

106. Emanuel D, Cunningham I, Jules-Elysee K, et al: Cytomegalovirus pneumonia after bone marrow transplantation successfully treated with the combination of ganciclovir and high-dose intravenous immune globulin. *Ann Intern Med* 1988; 109:777–782.

107. Lehoang P, Girard B, Robinet M, et al: Foscarnet in the treatment of cytomegalovirus retinitis in acquired immune deficiency syndrome. *Ophthalmology* 1989; 96:865–874.

108. Jacobson MA, O'Donnell JJ, Mills J: Foscarnet treatment of cytomegalovirus retinitis in patients with the acquired immunodeficiency syndrome. *Antimicrob Agents Chemother* 1989; 33:736–741.

109. Klintmalm G, Lonnqvist B, Oberg B, et al: Intravenous foscarnet for the treatment of severe cytomegalovirus infection in allograft recipients. *Scand J Infect Dis* 1985; 17:157–163.

110. Ringden O, Lonnqvist B, Paulin T, et al: Foscarnet for cytomegalovirus infections. *Lancet* 1985; 1:1502–1504.

111. Drugs for treatment of fungal infections. *Med Lett Drugs Ther* 1990; 32:58–60.

112. Bodey GP: Topical and systemic antifungal agents. *Med Clin North Am* 1988; 72:637–640.

113. ATS Board of Directors: Medical Section of the American Lung Association. Chemotherapy of the pulmonary mycoses. *Am Rev Respir Dis* 1988; 138:1078–1081.

114. Lepper MH, Kofman S, Blatt N, et al: Effect of eight antibiotics used singly and in combination on the tracheal flora following tracheotomy in poliomyelitis. *Antibiot Chemother* 1954; 4:829–843.

115. Greenfield S, Teres D, Bushnell LS, et al: Prevention of gram-negative bacillary pneumonia using aerosol polymyxin as prophylaxis. I. Effect on the colonization pattern of the upper respiratory tract of seriously ill patients. *J Clin Invest* 1973; 52:2935–2940.

116. Klick JM, du Moulin GC, Hedley-Whyte J, et al: Prevention of gram-negative bacillary pneumonia using polymyxin aerosol as prophylaxis. II. Effect on the incidence of pneumonia in seriously ill patients. *J Clin Invest* 1975; 55:514–519.

117. Feeley TW, du Moulin GC, Hedley-Whyte J, et al: Aerosol polymyxin and pneumonia in seriously ill patients. *N Engl J Med* 1975; 293:471–475.

118. Bodey GP, Keating MJ, McCredie KB, et al: Prospective randomized trial of antibiotic prophylaxis in acute leukemia. *Am J Med* 1985; 78:407–416.

119. van Saene HKF, Stoutenbeek CP, Gilbertson AA: Review of available trials of selective decontamination of the digestive tract (SDD). *Infection* 1990; 18(suppl 1):S5–S9.

120. Stoutenbeek CP, van Saene HKF, Miranda DR, et al: The effect of oropharyngeal decontamination using non-absorbable antibiotics on the incidence of nosocomial respiratory tract infections in multiple trauma patients. *J Trauma* 1987; 27:357–364.

121. Chin NX, Neu HC: Cefotaxime and desacetylcefotaxime: An example of advantageous antimicrobial metabolism. *Diagn Microbiol Infect Dis* 1984; 2:21S–31S.

122. Stoutenbeek CP, van Saene HKF, Miranda DR, et al: The effect of selective decontamination of the digestive tract on colonization and infection rate in multiple trauma patients. *Intensive Care Med* 1984; 10:185–192.

123. Stoutenbeek CP, van Saene HKF, Miranda DR, et al: A new technique of infection prevention in the intensive care unit by selective decontamination of the digestive tract. *Acta Anaesthesiol Belg* 1983; 34:209–221.

124. Unertl K, Ruckdeschel G, Selbmann HK, et al: Prevention of colonization and respiratory infections in long-term ventilated patients by local antimicrobial prophylaxis. *Intensive Care Med* 1987; 13:106–113.

125. Ledingham IM, Eastaway AT, McKay IC, et al: Triple regimen of selective decontamination of the digestive tract, systemic cefotaxime, and microbiological surveillance for prevention of acquired infection in intensive care. *Lancet* 1988; 1:785–790.

126. Hartenauer U, Thulig B, Lawin P, et al: Infection surveillance and selective decontamination of the digestive tract (SDD) in critically ill patients—results of a controlled study. *Infection* 1990; 18(suppl 1):s22–s30.

127. Kerver AJH, Rommes JH, Mevissen-Verhage EAE, et al: Prevention of colonization and infection in critically ill patients: A prospective randomized study. *Crit Care Med* 1988; 16:1087–1093.

128. Ulrich C, Harinck-de Weerd JE, Bakker NC, et al: Selective decontamination of the digestive tract with norfloxacin in the prevention of ICU-acquired infections: A prospective randomized study. *Intensive Care Med* 1989; 15:424–431.

129. Tetteroo GWM, Wagenvoort JHT, Castelein A, et al: Selective decontamination to reduce gram-negative colonization and infections after esophageal resection. *Lancet* 1990; 335:704–707.

130. Brun-Buisson C, Legrand P, Rauss A, et al: Interstinal decontamination for control of nosocomial multiresistant gram-negative bacilli. *Ann Intern Med* 1989; 110:873–881.

131. van Uffelen R, Rommes JH, van Saene HKF: Preventing lower airway colonization and infection in mechanically ventilated patients. *Crit Care Med* 1987; 15:99–102.

132. Clasener HAL, Vollaard EJ, van Saene HKF: Long-term prophylaxis of infection by selective decontamination in leukopenia and in mechanical ventilation. *Rev Infect Dis* 1987; 9:295–328.

133. Flaherty J, Kabins SA, Weinstein RA: New approaches to the prevention of infection in intensive care unit patients, in van Saene HKF, Stoutenbeek CP, Lawin P, et al (eds): *Update in Intensive Care and Emergency Medicine*. Heidelberg, Springer-Verlag, 1989, pp 184–188.

134. Wiesner RH, Krom RAF, Hermans P: Selective bowel decontamination to decrease gram-negative aerobic bacterial and candida colonization and prevent infection after orthotopic liver transplantation. *Transplantation* 1988; 45:570–574.

135. Johanson WG, Seidenfeld JJ, de los Santos R, et al: Prevention of nosocomial pneumonia using topical and parenteral antimicrobial agents. *Am Rev Respir Dis* 1988; 137:265–272.

136. Knaus WA, Draper EA, Wagner DP, et al: An evaluation of outcome from intensive care in major medical centers. *Ann Intern Med* 1986; 104:410–418.

137. Polk HC, Borden S, Aldrete JA: Prevention of respiratory infection in a surgical intensive care unit. *Ann Surg* 1973; 177:607–615.

138. Ziegler E, McCutchan J, Fierer J, et al: Treatment of gram-negative bacteremia and shock with human antiserum to a mutant Escherichia coli. *N Engl J Med* 1982; 307:1225–1230.

139. Baumgartner J, Glauser M, McCutchan J, et al: Prevention of gram-negative shock and death in surgical patients by antibody to endotoxin core glycolipid. *Lancet* 1985; 2:59–63.

140. Ziegler E, Fisher C, Sprung C, et al: Treatment of gram-negative bacteremia and septic shock with HA-1A human monoclonal antibody against endotoxin. *N Engl J Med* 1991; 324:429–436.

CHAPTER 2

Ethics in Cardiopulmonary Medicine

Deborah J. Cook, M.D., F.R.C.P., M.Sc.

Assistant Professor, Department of Medicine, Division of Critical Care and Department of Clinical Epidemiology and Biostatistics, McMaster University School of Medicine, McMaster University Medical Center, Hamilton, Ontario, Canada

Thomas A. Raffin, M.D.

Chief, Division of Pulmonary and Critical Care Medicine, Co-Director, Stanford University Center for Biomedical Ethics, Stanford University School of Medicine, Stanford University Medical Center, Stanford, California

Insight into the ethics of cardiopulmonary medicine requires an understanding of the development of the intensive care unit and the associated implications for the critical care physician, as well as an appreciation of biomedical ethical principles and a perspective on health care economics, health care rationing, and related legal issues.

THE INTENSIVE CARE UNIT AND THE TECHNOLOGIC IMPERATIVE

During the last century, dramatic changes have occurred in physicians' ability to prolong life. One hundred years ago, little more than rudimentary supportive care could be offered to most critically ill patients. Doctors now can provide effective therapy for many conditions in the modern intensive care unit (ICU) and can intervene to prolong survival in a large proportion of critically ill patients.

The objective of an ICU is to improve the short-term survival of patients with exigent, life-threatening illness. The ICU differs from general medical or surgical wards in several ways. The patients are more critically ill, often with cardiovascular instability, organ failure, and metabolic derangement. Invasive hemodynamic monitoring, such as is possible with the pulmonary artery catheter, means that more information is available to the clinician for management decisions. Life support systems, such as mechanical ventilation and dialysis, are widely used to sustain or prolong life.

Many physicians consider it their professional duty to prolong life under most circumstances. Although this appears to be time-honored, it actually is a modern phenomenon. According to Admundsen, the Hippocratic corpus described the three roles of medicine as (1) relieving suffering, (2) attenuating disease, and (3) refraining from treating hopelessly ill patients, lest physicians be considered charlatans.[1] However, with the development of improved diagnostic and therapeutic techniques and the creation of ICUs, life support became a primary obligation of medicine.[2]

Part of this obligation stems from the "technologic imperative," that is, the desires of physicians to do everything that they have been trained to do regardless of the cost-benefit ratio. This imperative is particularly compelling in the ICU, where patients are likely to die without aggressive management. Moreover, patients often cannot participate in medical discussions because they are intubated and/or sedated. Other factors also contribute to the tendency to treat aggressively in the ICU. Medical responsibility for the critically ill is often diffuse, divided among subspecialists who manage specific organ systems but fail to take a global point of view. In addition, fee-for-service and procedure-oriented payment encourages physicians to manage patients in the ICU. Physicians may practice "defensive medicine" in this setting, especially when iatrogenic insults have necessitated ICU admission.

ETHICAL PRINCIPLES/THEOLOGIC ISSUES

Ethically sound medical decisions in the ICU require that patients and physicians participate in discussions resulting in jointly acceptable decisions. However, in our pluralistic society, some significant differences exist among the major religions on critical issues in medical ethics. Fortunately, some ethical principles are shared and stem from values that transcend the capricious variations of time, culture, and environment. The four fundamental biomedical ethical principles are: beneficence, nonmaleficence, autonomy, and justice.

Beneficence.— In dealing with critically ill patients and their families, actions should be guided by the four fundamental biomedical ethical principles. The first is beneficence, which refers to the physician's responsibility to restore health, relieve suffering, and, fundamentally, preserve life. Respect for the sanctity of life has its roots in most religious traditions.

Nonmaleficence.—The second ethical principle is nonmaleficence, which echoes the tradition of "primum non nocere," or, above all, do no harm. This means that a health care provider should not deliver a therapy if the odds are greater that it might harm rather than benefit the patient. A good example of a violation of this ethical principle is when a practitioner provides nonindicated therapy that results in morbidity or mortality. In the ICU, this may be placing a nonindicated intravascular catheter that results in serious complications.

Autonomy.—The third ethical principle is autonomy, summarized as respect for the individuality of the patient. This is highlighted by the fact that patients are more than equal partners in arriving at decisions affecting their own lives and should be encouraged to assume the responsibility of this partnership. For example, it is paramount in the practice of medicine to provide, whenever possible, informed consent, so that patients understand the risks and benefits of a diagnostic or therapeutic procedure and can participate in their own care. It is a violation of the third principle, respect for the autonomy of the patient, that creates the ethical dilemma arising from the withdrawal of life support.

Justice.—The fourth ethical principle is justice. Unfortunately, at the present time in America, we do not have just allocation of medical resources. Disadvantaged Americans suffer greater morbidity and mortality from major illnesses and die younger in most disease-specific categories than do persons from the middle class.

These four ethical principles provide a basis for analyzing some of the complex biomedical ethical issues that have come to the forefront with ICU technology. One example of how these fundamental ethical principles can come into conflict can be appreciated in the current controversy regarding management of human immunodeficiency virus (HIV) infections. Ideally, we would like to prevent infections in persons unknowingly exposed to HIV. However, this conflicts with respecting the autonomy and privacy of HIV-infected individuals and the confidentiality of their HIV test results.

ECONOMIC ISSUES

The evolution of the American health care system has been characterized by a strong entrepreneurial influence, few cost controls, and a reliance on scientific progress and high technology to deliver the best possible care without regard to cost. There have been six major forces that have stimulated the growth and costs of our health care system: (1) technology, (2) the increasing price of services, (3) an aging population, (4) defensive medicine, (5) bureaucracy, and (6) the contribution of third-party payments.

It is primarily modern technologic advances that have afforded new diagnostic and therapeutic options for the critical care physician. However, the cost of these medical advances is substantial. Health care costs are projected to increase from 8% of the gross national product of Canada in 1980 to 15% by the year 2000,[3] and an increasing proportion of the health care dollar is being spent on a very small percentage of hospitalized patients in the last few days of life.[4, 5] Therefore, a considerable proportion of annual hospital expenditures is the cost associated with caring for patients in the ICU. Indeed, critical care contributes to the controversy of appropriate allocation of health care dollars.[6, 7]

There is great consternation over how to stabilize or decrease our health care costs, since it is apparent that we cannot afford our increasing fiscal commitment to health care. As a result, economic concerns often are an integral part of discussions concerning policies for life support and other ethical issues in the ICU.

HEALTH CARE RATIONING

Rationing has existed in health care and in the ICU for the past several decades.[8] Patients' income and the geographic location of medical services has restricted the availability of medical care for many Americans. Critical care physicians are on the front lines of patient care rationing decisions, since they must decide which patients are admitted or discharged from the ICU. Increasingly, urban center hospitals are being forced to make triage decisions when ICU resources are limited because there are too many critically ill patients, and other hospitals will not accept patients in transfer. Triage decision policies should be developed by institutional interdisciplinary commitees, as critical care physicians alone cannot be expected to act as economic gatekeepers. Unfortunately, because of the progressively more severe financial problems in our health care system, much more significant health care rationing is likely to occur in the next several years.

GOVERNMENT LEGISLATION: ADVANCE DIRECTIVES

In the early 1980s, state legislatures began to pass living will legislation that allowed citizens the right to dictate what type of health care they wanted to receive if they became legally incompetent. There are three types of living will or advanced directive documents passed by individual states. First, living wills, not necessarily endorsed by state legislatures, are available from the Society for the Right to Die or Concern for Dying.[9] It is not necessary for an individual completing a living will to list all of the specific management approaches that he or she would like taken if a specific illness befalls him or her. Rather, living wills are completed with general statements such as: "If I have, in essence, no chance to regain a reasonable quality of life, withhold or withdraw life support (including nutrition and hydration) from me so that I can die with peace and dignity." Second, there is another set of statutes known as natural death act directives. These instructional directives are documents created by patients that also can aid in decision-making.[10] Third, many states are beginning to pass legislation to support legal durable powers of attorney for health care. Proxy directives that empower others to decide medical issues for patients, such as the California Durable Power of Attorney for Health Care (1984), have been used extensively in California.

LEGAL PRECEDENTS

The American judicial system has been instrumental in shaping North American attitudes and social policy in the area of withholding and withdrawing life support from patients who are not brain-dead. In the process, U.S. courts have underscored the importance of privacy and the right to refuse treatment. They also have (1) contributed to the concept that human life is more than a biologic process, (2) defined how therapies may or may not benefit patients, (3) argued against a distinction between withholding and withdrawal of support, and (4) established guidelines for how support may be withheld or withdrawn.

Perhaps the best known judicial decision in this field was the case of Karen Ann Quinlan (1976). The father of the patient, who was in a persistent vegetative state, petitioned the court to appoint him her guardian with the power to discontinue mechanical ventilation. The lower court denied the petition, but the New Jersey Supreme Court reversed the decision. In doing so, the court reasoned that patients generally would accept or refuse medical treatment based on its ability to support sentient life, as distinguished from mere biologic existence. Having concluded that Ms. Quinlan would have decided to forego life support were she not in a persistent vegetative state, the court decided that her right to privacy would be abrogated if it prevented the exercise of this right on her behalf. The court, therefore, granted the father's petition, allowing him to exercise substituted judgment for his daughter, and stated that life support could be withdrawn if the physicians and the hospital ethics committee agreed that such support would not alter Ms. Quinlan's underlying condition.[11, 12]

In June 1990, the Supreme Court of the United States made its landmark ruling on the Nancy Cruzan case (which had been appealed by the State of Missouri).[13] This was the first case on which the Supreme Court ever ruled concerning the biomedical ethical issue of withholding and withdrawing life support. The Supreme Court upheld the State of Missouri in its position that a state can prohibit families from withdrawing life support from a legally incompetent loved one if there are not definite and convincing data that will support the fact that the loved one wanted life support to be withheld or withdrawn. Therefore, the Cruzan decision supported state rights to decide how to handle withholding and withdrawing life support, and it also upheld the importance of advance directives, which determine whether or not life support should be withheld or withdrawn from an incompetent patient.

Interestingly, most of the court cases regarding withholding or withdrawal of life support were brought by patients or their proxies against physicians and medical institutions for *failing to* withhold or withdraw support. Furthermore, most of the legislation has been advanced by the legal, not the medical, profession. There are certain to be future state and Supreme Court decisions concerning biomedical ethical issues germane to the practice of critical care medicine.

KEY PRACTICAL PRINCIPLES IN ETHICAL DECISION-MAKING

In dealing with ethical issues in cardiopulmonary medicine, in addition to the four general ethical principles, there are four key practical guidelines that should be followed.[14] These are discussed as follows.

Establish the Source of Authority for Decision-Making

Many of the ethical problems and controversies in critical care arise as a result of overt or covert violations of the first guideline. However, life support often is initiated under crisis conditions, when it is not possible to consult with the patient or the family. Thus, a temporary vacuum of authority is created that is filled by the health care team. During the early, aggressive management phase, patients may be intubated or have invasive lines inserted, and sophisticated monitoring equipment may be introduced. It is no surprise that, because of the emergent nature of many problems in ICU medicine, doctors often feel forced to embody authority and to proceed with diagnostic or therapeutic plans immediately.

Effectively Communicate With Patients and Family

There are several reasons why communication in the critical care setting is difficult for doctors. First, each case may be emotionally stressful, and the accumulated effect of many such cases exacts a high price from physicians in terms of emotional energy, personal fear of death, guilt, and anxiety. Moreover, effective communication in catastrophic situations requires time, a scarce commodity among doctors. Outside facilitators can be extremely valuable to the ICU health care team because of their well-developed communication skills and the time they have and make to exercise them. In optimizing communication, an appropriate setting is crucial (i.e., a noisy hospital corridor may hinder effective decision-making). Stress often impairs the reasoning ability of families, so communication should be helpful rather than overwhelming. Esoteric jargon should be avoided. Patients and families should be encouraged to speak about their feelings. It often is helpful to ask patients and families to summarize what has been said in order to correct misunderstandings, should they exist.

A classic example of poor communication in the ICU setting would be when a physician tells a family that their critically ill loved one is "stable," without much in the way of further explanation. Perhaps a more truthful report would be, "Your husband is as sick as any person could be, and the odds are overwhelming that he will not survive. His condition has not changed in the last 24 hours, and if he does not improve over the next several days, we might have to begin to discuss decreasing our level of support."

Determine Early and Frequently Review Patient Wishes

The early determination and ongoing review of patient desires is crucial, so that the health care team does not make erroneous assumptions. Patients may bring the subject up first with the nursing staff. Sometimes family members come forward with such information. It is the responsibility of each physician to try to learn the wishes of each patient regarding the extent to which they are being fulfilled in relation to the type and extent of medical care being delivered.

Recognize Patient Rights

The fourth practical guideline in ethical decision-making in critical care medicine is the recognition that patients have rights. The American Hospital Association has developed a code of patients' rights,[15] which has been enacted into law in several states. If critical care physicians observe the spirit of these rights, then ethical decision-making will not be a major difficulty. Some of these rights include the right (1) to receive considerate and respectful care, (2) to receive appropriate information in understandable terms, (3) to participate actively in decision-making, and (4) to have the patients' rights applied to the person who may have legal responsibility to make decisions on behalf of the patient.

BRAIN DEATH AND ORGAN TRANSPLANTATION

The development of organ transplantation has been one of the most exciting advances in modern scientific medicine. Transplantation of kidneys, hearts, lungs, and bone marrow is becoming established effective therapy for specific end-stage diseases.[16] In the early days of the development of organ transplantation, the definition of death was intact; death was recognized by the cessation of heart and lung function.

In 1968, the Ad Hoc Committee of the Harvard Medical School published their landmark report, "To Define Irreversible Coma as a New Criterion for Death."[17] To identify brain death, one must demonstrate irreversible loss of cerebral hemispheric and brain stem function including ventilatory reflexes. The effects of hypothermia and drugs must be excluded. Brain death, therefore, is a clinical diagnosis. However, family or surrogate approval is mandatory before retrieval of organs for transplantation takes place. Because one of the major limitations to widespread transplantation in the United States is the scarcity of donor organs, it is extremely important that health care workers discuss this issue with family members or surrogates of patients who are brain-dead or near brain death, if they are prospective organ donors.

WITHHOLDING AND WITHDRAWING BASIC LIFE SUPPORT

Providing basic life support such as food, water, and supplementary oxygen is difficult to forego in general medical practice because it is perceived as basic minimal care. However, basic life support is not always in the patient's best interest. For example, patients who are terminally ill, suffering, and awaiting death might be better served by not having infections treated with antibiotics or cerebral edema treated with steroids. It can be difficult to observe comatose, hopelessly ill patients being held back from a painless death to live out an extra few days in indignity.

Once intravenous lines or feeding tubes are in place, it becomes harder to stop hydrating, treating electrolyte abnormalities, or feeding. Withholding basic life support such as hydration or nutrition is controversial and is a problem frequently faced by ICU physicians. As always, the key to resolving ethical problems in this area lies in clarifying what is in the patient's interest. In the situation where a patient becomes comatose after a prolonged cardiopulmonary arrest, for example, such a dilemma may arise. In the presence of truly informed consent and sensitive, open communication, most decisions about withholding or withdrawing basic life support can be made less painful. Families need assurances that comfort and care will be maintained, and that care providers will not abandon the patient.

WITHHOLDING AND WITHDRAWING ADVANCED LIFE SUPPORT

Withholding and withdrawing life support are the processes by which various advanced medical interventions either are not given to or are removed from patients, with the expectation that they probably will die soon without such interventions. Because advanced life support often is extended to the critically ill population, the question of whether to withhold or withdraw such support comes up frequently in the ICU. The focus of the remainder of this chapter will be on these issues.

Unfortunately, the quality of life so skillfully sought by critical care physicians can range from acceptable to tolerable to miserable. This issue underscores the importance of an ethical framework for making decisions about the initiation and withdrawal of advanced life support.[18]

Withholding Advanced Life Support

Despite increasing public and medical interest in withholding and withdrawal of life support from critically ill patients, little is known about how much support actually is withheld or withdrawn. Most studies have focused on the circumstances in which "do not resuscitate" (DNR) orders are written and what happens to patients subseqently.[19–23] In general, these studies have demonstrated that DNR orders are written relatively late in a patient's admission, even when they are hospitalized in the ICU. Justification for the orders and treatment goals after the orders are written frequently are lacking. The brief interval between writing orders and death or ICU discharge suggests that the orders often represent a decision point for placing broader limits on therapy. Although many ethicists and physicians consider DNR status as compatible with aggressive medical judgment in actual practice, the writing of DNR orders usually leads to less intensive care.

Withdrawing Advanced Life Support

Physicians attempt to fulfill two basic interwoven ethical obligations in the care of patients: to restore health and relieve suffering. Ideally, the two may be achieved simultaneously. However, in practice, these obligations often conflict, as in the care of a chemotherapy-treated patient with advanced cancer and septic shock. This conflict reaches its pinnacle in the care of the critically ill, who may linger in the ICU on advanced life support for many days with little or no chance of regaining a reasonable quality of life, cognition, or sapience. As hope of recovery fades, the physician confronts a third obligation: to help the dying achieve a peaceful and dignified death.

One study at the University of California, San Francisco, and the San Francisco General Hospital[24] demonstrated that withholding or withdrawing life support is relatively uncommon among ICU patients (24 of 648 patients), perhaps because of restrictions on ICU admissions in the first place. Patients from whom life support was withheld or withdrawn most often had multiple organ failure, end-stage respiratory disease, intracranial disorders, or cancer. Withholding or withdrawing support occurred earlier in brain-dead patients, although the timing was not influenced by a previous wish to limit care. Mechanical ventilation was the therapy most often withheld or withdrawn, although dialysis, vasopressors, supplemental oxygen, antibiotics, and, rarely, fluid and nutrition also were withdrawn. A poor prognosis was the reason identified in the majority of cases. Information for this study was obtained from chart review and nonsystematic interviews with nurses, physicians, and families.

The impact of withdrawal of life support has been studied on surviving relatives of patients who died when chronic dialysis was discontinued.[25] Relatives felt that the family members most often are the initiators of the discussion that led to withdrawal of life support, and that patients and family members tended to make the final decisions. Other authors support this contention.[26, 27] The relatives expressed disappointment with physicians who were unwilling to talk to them, were overly optimistic, or continued with treatment too long; in general, relatives wished for more openness and truthfulness.

A Look Into the Future

The American College of Chest Physicians and the Society of Crtical Care Medicine in the United States held a consensus conference in 1989 to determine ethical and moral guidelines for the initiation, continuation, and withdrawal of intensive care.[28] Their charge was to examine the characteristics that would identify appropriately an adult patient for admission to an ICU and to recommend criteria for the initiation, continuation, or withdrawal of intensive care. Few of these onerous tasks were completed successfully; however, a conceptual framework for making decisions about intensive care resulted, and issues to be addressed in the future were identified.

The decision to withdraw advanced life support is one of the most difficult to face the critical care physician. Despite the fact that this challenge has been part of ICU medicine for many years, there has been little research into the patient and physician factors that play a role in the decision. Given the escalating cost of medical care and the increasing pressure on acute care units, policies for ICU physicians regarding life support withdrawal are being considered in some institutions. Although it is clear that individual patient assessment is needed in most situations and that the principles of biomedical ethics should be central to this process, there remains a need to learn about the general perspective on this issue.

It would be worthwhile to assess the independent contribution and interaction of patient and physician factors in the decision to withdraw life support. Patient factors may include age, sex, prognosis, occupation, employment status, prior cognitive function, psychiatric history, history of self-destructive behavior, sexual orientation, marital status, degree of family support, and directives from the patient and family. Physician factors may include age, sex, year of medical school graduation, country of graduation, years since completion of training, training program, country of birth, religion, and current status in the medical system.

We believe that understanding the factors that determine physicians' decisions to withhold or withdraw life support is crucial and needs to be evaluated on a large scale before widespread policies are implemented without an adequate assessment of the North American perspective on this issue.

Ethics Consultations

When critical care practitioners are confronted by a thorny ethical dilemma in the ICU or a tense, and possibly adversarial, relationship with a patient, family member, or surrogate, it is wise to enlist the aid of a facilitator as soon as possible. A facilitator could be a representative from an organized religion who is trained in ethics and legalities of critical care medicine, a social worker, an ethicist, or a psychotherapist. Most hospitals have ethics committees that act in a consultative capacity. Sometimes the whole ethics committee deliberates over the case; in other situations, a single experienced consultant from the panel is used.[29]

The use of ethics consultations is increasing.[30, 31] La Puma and colleagues reported on the prospective evaluation of a newly established ethics consultation service in a teaching hospital. A physician-ethicist interviewed and examined patients, interviewed families, and wrote a note in the medical records. Fifty-one consultation requests were received from 45 physicians from July 1986 to June 1987. Thirty percent of consults were in the ICU, and 37% of patients were oriented at the time of consultation. Questions concerning cardiopulmonary resuscitation were addressed in 37% of cases, and legal issues were addressed in 31%. In 71% of cases, the requesting physician stated that the consultation was very important in assisting management. The help was embodied in (1) encouragement of frank discussion about quality of life issues, (2) facilitation of patient-family participation in decision-making, and (3) reassurance of all parties that patients can be allowed to die without this being equated to abandonment.

When the fundamental principles of biomedical ethics are used as guidelines for critical care and life support decisions, patients, their families, and the medical staff all benefit. Respect for the autonomy of the critically ill individual, regard for the emotional needs of the survivors, and understanding of the medicolegal bases for decisions to withhold or withdraw care, especially if a substituted judgment is required, should be woven into the fabric of physician education and become intrinsic features of the art and practice of medicine in the 1990s.

REFERENCES

1. Admundsen D: The physicians' obligation to prolong life: A medical study without classical roots. *Hastings Cent Rep* 1978; 8:23–24.

2. Loewy EH: Treatment decisions in the mentally impaired—limiting but not abandoning treatment. *N Engl J Med* 1987; 317:1465–1468.

3. Enthoven A, Kronik R: A consumer-choice health plan for the 1990s: University health insurance in a system designed to promote quality and economy. *N Engl J Med* 1989; 320:29–37.

4. Schroeder SA, Showstack JA, Roberts JE: Frequency and clinical description of high-cost patients in 17 acute care hospitals. *N Engl J Med* 1979; 300:1306–1309.

5. Zook CJ, Moore FD: High-cost users of medical care. *N Engl J Med* 1980; 302:996–1002.

6. Evans R: Health care technology and the inevitability of resource allocation and rationing decisions. *JAMA* 1983; 249:2047–2053.

7. Singer D, Carr P, Mulley A: Rationing intensive care—physician responses to a resource shortage. *N Engl J Med* 1983; 309:1155–1160.

8. Relman AS: Is rationing inevitable? *N Engl J Med* 1990; 322:1809–1810.

9. Society for the Right to Die: *The Physician and the Hopelessly Ill Patient.* New York, Society for the Right to Die, 1985.

10. Raffin TA: Value of the living will. *Chest* 1986; 90:444–446.

11. Gilfix M, Raffin TA: Withholding and withdrawing extraordinary life support—optimizing rights and limiting liability. *West J Med* 1984; 141:387–394.

12. Suber DG, Tabor WJ: Withholding of life-sustaining treatment from the terminally ill, incompetent patient: Who decides? *JAMA* 1982; 248:2250–2251.

13. Lo B, Rouse F, Dornbrand L: Family decision making on trial: Who decides for incompetent patients? *N Engl J Med* 1990; 322:1228–1232.

14. Raffin TA: Perspectives on clinical medical ethics, in Hall JB, Schmidt GA, Wood LDH (eds): *Principles of Critical Care Medicine.* New York, McGraw Hill, Inc, in press.

15. Title 22, Section 70707, California Administrative Code.

16. Stevens JH, Raffin TA, Baldwin JC: The status of transplantation of the human lung. *Surg Gynecol Obstet* 1989; 169:179–185.

17. Guidelines for determination of death: Report of the medical consultants on the diagnosis of death to the President's Commission for the Study of Ethical Problems in Medicine and Biomedical and Behavioral Research. *JAMA* 1981; 246:2184–2186.

18. Ruark JE, Raffin TA, and the Stanford University Medical Center Committee on Ethics: Initiating and withdrawing life support: Principles and practices in adult medicine. *N Engl J Med* 1988; 318:25–30.

19. Lo B, Saika G, Strull W, et al: "Do not resuscitate" decisions—a prospective study at three teaching hospitals. *Ann Intern Med* 1985; 145:1115–1117.

20. Bedell SE, Pelle D, Maher PL, et al: Do-not-resuscitate orders for critically ill patients in the hospital—how are they used and what is their impact. *JAMA* 1986; 256:233–237.

21. Younger SJ, Lewandowski W, McClish DK, et al: "Do not resuscitate" orders—incidence and implications in medical intensive care units. *JAMA* 1985; 253:54–57.

22. Zimmerman JE, Knaus WA, Sharpe SM, et al: The use and implications of do not resuscitate orders in intensive care units. *JAMA* 1986; 255:351–356.

23. Lipton HL: Do-not-resuscitate decisions in a community hospital—incidence, implications, and outcomes. *JAMA* 1986; 255:1164–1169.

24. Smedira NG, Evans BH, Cohen NH, et al: Withholding and withdrawing life support from the critically ill (abstract). *Am Rev Respir Dis* 1988; 137:475.

25. Roberts JC, Snyder R, Kjellstrand CM: Withdrawing life support—the survivors. *Acta Med Scand* 1988; 224:141–148.

26. Neu S, Kjellstrand CM: Stopping long-term dialysis: An empirical study of life-supporting treatment. *N Engl J Med* 1986; 314:14–20.

27. Munoz-Silva JE, Kjellstrand CM: Withdrawing life support. Do families and physicians decide as patients do? *Nephron* 1988; 48:201–205.

28. Bone RC, Rackow EC, and the ACCP/SCCM Consensus Panel: Ethical and moral guidelines for the initiation, continuation, and withdrawal of intensive care. *Chest* 1990; 97:949–958.

29. Rosner F: Hospital medical ethics committees: A review of their development. *JAMA* 1985; 253:2693–2697.

30. La Puma J, Stocking CB, Silverstein MD, et al: An ethics consultation service in a teaching hospital: Utilization and evaluation. *JAMA* 1988; 260:808–811.

31. Brennan TA: Ethics committees and decisions to limit care: The experience of the Massachusetts General Hospital. *JAMA* 1988; 260:803–807.

CHAPTER 3

Modes of Mechanical Ventilation

Theodore W. Marcy, M.D.

Assistant Professor of Medicine, University of Minnesota, Pulmonary and Critical Care Section, St. Paul-Ramsey Medical Center, St. Paul, Minnesota

John J. Marini, M.D.

Professor of Medicine, University of Minnesota, Pulmonary and Critical Care Section, St. Paul-Ramsey Medical Center, St. Paul, Minnesota

Mechanical ventilation first became practical life support therapy for respiratory failure during the polio epidemics of the 1930s with the advent of the Drinker ventilator or iron lung.[1] Since then, a variety of modes of ventilation have evolved, accompanied by impressive advancements in ventilator equipment and microprocessor-based monitoring and control systems.[1] These different modes can support critically ill patients who are unable to meet their gas exchange requirements because of neuromuscular impairment, cardiovascular collapse, diffuse lung disease, or disordered central respiratory drive. However, technologic improvements frequently have outpaced our understanding of their optimal use.[2] In this chapter, we review general considerations regarding ventilatory support. We then explore ventilatory modes and strategies for the different forms of respiratory failure for which they are employed.

GENERAL CONSIDERATIONS IN MECHANICAL VENTILATION

Goals

The primary goals of mechanical ventilation are improving arterial blood oxygenation, decreasing or eliminating energy consumption of the respiratory muscles, and preserving acid-base homeostasis. To accomplish ventilation, mechanical ventilators move volumes of gas into and out of the lung by generating phasic changes in transpulmonary pressure. To accomplish oxygenation, ventilators deliver oxygen-enriched gas to alveoli and, in certain situations, increase lung volume to reexpand areas of lung not participating in gas exchange. As ventilatory requirements rise with increasing CO_2 production or with an increased physiologic dead space, the phasic changes in pressure must be greater or occur at a higher frequency. Refractory arterial hypoxemia due to pulmonary arteriovenous shunting also requires adjustments in the ventilator's pattern of applied pressure (and volume). Pressure applied at the airway not only must recruit nonaerated alveoli, but also must prevent alveolar collapse at end expiration.

Hazards

Barotrauma
Unfortunately, pressure and volume cannot be applied with impunity. Extremes of pressure and volume have many deleterious effects, particularly when the lung injury is not distributed uniformly. When there is significant atelectasis, or when lung units exhibit heterogeneity in their mechanical characteristics, the magnitude of pressure required to accomplish oxygenation and ventilation at normal tidal volumes may overdistend and rupture the fragile membranes of normally compliant alveoli. Gas then extravasates from torn alveoli into the bronchovascular adventitia, which may be visible radiographically as pulmonary interstitial emphysema. Gas then can dissect along the bronchovascular sheath into the mediastinum, and from there through different fascial planes into the subcutaneous tissue and retroperitoneum.[3-6] Gas can enter the pleural space through disruptions of the mediastinal parietal pleura or from rupture of subpleural air cysts—pockets of interstitial gas collecting adjacent to the visceral pleura.[7]

Certain forms of extra-alveolar gas will result in severe systemic complications. Pneumothoraces under tension cause hemodynamic compromise or collapse as highly positive intrapleural pressures impede venous return and compress central vascular structures.[3] In addition, interstitial gas under pressure may rupture into pulmonary venules and enter the systemic circulation, causing unexpected (and possibly unrecognized) myocardial and cerebrovascular damage.[8, 9]

The rupture of alveoli with extravasation of alveolar gas may not be the only manifestation of tissue injury from pressure applied at the airway. Several investigators have provoked an injury indistinguishable from that of the adult respiratory distress syndrome (ARDS) in experimental animals ventilated with moderately high peak airway pressures (30 to 50 cm H_2O).[10-16] Although not yet confirmed in patients, these studies suggest that lung injury may be extended by the very technique designed to compensate for it.

Hemodynamic Consequences

The hemodynamic consequences of mechanical ventilation are due primarily to changes in intrapleural pressure and lung volume. These concepts have been reviewed recently,[17, 18] and will be discussed in more depth in the section of this chapter on cardiovascular compromise.

Risks of Artificial Airways

Even if the pressures required for adequate oxygenation and ventilation are not excessive, establishing an airway for ventilation with either an endotracheal tube or a tracheostomy can lead to serious complications.[19, 20] During translaryngeal intubation, the mucosal surfaces of the upper airway may hemorrhage or become edematous. Prolonged attempts at intubation can lead to cardiac arrest or seizures, and intubation of the right main bronchus may cause atelectasis or a pneumothorax. Once in place, a variety of endotracheal tube malfunctions—dislodgment, tube occlusion, cuff laceration—occur approximately 6% of the time.[20] In nasally intubated patients, paranasal sinusitis may present as a source of fever and sepsis.[21] Tracheal ulceration and ischemic injury from excessive cuff pressures predispose patients to eventual tracheomalacia or stenosis.[20, 22] Tracheostomy poses its own risks from operative hemorrhage, tube displacement, fistula formation, and tracheal stenosis.[20]

Both endotracheal tubes and tracheostomies violate an anatomical barrier guarding against contamination of the usually sterile lower respiratory tract, and thereby serve as a conduit for colonizing the lower respiratory tract with pathogenic organisms. The incidence of nosocomial pneumonias is significantly higher in intubated than in nonintubated patients in the intensive care unit, and is related linearly to the duration of mechanical ventilation.[23, 24] There is increasing recognition that nosocomial pneumonias are an important cause of mortality in patients with ARDS and other problems requiring mechanical ventilation.[25, 26]

General Approach to Ventilatory Support

The appropriate mode and strategy of mechanical ventilation is that which minimizes adverse consequences while still accomplishing the goals of ventilatory support. However, which mode and ventilatory strategy is best depends on the clinical problem for which it is required. When respiratory failure is from diffuse lung injury or exacerbations of airflow obstruction, minimizing adverse consequences associated with pressure and volume becomes paramount. By contrast, in patients with failure of neuromuscular function, the preferred mode of ventilation may be that which permits assisted ventilation without the consequences of an artificial airway. In patients recovering from respiratory muscle fatigue, the best method of ventilation may be that which facilitates the resumption of spontaneous ventilation ("weaning").

The selection of appropriate end points (pH, $Paco_2$, Pao_2) during mechanical ventilation is as important as the choice of ventilatory mode or strategy. Under certain circumstances, achieving normal levels of oxygenation or acid-base status with mechanical ventilation may be unnecessarily dangerous. It may be prudent and desirable to accept oxygen saturations of less than 85% or some respiratory acidosis to balance the physiologic consequences of hypoxemia and acidosis against the mechanical and hemodynamic consequences of high applied pressures and volumes.[27, 28]

AIRFLOW OBSTRUCTION

Pathophysiology

Diseases associated with acute or chronic airflow obstruction—asthma, chronic bronchitis, emphysema, bronchiectasis—impose a significant mechanical burden on the respiratory system. Airway diameter is variably narrowed by bronchospasm, mucosal edema, exudates of inflammatory cells and mucus, and dynamic expiratory airway collapse. Estimates of the inspiratory resistance of the respiratory system in patients on mechanical ventilation for airflow obstruction average fivefold higher than those of normal anesthetized subjects.[29–31] When patients with severe airflow obstruction experience expiratory flow limitation during tidal respiration, increasing expiratory effort simply raises alveolar pressure without improving expiratory airflow. If minute ventilation increases above a certain value, or if expiratory time decreases sufficiently, the lung cannot deflate to its usual resting equilibrium volume between breaths. Several important consequences arise from the associated changes in lung volume and pleural pressure. As lung volumes become higher, respiratory system compliance decreases.[32] End-expiratory alveolar pressure becomes positive relative to airway opening pressure, a phenomenon termed autoPEEP that can be defined as a positive flow-driving difference between pressures in the alveolus and the airway opening pressure at end-exhalation.[33, 34] Thus, end-expiratory pressure is the sum of PEEP and autoPEEP (Fig 1). In the presence of autoPEEP, a negative intrapleural pressure equal in magnitude to the level of autoPEEP must be generated by the respiratory muscles before inspiratory flow will begin or a ventilator-assisted machine cycle can be triggered (Fig 2).

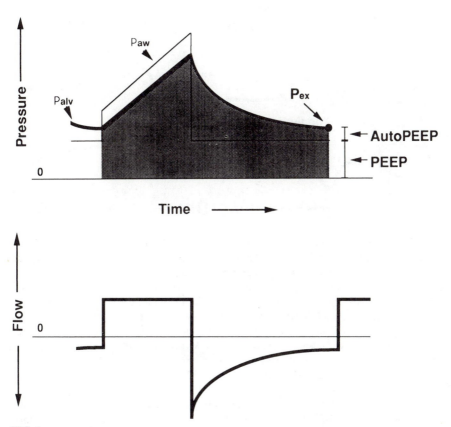

FIG 1.
Schematic diagram of flow and airway *(Paw)* and alveolar *(Palv)* pressures during a volume-cycled positive-pressure breath delivered to a passively ventilated patient with expiratory airflow obstruction. The diagram illustrates that positive end-expiratory alveolar pressure *(Pex)* is the sum of applied positive end-expiratory pressure *(PEEP)* and the positive end-expiratory pressure due to dynamic hyperinflation *(AutoPEEP)*.

Therefore, autoPEEP represents a threshold inspiratory load on the muscles of the respiratory system.[35, 36] Despite the positive end-expiratory alveolar pressure, mean pleural pressure in the spontaneously breathing patient with acute airflow obstruction often is more negative than normal due to exaggerated inspiratory efforts.[37] For this reason, cardiovascular compromise from autoPEEP usually does not occur during spontaneous breathing.

The mechanical consequences of airflow obstruction (decreased compliance at high lung volumes, high respiratory system resistance, and the development of autoPEEP) increase the work of breathing and the energy required for any level of minute ventilation. The work of breathing itself will increase CO_2 production, and thus the minute ventilation requirement. A further increase in energy expenditure is necessary because the associated gas exchange derangements require increased minute ventilation to compensate for additional physiologic dead space. Unfortu-

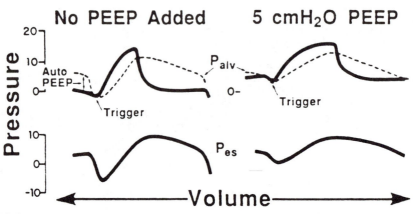

FIG 2.
Schematic diagram illustrating the impact of positive end-expiratory pressure due to dynamic hyperinflation *(AutoPEEP)* on the inspiratory effort required to trigger an assisted breath. The *solid line* in the upper tracings represents the airway opening pressure. To trigger a machine cycle, alveolar pressure *(Palv, broken line)* must fall by the amount of autoPEEP plus the set trigger sensitivity. The large dip in esophageal pressure *(Pes)* reflects this effort. The addition of PEEP downstream from dynamically collapsing airways reduces the alveolar-airway pressure gradient, and attenuates the breathing work load without a significant increase in end-inspiratory Palv. (From Marini JJ: Ventilatory management in chronic obstructive pulmonary disease, in Cherniack NS (ed): *Chronic Obstructive Pulmonary Disease*. Philadelphia, WB Saunders, 1990 p 502. Used by permission.)

nately, the respiratory muscles performing this work also are placed at a disadvantage. The outward displacement of the diaphragm and other muscles of the thoracic cage by lung hyperinflation not only positions the muscle fibers on a disadvantageous portion of their length-tension curve, but the altered orientation of the diaphragm to the thoracic cage reduces its mechanical efficiency.[38–42] With extreme hyperinflation, diaphragm contraction paradoxically may decrease the circumference of the lower thorax. Respiratory muscle strength can be compromised further by malnutrition, chronic corticosteroid use, and hypercapnia.[43]

Respiratory failure occurs when the respiratory muscles are unable to compensate and maintain sufficient minute ventilation to prevent respiratory acidosis. An alternative explanation for the failure of the respiratory system to meet ventilatory requirements is that the central nervous system responds to the high respiratory muscle workload and potential muscle fatigue by decreasing central respiratory drive and avoiding irreversible muscle injury.

Ventilatory Strategies for Airflow Obstruction

The primary indication for ventilatory support in patients with acute airflow obstruction is progressive respiratory acidosis that fails to respond to initial medical interventions, or that presents with a decreased level of consciousness or hemodynamic collapse. In some cases, ventilatory support may be initiated for progressive dyspnea or evidence of impending respiratory muscle fatigue, even in the absence of significant respiratory acidosis.[44] Oxygenation crises during acute exacerbations of airflow obstruction are unusual, and rarely are an indication for mechanical ventilation. These patients respond to relatively small increments of fractional inspired oxygen concentration (FIO_2), as the mechanism for hypoxemia usually is either hypoventilation or $\dot{V}/\dot{Q}$ mismatching.[45, 46]

Once initiated, the immediate goal of ventilatory support is to reverse life-threatening acidosis. Following this, mechanical ventilation assists in maintaining adequate acid-base homeostasis while reversible causes of airflow obstruction are treated and the respiratory muscles are allowed to recover from fatigue.

Formulating the appropriate ventilatory strategy for patients with airflow obstruction can be quite challenging. As was the case prior to intubation, the ventilated patient may be flow-limited during expiration, developing dynamic hyperinflation and autoPEEP if minute ventilation exceeds a certain volume or if expiratory time is short. Unlike the spontaneously breathing patient with autoPEEP, the patient with airflow obstruction ventilated with positive pressure may suffer significant hemodynamic consequences of dynamic hyperinflation.[34, 37] In this situation, mean intrapleural pressure rises, decreasing venous return (preload). Lung hyperinflation increases pulmonary vascular resistance, raising right ventricular afterload.[17] Increased intrapleural pressures will elevate the pressures measured by pulmonary artery catheters, even though the transmural left ventricular pressure (wedge pressure–juxtacardiac pressure) may fall.[47] Unless the presence of autoPEEP is recognized, clinicians may misinterpret the hypotension, elevated wedge pressure, and decreased cardiac output as evidence of cardiogenic shock. Another consequence of lung hyperinflation is an increased risk of barotrauma.[3, 5, 6]

In the passively ventilated patient, the degree of dynamic hyperinflation can be quantitated by measuring with a spirometer the total volume exhaled during a period of apnea sufficiently long to permit the lung to reach the relaxed equilibrium point (up to 50 seconds).[48] Alternatively, and perhaps more readily, autoPEEP can be measured in the patient who is not making active expiratory efforts by transiently stopping flow at end-expiration, allowing equilibration of pressure throughout the circuit, and detecting end-expiratory alveolar pressure by the ventilator's manometer.[47] The magnitude of autoPEEP is a function of expiratory resistance to airflow (Rx), the compliance of the respiratory system (C), the expiratory time (TE), and the tidal volume (VT). Assuming passive exhalation, uni-exponential deflation, constant values for Rx and C, and no applied PEEP, the expression linking these variables is[49]:

$$\text{AutoPEEP} = \frac{V_T}{C(e^{TE/RXC} - 1)}$$

AutoPEEP and dynamic hyperinflation can occur even in the absence of expiratory flow limitation if the minute ventilation is high or the expiratory time is short. Thus, autoPEEP may occur in patients with ARDS who have high ventilatory requirements or are on modes of ventilation with long inspiratory and short expiratory times (see section on ARDS following).[49]

It is hazardous to correct completely the respiratory acidosis of many patients with airflow obstruction because dynamic hyperinflation increases with minute ventilation. When the ventilator assumes the work load of breathing from the respiratory muscles, the ventilatory requirement falls as the metabolic rate of these muscles decreases. Nonetheless, patients with severe airflow obstruction often cannot be ventilated at a minute ventilation sufficient to achieve a normal pH without generating dangerous levels of dynamic hyperinflation. We have seen hemodynamic collapse occur in the setting of overexuberant ventilation of patients with asthma or chronic obstructive pulmonary disease (COPD) that reversed dramatically during temporary cessation of mechanical ventilation. For this reason, during the initial management of these patients, we tolerate a level of respiratory acidosis corresponding to a pH of ≈ 7.25 or even lower until we are certain that a higher minute ventilation can be achieved without significant dynamic hyperinflation (autoPEEP < 8 cm H_2O).

Asthma

Patients requiring intubation for asthma can be classified into three groups[50]:(1) patients with an abrupt (less than 8 hours) decompensation that resembles an acute asphyxic event; (2) patients with a subacute exacerbation of their asthma that presents with respiratory acidosis unresponsive to initial medical management, or that is associated with cardiovascular collapse or coma; and (3) patients with a more gradual deterioration that eventually results in severe respiratory muscle fatigue. Recent experience suggests that a large proportion of patients presenting with severe asthma and hypercapnia do not require mechanical ventilation. Even patients with marked acidosis (pH as low as 6.90) and hypercapnia ($Paco_2$ as high as 117 mm Hg) have been reported to respond to medical therapy alone.[51, 52] A significant portion of the patients who are intubated have had a preceding cardiac arrest or coma. In Braman's series, some of these patients did not require mechanical ventilation and could be extubated once they had been resuscitated.[51]

Early experience with mechanical ventilation in asthma was marked by a significantly higher complication rate than that seen in other intubated patients. The mortality rate in the early reports of asthmatic patients requiring mechanical ventilation was as high as 38%.[53] Up to one third of these deaths could be attributed to ventilator-associated complications: hypotension, pneumothoraces, or tube malfunction. In large part, such problems probably were related to dynamic hyperinflation. More recent series from institutions incorporating ventilator strategies that limit dynamic hyperinflation report a mortality rate approaching zero.[48, 51, 52, 54]

Practically every patient with asthma who requires mechanical ventilation should be both sedated and paralyzed initially. This allows precise regulation of the patient's minute ventilation and prevents the uncontrolled increase in dynamic hyperinflation that occurs with agitation and breath stacking.

Once the patient has been paralyzed and sedated, the ventilator is set on volume-cycled ventilation at a relatively low tidal volume of 6 to 8 mL/kg and a low respiratory rate of 6 to 8 breaths per minute. The respiratory rate is increased steadily during the initial evaluation period, but only if the autoPEEP level is less than 8 cm H_2O. In our practice, we tolerate the respiratory acidosis inherent with this technique, particularly in young individuals with good cardiovascular reserve. In the setting of possible ischemia or hemodynamic compromise, we infuse bicarbonate or tromethamine (Tris or Tham buffer) to speed metabolic compensation for the respiratory acidosis.

There is a debate regarding the appropriate inspiratory flow rate in these patients. Darioli and Perret have advocated inspiratory flow rates that maintain peak dynamic airway pressure less than 50 cm H_2O.[54] They reasoned that higher peak pressures may be transmitted to those lung units in which the airways are not as severely obstructed, potentially increasing the risk of barotrauma. In lung units with significant ball-valving (expiratory resistance very much greater than inspiratory resistance), theoretically the mean alveolar pressure may approach the peak dynamic airway pressure. However, barotrauma in patients with airflow obstruction is not associated as closely with high peak airway pressures as it is in patients with ARDS.[3]

The adverse consequence of a slow inspiratory flow rate is a short expiratory time that may increase dynamic hyperinflation dramatically. In Tuxen and Lane's studies of mechanically ventilated patients with airflow obstruction, progressive decreases in flow rate at any given minute ventilation caused significant additional air trapping (Fig 3).[48] Hypotension occurred with low inspiratory flow rates at high minute volumes despite modest peak dynamic airway pressures (approximately 50 cm H_2O). While peak airway pressures were elevated at the higher inspiratory flow rates, average lung volume was significantly lower. In a related study, Connors observed that higher flow rates improved gas exchange in patients mechanically ventilated for chronic airflow obstruction, presumably because of decreased alveolar gas trapping.[55] Currently, we allow maximum flow to approach 100 L/min and peak *airway* pressures to approach 60 to 70 cm H_2O when necessary to avoid serious air trapping, achieve synchrony, or establish patient comfort. Peak *alveolar* (plateau) pressures are not allowed to exceed 40 cm H_2O. In patients who are triggering the ventilator, increased ventilator flow rates may reduce inspiratory muscle work and CO_2 production.

Anecdotal reports suggest that applied PEEP may benefit mechanically ventilated patients with asthma.[56, 57] Despite these reports, there are both few data to support this strategy in passively ventilated patients and theoretic objections to its use. Applied PEEP will increase lung volume unless it significantly reduces expiratory resistance by recruiting collapsed airways or dilating flow-limited segments.[33] Careful studies by Tuxen in a series of patients composed primarily of ventilated asthmatics demonstrated that lung volume increased at all levels of applied PEEP.[58] While oxygenation improved, this usually unnecessary advantage was negated overwhelmingly by the associated hemodynamic deterioration and

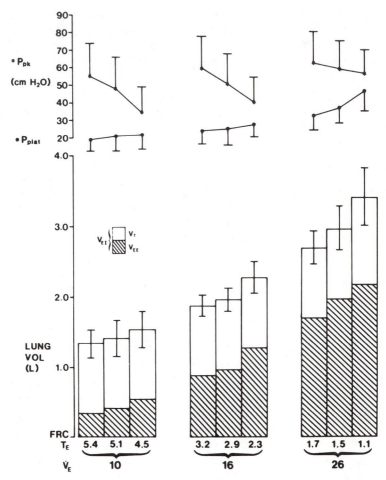

FIG 3.
The effect of different flow rates and respiratory rates on the peak *pressure (Ppk)*, the inspiratory plateau airway pressures *(Pplat)*, and lung volume at end-inspiration *(V_{EI})*. V_{EI} consists of the sum of tidal volume *(Vt)* and the volume of the lung above functional residual capacity *(FRC)* at end-expiration *(V_{EE})*. The expiratory time $T\dot{E}$ is a function of the inspiratory flow rate and the minute ventilation *($\dot{V}E$)*. The volume of air trapped in the lung (dynamic hyperinflation) is less at the higher flow rates and lower $\dot{V}E$. Note that the Ppk does not reflect the degree of dynamic hyperinflation. (From Tuxen D, Lane S: *Am Rev Respir Dis* 1987; 136:872–879. Used by permission.)

the additional risk of barotrauma from further lung inflation. With reversal of airflow obstruction these patients typically resume spontaneous ventilation without difficulty and can be removed from the ventilator.

Gluck and colleagues recently reported that seven intubated asthma patients appeared to improve when ventilated with helium-oxygen gas mixtures.[59] Helium, an inert gas, has a lower density than oxygen or ambient air, and a higher kinematic viscosity (the ratio of viscosity to density). Because of these properties, helium-oxygen mixtures remain in laminar flow under conditions and flow rates that cause turbulence with air or oxygen. Lower pressures are required to deliver the same volume at the same inspiratory flow rate under laminar as opposed to turbulent conditions because the resistive-pressure loss is less. Turbulent flow almost certainly occurs at the level of the endotracheal tube in intubated patients. However, in acutely ill patients, the site of maximal flow limitation usually is much more peripheral, where airflow is assumed to be laminar. Therefore, helium-oxygen mixtures would have little effect on airflow resistance at this level. Nonetheless, this technique could be useful if ventilation cannot be accomplished because of pressure limitations. Further work is required to determine if helium-oxygen mixtures also improve gas flow and gas exchange in the periphery of the lung during asthma exacerbations. Helium-oxygen ventilation in asthma remains an experimental technique.

Chronic Obstructive Pulmonary Disease

The indications for mechanical ventilation in the initial management of patients with acute exacerbations of COPD are similar to those for patients with asthma. However, in comparison with patients with asthma, COPD patients often have less structural airflow obstruction at the point when they require ventilatory support, and require more prolonged treatment before recovery. Even when COPD patients are clinically stable, the force reserve and fatigue threshold of their diaphragms are decreased significantly, and small departures from the spontaneous breathing pattern will lead to evidence of diaphragmatic failure.[60–64] Even moderate mechanical loads will overwhelm the chronically disadvantaged respiratory muscles of these patients.

With these differences in mind, we alter our ventilatory strategy for COPD patients in the following way. We do not use paralytics routinely unless spontaneous respiratory efforts cause uncontrolled increases in dynamic hyperinflation. Paralytic medications interfere with the clearance of lower respiratory tract secretions that contribute to atelectasis and impaired gas exchange. In addition, protracted paralysis accelerates atrophy and catabolism of the already disadvantaged respiratory muscles.[65]

As in asthma, adding PEEP to the passively ventilated patient with COPD may increase dynamic hyperinflation. However, in patients with dynamic collapse of the small airways during tidal breathing (perhaps the majority), low levels of PEEP may dilate collapsed or severely narrowed airways, decompress lung units, and, therefore, not raise lung volume or alveolar pressure significantly.[32, 33, 35] Expressed differently, when there is dynamic airway collapse, the end-expiratory alveolar pressure is not the sum of the original level of autoPEEP and the applied PEEP. Under these conditions, applied PEEP narrows the difference between airway pressure and end-expiratory alveolar pressure, reducing autoPEEP and the threshold load on the inspiratory muscles that must overcome this pressure difference before inspiratory flow can begin. Small amounts of applied PEEP (less than the original level of autoPEEP) then may reduce the work of breathing of COPD patients who are beginning to resume spontaneous respirations, but who continue to have dynamic airway collapse during tidal breathing.[32, 35] Continuous positive airway pressure (CPAP) applied to spontaneous breathing cycles appears to benefit patients the same way as PEEP does during machine-assisted cycles.[66]

Over the years, there have been many attempts to reverse respiratory failure in COPD patients by alleviating respiratory muscle fatigue with ventilatory assist devices that do not require intubation. Several investigators have reported that intermittent negative-pressure ventilation with a tank ventilator, cuirass, or poncho wrap improved respiratory muscle function and $Paco_2$ in patients with chronic hypercapnia.[67-69] However, this technique is not consistently effective in patients with airflow obstruction[70] and has not been used widely because of poor patient tolerance and the difficulty of adjusting the equipment so that the respiratory muscles decrease their activity.

Recently, positive-pressure ventilation has been applied by either face or nasal mask in patients with acute exacerbations of COPD.[71-73] Modes of ventilation used include pressure-cycled ventilation sensitive to the patient's respiratory efforts (pressure support ventilation, or PSV) and assisted volume-cycled ventilation. Many patients recently have been reported to have significant and lasting improvement in gas exchange and other clinical parameters, suggesting that this intervention prevented the need for intubation. Problems that limit the use of these modes include poor patient cooperation, gastric distention, and leakage of pressure around the mask or, in the case of nasal masks, through the mouth. Nonetheless, these techniques have promise in preventing some of the complications associated with mechanical ventilation in selected patients with acute respiratory failure from COPD, and for long-term intermittent use (e.g., nocturnal ventilation).

ADULT RESPIRATORY DISTRESS SYNDROME

Pathophysiology

One of the defining characteristics of ARDS is diffuse pulmonary infiltrates on the chest radiograph.[74] However, the distribution of lung injury, gas exchange abnormalities, and mechanical alterations do not appear to be homogeneous early in the course of ARDS.[75] Within the first 10 days after onset, there is marked heterogeneity in the radiographic density of the lung on computed tomographic (CT) scans.[76, 77] CT cross-sections reveal areas that have the density of normally aerated tissue, as well as areas that appear poorly aerated or consolidated. Analyses of gas exchange using inert gas techniques demonstrate that, despite the marked increases in shunt and dead space, a significant proportion of lung units retain normal ventilation to perfusion ($\dot{V}/\dot{Q}$) ratios.[78, 79] Another indication that many lung units are uninvolved (or at least mechanically normal) is that the compliance of the lung corrected for aerated lung volume (the specific compliance) is comparable to that of anesthetized normal subjects.[80, 81]

The aerated lung volume at functional residual capacity (FRC) is significantly smaller in patients with ARDS because a large number of alveoli—perhaps as much as one half to three fourths of them—are atelectatic, flooded with edema fluid, or filled with inflammatory debris.[76, 80] Some of these collapsed or fluid-filled alveoli can be reexpanded and aerated, improving gas exchange. When the static pressure-volume relationships are studied in patients early in their disease course, the inflation portion of the pressure-volume curve is typically flat until reaching an inflection point at low lung volumes (Fig 4).[80, 82, 83] Significant hysteresis tends to be present, that is, the volume of aerated lung is greater during deflation than during inflation at the same transpulmonary pressure. Increments of applied PEEP often decrease hysteresis and abolish this inflection point.[80] These observations are consistent with collapse and reopening of airways and alveoli during the different phases of the respiratory cycle. However, with time, the infection points and hysteresis become less evident, presumably because recruitable units either normalize or consolidate as the disease progresses.

These findings suggest that the functioning lung in ARDS is not so much stiff as it is small. While certain lung units are not aerated due to edema or atelectasis, other lung units are normally aerated and have normal compliance and V̇/Q̇ ratios. Increased airway pressures are required to deliver a tidal volume of "standard size" (10 mL/kg) into these small lungs, or to recruit poorly aerated alveoli. The higher applied pressures place normally compliant alveoli at risk for overdistention, rupture, or injury. Recent work by several independent investigators has demonstrated that normal lung units and small bronchi can be injured by transpulmonary pressures greater than 30 to 35 cm H_2O.[11–14, 16]

Ventilatory Strategies in the Adult Respiratory Distress Syndrome

The ideal ventilatory strategy in ARDS would assure adequate minute ventilation, recruit collapsed or flooded alveoli, and prevent recollapse of these airways and alveoli during exhalation, without causing barotrauma or adverse hemodynamic effects. Unfortunately, it is not possible to dissociate entirely the adverse effects of high applied pressure from the pressure-dependent objectives of maintaining adequate alveolar ventilation and oxygenation. Instead, the pattern and magnitude of applied pressure must be manipulated to optimize gas exchange with a minimum of alveolar hyperinflation and adverse hemodynamic consequences. Understanding the relationship between applied pressure and alveolar recruitment may help guide these manipulations.

During positive-pressure ventilation of a passive subject, mean airway pressure (MAP) is the pressure measured at the Y-connector of the ventilator circuit aver-

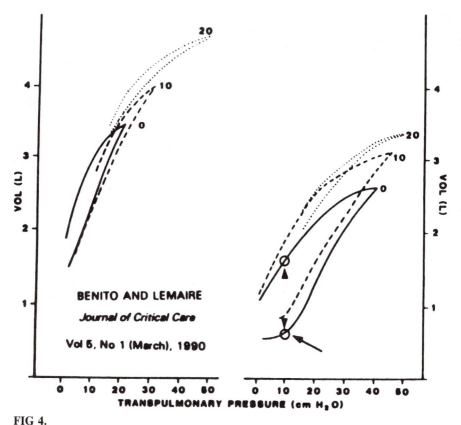

FIG 4.
Static pressure-volume curves of the respiratory system for two patients on mechanical ventilation at 0, 10, and 20 cm H_2O of positive end-expiratory pressure (PEEP). The curves on the left are from a patient with a normal chest radiograph who was intubated for coma. There is little hysteresis and the functional residual capacity is normal. The curves on the right are from a patient early in the course of the adult respiratory distress syndrome. Without PEEP applied, the pressure-volume curve demonstrates marked hysteresis *(arrowheads)* and an inflection point on the inflation limb *(right arrow)*. At the highest level of PEEP (20 cm H_2O), the inflection point is lost and the pressure-volume curve assumes a monotonic profile with a pressure-volume slope (compliance) similar to that of patients with normal lungs. (Adapted from Benito S, Lemaire F: *J Crit Care* 1990; 5:27–34. Used by permission.)

aged over the entire respiratory cycle, and reflects the average pressure applied by the ventilator. Under the same conditions, mean alveolar pressure is the average pressure acting to distend the alveoli against the combined recoil of lung and chest wall.[84, 85] In the setting of lung edema, mean alveolar pressure corresponds directly to alveolar recruitment, shunt reduction, and blood oxygenation. Although mean alveolar pressure cannot be measured directly during the tidal cycle, it is related closely to changes in the MAP of the passively ventilated patient.[49] As a

TABLE 1.

Ventilator Guidelines for Patients With the Adult
Respiratory Distress Syndrome (ARDS)

Targets	
Pa_{CO_2}	< 65 mm Hg
pH	> 7.25
O_2 saturation	> 85%
F_{IO_2}	< 0.65
Machine settings	
Tidal volume	6–8 mL/kg
Minimum end-expiratory alveolar pressure	7–10 cm H_2O
Maximum transpulmonary pressure	< 30–35 cm H_2O
Peak alveolar pressure	< 35–45 cm H_2O
Mean airway pressure	Minimum value associated with adequate oxygenation

result, MAP is a major determinant of both oxygenation and hemodynamic compromise.[86, 87] MAP, in turn, is a function of minute ventilation, the amount of applied PEEP, and the pattern of applied airway pressure. Common objectives of the different ventilatory strategies in ARDS are increasing MAP to the minimum amount that achieves adequate lung recruitment and ventilation; maintaining a minimum effective level of positive alveolar pressure throughout the respiratory cycle, thereby preventing collapse of unstable lung units; and minimizing peak alveolar pressures to decrease the incidence of barotrauma (Table 1).

Conventional Volume-Cycled Ventilation with Positive End-Expiratory Pressure

The conventional approach to ventilatory support in ARDS is volume-cycled ventilation with tidal volumes of 10 mL/kg and flow rates that maintain an inspiratory:expiratory (I:E) ratio considerably lower than 1:1. PEEP is added to recruit nonaerated alveoli and to prevent airway closure and alveolar collapse at end-expiration.[88] Once the diagnosis of ARDS is established, we initiate conventional volume-cycled ventilation with the assist-control mode using tidal volumes of 7 to 10 mL/kg. We add a minimum of 7 cm H_2O of PEEP, since the supine position alone is associated with a substantial fall in lung volume that PEEP helps to restore. Increments of PEEP are added as needed to reduce F_{IO_2} requirements to safe levels. To minimize applied pressures in a patient with adequate cardiovascular reserves, we accept an F_{IO_2} and a PEEP level that provide an arterial oxygen saturation of 85%. If the PEEP exceeds 10 cm H_2O, cardiac outputs are monitored with a pulmonary artery catheter.

We aggressively control respiratory infections, work to clear secretions, and reposition the patient frequently (if tolerated) to maximize volume recruitment and minimize alveolar collapse.[90, 91] Tidal volume is adjusted to maintain peak alveolar (plateau) pressures at or below 40 cm H_2O. This corresponds in most patients to a maximal transpulmonary pressure of less than 35 cm H_2O. Occasionally, higher maximal alveolar pressures may be appropriate in a patient with a very stiff chest wall. Animal experiments suggest even lower peak alveolar pressures may be necessary to avoid lung injury altogether. To limit cycling pressures and lung injury, it may be desirable and necessary to decrease the minute ventilation while using small tidal volumes (6 to 8 mL/kg) and higher cycling frequencies. To stay within acceptable pressure limits, pH may need to be maintained at 7.35 or even lower.[28]

Sedatives, supplemented with a paralytic agent as needed, are used if patients have high cycling pressures, are not breathing synchronously with the ventilator, or have refractory hypoxemia despite PEEP. Sedation and paralysis may improve the effectiveness of PEEP by eliminating expiratory muscle activity (thereby increasing FRC), by improving the distribution of ventilation to perfusion, or by decreasing oxygen consumption and raising the oxygen saturation of venous blood.[92] Paralytics are discontinued as soon as feasible and are withdrawn temporarily at least 1 to 2 times a day to assess neurologic status and minimize muscle atrophy.

However, for a constant tidal volume and respiratory compliance, with progressive increments in PEEP often elevates peak alveolar pressures to unacceptable levels, increasing the risk of disrupting or damaging fragile lung units with normal compliance. In addition, at constant tidal volume and MAP, increased PEEP increases dead space and raises the minute ventilation required to maintain $Paco_2$ constant.[89]

Pressure-Controlled Ventilation

During pressure-controlled modes of ventilation (PCV), a rectangular ("square") wave of predetermined pressure is applied at the airway opening for a specific duration (usually expressed as a fraction of the total respiratory cycle, or as the ratio to expiratory time). Initial inspiratory flow is high, reflecting the large gradient between alveolar and airway pressure; it then decreases as the pressure gradient falls (Fig 5). There are several potential advantages to this mode. First, the set pressure represents a maximum pressure that alveolar pressure cannot exceed under conditions of passive ventilation, thereby preventing uncontrolled and dangerous increases in alveolar pressure. Second, gas exchange may improve with decelerating flow.[93–95] Theoretically, for the same tidal volume, inspiratory time, and impedance characteristics of the lung, constant pressure ventilation results in a higher mean alveolar pressure than constant or sinusoidal flow when respiratory system compliance is low.[96] Rapid expansion of alveoli may facilitate collateral ventilation or improve gas exchange by other mechanisms. Abraham and Yoshi-

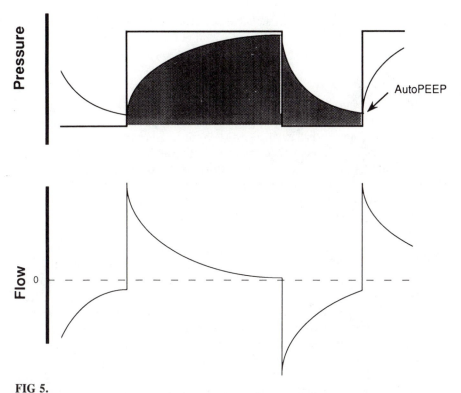

FIG 5.
Schematic diagram of flow and airway and alveolar pressures during pressure-controlled ventilation. Airway pressure is indicated by the *thick line;* alveolar presure is indicated by the *fine line* and *shaded area.* In this diagram, pressure-controlled inverse-ratio ventilation (PC-IRV) is illustrated; the time during which pressure is applied at the airway opening (inspiratory time) exceeds the expiratory time. Note that in this example there is expiratory flow and positive alveolar pressure *(autoPEEP)* at the end of the expiratory phase. (Adapted from Marcy TW, Marini JJ: *Chest* 1991; 100:494–504. Used by permission.)

hara found that oxygenation of patients with ARDS improved when they were converted from volume-cycled ventilation to PCV, even when inspiratory time and MAP remained the same.[97]

As with any pressure-limited mode of ventilation, the volume delivered varies with respiratory system compliance and resistance.[49] Furthermore, any inadvertent end-expiratory pressure generated by dynamic hyperinflation will exert a direct (and possibly undetected) opposing pressure. Therefore, careful monitoring of exhaled volume and minute ventilation is mandatory. Increments of applied PEEP also will decrease delivered tidal volume unless the set pressure is increased. If minute ventilation is inadequate, it may seem logical to raise respiratory frequency. However, minute ventilation does not increase linearly with frequency during PCV and actually reaches a plateau.[49] Alveolar ventilation reaches a peak and then actually falls with further increases in frequency. Finally, not all adult ventilators are able to provide PCV, and not all clinicians are familiar with its use or complexities.

Extended Inspiratory Time Ventilatory Modes (Inverse Ratio Ventilation)

One approach to ventilator management in ARDS patients may be use of inspiratory flow patterns that augment MAP by increasing the inspiratory time.[98] These methods include controlled volume-cycled ventilation applied with either low inspiratory flow rates, an end-inspiratory pause, or decelerating flow (VC-IRV) (Fig 6).[98, 99] PCV can also be used with prolonged inspiratory times (PC-IRV).[100–103] Based on work by Reynolds nearly 2 decades ago, neonatologists have employed successfully variations of these methods in neonates with the infant respiratory distress syndrome.[84, 85, 104]

In concept, prolonging the inspiratory time can maintain the same tidal volume and MAP using less PEEP and at lower peak alveolar pressure, provided that excessive gas trapping does not occur. Sustained elevations in airway pressure may recruit lung units more effectively than transient increases since nonaerated alveoli may require sustained traction to open, and some lung units with prolonged ventilatory "time constants" may require a longer inspiratory time to inflate fully.[30] Sustained alveolar inflation also appears to decrease dead space, perhaps by enhancing the efficacy of collateral ventilation or by facilitating the mixing of gas between well- and poorly perfused regions.[105, 106] Reducing dead space decreases minute ventilation requirements, allowing lower tidal volumes and lower peak cycling pressures.

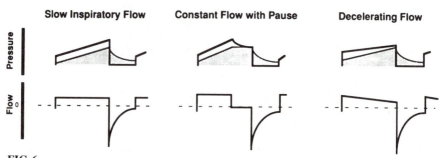

FIG 6.
Schematic diagram of flow and airway and alveolar pressures during three different forms of volume-controlled inverse-ratio ventilation (VC-IRV): slow inspiratory flow, constant flow with an end-inspiratory pause, and decelerating flow. Airway pressures are indicated with the *thick line*. Alveolar pressure during the respiratory cycle is indicated by the *shaded area*. For equivalent tidal volume, frequency, and inspiratory:expiratory ratio, the constant flow with an end-inspiratory pause provides the highest mean airway pressure. As during PC-IRV, there may be expiratory flow and positive alveolar pressure (autoPEEP) at the end of the expiratory phase. (From Marcy TW, Marini JJ: *Chest* 1991; 100:494–504. Used by permission.)

As expiratory time is shortened, development of autoPEEP acts in concert with applied PEEP to prevent end-expiratory collapse of unstable alveoli and airways. In patients with ARDS (patients who do not usually experience dynamic airway collapse during tidal breathing), increments of applied PEEP increase end-expiratory pressure above that due to autoPEEP. Unlike in patients with dynamic airway collapse, PEEP and autoPEEP are additive.[33] As end-expiratory alveolar pressure increases, either peak alveolar pressure will rise during VC-IRV or tidal volume will fall during PC-IRV. However, recognizing the need to prevent alveolar collapse at end-expiration, the total end-expiratory pressure (determined by end-expiratory port occlusion) should be monitored and maintained between 10 and 15 cm H_2O by altering the level of applied PEEP.

There are several real or theoretic problems associated with IRV. As expiratory time falls, there may be air-trapping in lung units with high expiratory resistance. In one uncontrolled study of PC-IRV in ARDS patients, pneumothoraces occurred during 23% of the IRV attempts.[103] Prolonged inflation times or excessive air trapping may have exacerbated the tendency for lung rupture. However, the incidence of pneumothoraces may have been high chiefly because large tidal volumes (15 to 20 mL/kg) were delivered. The incidence of pneumothoraces has not been as high in other studies of IRV that used smaller tidal volumes.[100, 102] Whether produced by IRV or by other mechanisms, increases in MAP and inspiratory time may worsen barotrauma that already has occurred. Therefore, when using either PC-IRV or VC-IRV, the ventilator should be adjusted to provide the least MAP and shortest inspiratory time adequate for oxygenation.

The second potential problem with IRV is that cardiac output may fall as MAP and autoPEEP increase. It usually is possible to select I:E ratios that improve gas exchange without adverse hemodynamic consequences. In ten patients with ARDS placed on VC-IRV, Cole and colleagues observed a decrease in cardiac output and oxygen delivery with I:E ratios of 4:1, but not with I:E ratios of 1.1:1 or 1.7:1.[99] Similarly, Abraham and Yoshihara did not observe hemodynamic changes when they converted nine ARDS patients from conventional ventilation to PC-IRV with I:E ratios of 2:1.[100]

A third problem with IRV is that most patients do not tolerate ratio inversion without sedation. Some critically ill patients require both deep sedation and paralytic medications. This is particularly important in VC-IRV, because alveolar pressures will rise dangerously if the patient triggers the ventilator above the set rate. For these reasons, respiratory efforts must be silenced during VC-IRV even though sedation and paralysis add the risks of apnea during ventilator disconnection, adverse pharmacologic effects, impaired secretion clearance, regional atelectasis, enhanced muscle catabolism, and inability to monitor neurologic status.[65]

Fourth, the delivered tidal volume is relatively small when peak alveolar pressure is kept below 35 to 40 cm H_2O and end-expiratory pressure is set above 7 to 10 cm H_2O. Therefore, it often is necessary to deliberately maintain controlled hypercapnia in these patients, achieving an adequate acid-base status (pH $\geq$ 7.30) with judicious use of bicarbonate or tromethamine (Tris or Tham buffer) infusions, if necessary.

Although there are many anecdotal reports comparing outcome for ARDS patients treated with IRV as opposed to conventional ventilation, there are no controlled studies. Further, we do not know if IRV has any physiologic advantages over conventional ventilation if MAP is held constant during the two ventilatory strategies. Reports of the clinical application of IRV are limited to observations of gas exchange and, in some studies, oxygen delivery. Three studies did not control for the effects of sedation and paralysis instituted at the time of conversion to IRV.[102, 103, 107] Only one of two studies that controlled for the effects of sedation and paralysis reported a significant increase in oxygen delivery. No study has determined whether IRV alters survival of patients with ARDS.[99, 100]

We consider the process of prolonging the inspiratory time to be a continuum aimed at raising MAP to the minimum effective level. Some patients may not require inversion of their I:E ratio. Unfortunately, in many cases, the benefits of IRV do not justify its hazards. In such cases, IRV is discontinued after an evaluation period. Increasing the I:E ratio is likely to be most effective early in the disease process when there are still recruitable lung units. There is little rationale, theoretic or empiric, for raising MAP if alveolar recruitment does not occur; tissue oxygen delivery actually will decline if increases in MAP compromise cardiac output.

Airway Pressure-Release Ventilation

Airway pressure-release ventilation (APRV) is a form of partial ventilatory support intended to provide a portion of the energy required for ventilating patients with ARDS.[108] APRV elevates mean airway pressure by continuously maintaining a moderately high level of continuous positive airway pressure. Periodically, the airway is allowed to depressurize rapidly but transiently, exhausting waste gas from the functional expiratory reserve volume before replacing it with fresh gas as the airway pressure is restored to the baseline level of CPAP.

Although the airway pressure profile of APRV closely resembles that of IRV, the key difference is that APRV allows the patient to breathe spontaneously, lowering the peak and main alveolar pressures associated with a given level of ventilation. A reduction in mean alveolar pressure decreases the adverse hemodynamic effects associated with positive-pressure ventilation. In addition, gas exchange may be more efficient during spontaneous ventilation than during positive-pressure ventilation. Finally, overdistention and barotrauma may be reduced, as peak airway pressure is limited to the CPAP applied. However, a vigorously breathing subject may be exposed intermittently to *transpulmonary* inflation pressures considerably higher than CPAP, as peak transpulmonary pressure is the difference between CPAP and intrapleural pressure.

APRV has a well-defined set of potential problems. In order to apply a sufficient pressure difference to assist ventilation during the release-repressurization cycles, CPAP first must be raised to a moderately high level. If chest compliance is high, the respiratory muscles will be placed at a disadvantage by hyperinflation, leading to an increased sensation of dyspnea. Second, as the number and duration of release cycles increase, mean airway pressure will fall. CPAP then may need to be raised to compensate for this. Third, maximizing ventilatory support requires that the release cycle be synchronized with the patient's exhalation. If not designed properly, APRV circuits may impose an excessive breathing work load on spontaneously breathing patients.

APRV is designed as a partial assist for patients with only moderately severe acute respiratory failure. It is unlikely to be successful or helpful in patients where it is most needed—those with extreme weakness, very high breathing work loads, unstable respiratory drive, or severe airflow obstruction. Although APRV can be used successfully in postoperative and mildly affected patients, eventually it may prove to have few absolute indications, and a quite restricted place in the management of patients with ARDS.

Extrapulmonary Gas Exchange

Because of the spectrum and severity of injury associated with ventilation of the lung, there has been renewed interest in supplementing pulmonary gas exchange with methods exposing some of the total blood flow to fresh gas across semipermeable artificial membranes. The first such approach utilized a venoarterial bypass that diverted venous blood through extracorporeal circuits designed to accomplish oxygen transfer (extracorporeal membrane oxygenation, ECMO).[109] Unfortunately, a large fraction of the total cardiac output must be diverted to improve oxygenation because of the inability to oxygen-load the blood significantly as hemoglobin approaches full saturation. In addition, ECMO requires extensive resource commitment and technical support. Sepsis and bleeding are common sources of morbidity, and the pulmonary ischemia caused by venoarterial bypass may delay or prevent lung repair. The dismal results of a trial of ECMO sponsored by the National Institutes of Health in very severe ARDS led to its virtual abandonment in North America.[110] However, ECMO has been used impressively in neonates with the infant respiratory distress syndrome; recent reports indicate 80% survival.[110]

An alternative strategy is venovenous extracorporeal CO_2 removal ($ECCO_2R$) which eliminates CO_2 using a much smaller blood flow than ECMO—approximately 25% of the total cardiac output—possible because of the difference between the O_2 and CO_2 dissociation curves (Fig 7).[112] Unlike during ECMO, the majority of oxygen exchange is in the patient's lung. $ECCO_2R$ is extremely effective for reducing the ventilatory requirements, and perhaps for reducing adverse effects of positive-pressure ventilation as well. Patients on $ECCO_2R$ receive small numbers ($\approx$ 4 breaths per minute) of PCV breaths to prevent atelectasis. Oxygenation is maintained with continuous insufflation of O_2 through a tracheal catheter and positive end-expiratory airway pressure.

Techniques for implementing $ECCO_2R$ have improved substantially in recent years, especially with the advent of percutaneous femoral catheterization.[113] How-

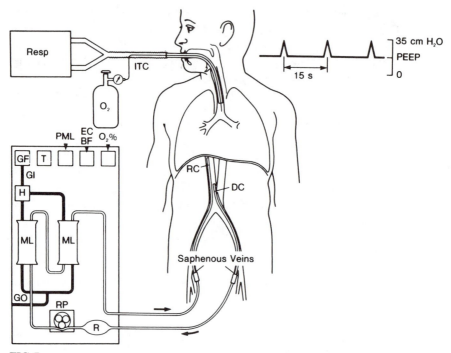

FIG 7.
Schematic illustrating the cannulation and perfusion circuit of extracorporeal CO_2 removal (ECCO$_2$R). Venous blood is drawn from the saphenous vein through a drainage catheter *(DC)* with a venous reservoir *(R)* by means of a roller pump *(RP)*. The blood is circulated through two membrane lungs *(ML)* in series and then returned through a blood-return catheter *(RC)*. Gas is circulated through the membrane lungs by another circuit (*GI* = gas inlet; *H* = humidifier; *GO* = gas outlet). Monitors on the membrane lung apparatus measure gas flow *(GF)* to the membrane lung, extracorporeal blood flow *(EC BF)*, membrane lung pressure *(PML)*, temperature *(T)*, and venous blood oxygen saturation *(O$_2$%)*. The patient's native lung is ventilated at a slow respiratory rate with applied positive end-expiratory pressure *(PEEP)*, and with continuous flow oxygen via an intratracheal catheter *(ITC)*. (From Gattinoni L, Pesenti A, Mascheroni D, et al: *JAMA* 1986; 256:881–886. Used by permission.)

ever, there remain risks of circuit disruption, air embolism, and, perhaps most important, hemorrhage related to the need for systemic heparinization. Continued evolution of ECCO$_2$R (for example, the development of regional heparinization of the membrane lung) may reduce these complications. Pioneering studies by Kolobow, Gattinoni, and others have suggested that ECCO$_2$R may improve survival in ARDS significantly. A controlled trial of ECCO$_2$R in adult patients with ARDS currently is under way.

Another variant of extrapulmonary gas exchange employs a large-diameter vena caval catheter comprised of numerous hollow fibers (Fig 8).[114] The narrow hepa-

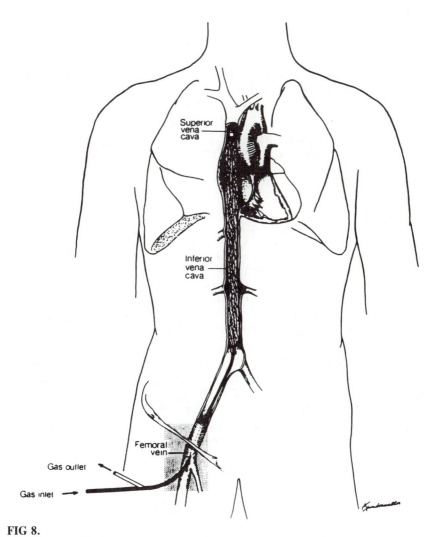

FIG 8.
Diagram of an IVOX catheter, an intravenous, extrapulmonary gas exchange device. The catheter is introduced through a venotomy in the right common femoral vein, and is advanced so that its tip lies in the superior vena cava. The crimped hollow fibers lie free in the vena caval blood stream. The double-lumen gas conduit connects to the potted manifolds at the ends of the hollow fibers. The inner (inlet) gas conduit is connected to an oxygen source; the outer (outlet) gas conduit is connected to a vacuum pump that pulls the gas through the hollow fibers at controlled subatmospheric pressures. (From Mortensen JD, Berry G: *Int J Artif Organs* 1989; 12:384–389. Used by permission.)

rin-bonded fibers fill the lumen of the vena cava without substantially impeding blood flow. As oxygenated gas is drawn through these fibers and past venous blood, gas exchange takes place across the gas-permeable walls of each filament. The gas exchange efficiency of the device varies with the size of the catheter, venous gas tensions, and blood flow. This technique may reduce substantially the requirement for ventilation across the lung. Systemic anticoagulation still is required despite heparin bonding of the fibers, and the device in its current configuration requires a venotomy for placement. Human studies are limited, but animal studies are promising. If successful, this form of gas exchange not only may limit barotrauma in patients with ARDS, but also may obviate mechanical ventilation for less severely ill patients with either ARDS or exacerbations of airflow obstruction.

CARDIOVASCULAR COMPROMISE

Interactions between the respiratory and cardiovascular systems are complex, making it difficult to predict the hemodynamic consequences of different modes of ventilation. Sometimes a specific method of ventilation will affect patients differently because their left ventricular function, intravascular volume status, and lung function differ. This complexity arises because the cardiovascular system consists of several vascular compartments, including the abdomen, the right heart, alveolar and extra-alveolar pulmonary vascular beds, the left heart, and systemic arterial and venous beds. These compartments are linked in series and, in some cases, in parallel, and several are located within the thorax. Flow from each compartment is affected by changes in the surrounding pressure, the compliance of the compartment, and the afterload, as well as by variations in the outflow from compartments "upstream." Changes in intrathoracic (pleural) pressure and lung volume related to mechanical ventilation significantly alter these variables in vascular compartments within the thorax. In addition, the abdominal vascular beds are affected by increased abdominal pressure created by movement of the diaphragm.[18]

Though various autonomic reflexes are triggered with increased lung volume, the predominant hemodynamic effects of varying lung volumes are related to the mechanical changes in the pulmonary vasculature and cardiac chambers.[17, 18] Due to the different effects of volume on extra-alveolar and alveolar vessels, lung volumes either significantly lower or higher than FRC can elevate pulmonary vascular resistance, thereby increasing right ventricular (RV) afterload. As RV afterload rises, RV volume usually increases to maintain cardiac output. As it does so the interventricular septum shifts and increases pericardial pressure, impairing left ventricular (LV) compliance.[115] In hypovolemic states, an increased lung volume reduces LV preload, since the capacitance of the pulmonary vasculature increases, while in conditions associated with pulmonary vascular congestion, similarly increased lung volume augments LV filling as blood is "squeezed" out of alveolar vessels.[18] Finally, inflation of the lungs eventually can compress the heart, reducing the compliance of both ventricular compartments.[116]

Changes in intrathoracic pressure affect both systemic venous return to the RV, and systemic LV outflow independent of ventricular contractility.[17, 18, 117] During positive-pressure ventilation, increased intrathoracic pressure reduces the venous gradient for right atrial filling, decreasing RV preload and, thus, impairing cardiac output in situations where ventricular function is sensitive to changes in preload. On the other hand, by increasing intrathoracic pressure, mechanical ventilation applies pressure to the outside of the LV, reducing the transmural ventricular pressure necessary to maintain any given level of systemic blood pressure, in effect reducing LV afterload.[118–120] A corollary to this is that markedly negative swings in intrathoracic pressure, as during respiratory distress, may increase LV afterload.[37] The net result of elevated intrathoracic pressure on cardiac output depends on the patient's LV function and the intravascular volume status.

Ventilatory Strategies for Hemodynamic Disorders

Patients with impaired LV function often present with acute respiratory insufficiency due either to their cardiac disease (cardiogenic pulmonary edema) or to other intercurrent diseases (pneumonia, COPD exacerbation). Oxygen consumption by the respiratory muscles ($\dot{V}O_2resp$) rises with the increased ventilatory requirements and the added work of breathing, imposing a significant burden on an already compromised cardiovascular system.[121] In comparison to normal subjects, in whom less than 5% of the total O_2 requirement is consumed by the respiratory muscles, patients with acute cardiorespiratory disease may have a $\dot{V}O_2resp$ that averages 20% of their total oxygen requirement (and may approach 60% in some patients).[122] When total oxygen delivery is limited by hemodynamic compromise, either the respiratory muscles will fail from inadequate oxygen supplies, or other organs will be deprived, including the myocardium.[121]

These observations support the early use of mechanical ventilation for patients with cardiovascular compromise and substantial breathing work loads. Mechanical ventilation can reduce the electromyographic activity of the diaphragm to as low as 10% of that during spontaneous ventilation in patients with severe obstructive or restrictive disease, leading to a substantial reduction in oxygen requirements of the respiratory muscles and diversion of this portion of total oxygen delivery to other organ systems.[63, 122] In addition, the reversal of acidosis and hypoxemia with ventilatory support may improve cardiac performance, increase oxygen delivery, and decrease pulmonary vascular resistance. Finally, positive-pressure ventilation may improve LV performance by decreasing LV afterload, and may reduce pulmonary vascular congestion by decreasing systemic venous return.[120, 123, 124]

It is preferable to initiate ventilatory support of these patients with assist/control volume-cycled modes of ventilation that can perform much or all of the work necessary to maintain an adequate minute ventilation. Full-support modes guarantee a minimum minute ventilation, reduce the oxygen consumption of the respiratory muscles, and maintain a positive intrathoracic pressure, with its potential physiologic advantages. Increments of PEEP, or the use of pressure support ventilation (PSV), have been used to maintain a positive intrathoracic pressure during spontaneous breaths.[125, 126] However, progressive increases in intrathoracic pressure eventually will impair cardiac output by reducing systemic venous return. Ventilator settings must be selected to balance the opposing consequences of intrathoracic pressure, and they must be based on careful monitoring of the patient's cardiovascular status.

Pinsky and colleagues attempted cardiac augmentation by phasically increasing intrathoracic pressure during inspiration with abdominal and chest wall binders applied loosely enough to increase pleural pressure during inspiration but minimize end-expiratory pleural pressure.[118] Cardiac output of five of seven patients with profound cardiogenic or septic shock increased significantly. Investigators also have attempted to exploit the potential of positive intrathoracic pressure to unload the LV without intubating patients or placing them on mechanical ventilation. In-

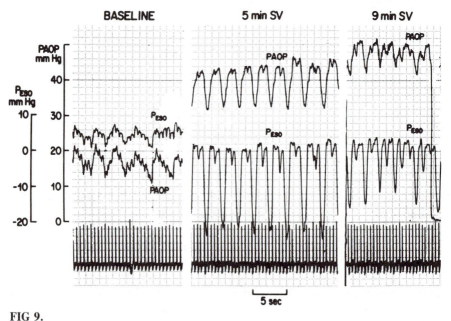

FIG 9.

Tracings of esophageal (P_{ESO}) and pulmonary wedge *(PAOP)* pressures from a patient with left ventricular dysfunction and respiratory failure during an attempt to convert from positive-pressure mechanical ventilation (baseline) to spontaneous ventilatory efforts *(SV)*. There is a progressive increase of PAOP from 14 mm Hg (baseline) to 50 mm Hg (9 min SV). The P_{ESO} is reduced during SV with marked negative inspiratory excursions. (From Lemaire F, Teboul J-L, Cinotti L, et al: *Anesthesiology* 1988; 69:171–179. Used with permission.)

creases in cardiac output have been observed with the use of CPAP masks in patients with cardiogenic pulmonary edema.[119]

Ventilatory support must be withdrawn carefully from patients with marginal cardiovascular reserve. Sudden transitions from positive-pressure ventilatory support to spontaneous breathing may precipitate hemodynamic deterioration and even myocardial ischemia. Lemaire and colleagues reported that patients with LV dysfunction may experience dramatically increased preload and LV afterload during unsuccessful attempts to discontinue mechanical ventilation (Fig 9).[127] Although the etiology undoubtedly was multifactorial, there was evidence of ventricular ischemia with consequent diastolic dysfunction. Permutt, in an accompanying editorial, speculated that a portion of the increased pulmonary vascular congestion during spontaneous respiration was related to increased abdominal pressure from the contraction of the diaphragm, causing a transfer of intravascular volume from the splanchnic circulation to the pulmonary vasculature.[128]

Evaluation of patients prior to "weaning" of ventilatory support should include a careful assessment of their intravascular volume status and cardiac function. Patients with marginal LV function may require further diuresis, inotropic agents, or afterload reduction before they can resume spontaneous ventilation successfully. The transition from full ventilatory support to spontaneous ventilation in these patients is done best gradually either with intermittent mandatory ventilation or with the use of PSV. During this transition, it may be necessary to monitor cardiac output and central vascular pressures with a pulmonary artery catheter.

NEUROMUSCULAR DISEASE, THORACIC CAGE DEFORMITY, AND DISORDERS OF CENTRAL RESPIRATORY DRIVE

While the previous sections of this chapter focused on disorders that primarily injure the lungs, there are a variety of diseases that affect the function of the "ventilatory pump," that part of the respiratory system responsible for gas movement into the lungs. This ventilatory pump consists of three major components: a rigid thoracic cage, the muscles that act as force (pressure) generators and the nerves that innervate them, and the central nervous system centers that control and coordinate the respiratory muscles. Impairment of any one of these components by disease can lead to respiratory failure.[38, 39, 41]

Respiratory failure in association with acute, reversible disorders of the ventilatory pump (e.g., drug overdosage, botulism, flail chest) is managed best with intubation and conventional modes of positive-pressure ventilation. Criteria for initiating ventilatory support are similar to those for patients with diseases affecting the lung parenchyma: depressed levels of consciousness, progressive respiratory acidosis, refractory hypoxemia, and hemodynamic instability. However, these criteria may not be sensitive enough for detecting impending respiratory failure in some situations, particularly in patients with neuromuscular disorders (e.g., Guillain-Barré syndrome). Intubation and ventilatory support are recommended when indices of muscle strength are markedly abnormal, even if the other criteria for intubation are absent.[129] On the other hand, a flail chest no longer is considered an absolute indication for ventilatory support, since many of these patients can be treated successfully with an aggressive approach to pulmonary toilet.[130] If ventilatory support is initiated in patients with ventilatory pump failure, the mode of ventilation is less a concern than determining when, and by what means, these patients can resume spontaneous ventilation. This approach will be discussed in the section on weaning.

The challenge is different when patients need ventilatory support for disorders that cause persistent or progressive ventilatory pump dysfunction. Patients with quadriplegia and diaphragmatic paralysis from high cervical cord injuries usually require continuous ventilatory support. Selected patients with kyphoscoliosis, neuromuscular disease, or central alveolar hypoventilation may benefit from intermittent (usually nocturnal) ventilatory support, particularly if they have evidence of cor pulmonale or hypercapnia.[72, 131–145] In these patients, the tracheostomy required for conventional volume-cycled ventilation adds significantly to morbidity, and the size of the ventilator may limit mobility, so a variety of noninvasive modes of ventilation have been attempted.

Factors determining whether patients with these disorders will develop respiratory failure are complex and not well understood. In chronic neuromuscular diseases, the development of respiratory failure appears to correspond to evidence of significant respiratory muscle weakness.[38, 41] In a study by Braun and colleagues of patients with polymyositis or other proximal myopathies, there was a greater chance of atelectasis, pneumonia, and hypercapnia in patients with inspiratory and expiratory maximal pressures less than 40% of normal or with a vital capacity less than 55% of predicted.[146] Experiments in normal subjects and patients with lung disease have demonstrated that the diaphragm will fatigue if the transmural pressure that must be generated for tidal breathing exceeds a certain proportion of the diaphragm's maximal generated transmural pressure.[64] Thus, both conditions that weaken the diaphragm and conditions that increase the work of breathing will lower the fatigue threshold.

The mechanisms by which nocturnal ventilatory support reverses chronic hypercapnia in these patients are not yet fully understood. Intermittent ventilatory support may improve sleep quality, reverse muscle fatigue by allowing intermittent rest and recovery,[63, 67] or help correct hypercapnia, which causes impaired muscle function.[43] Alternatively, abnormalities in central respiratory drive may contribute to the respiratory insufficiency, and intermittent ventilation may "reset" the respiratory control centers so that they are more responsive to elevations in $Paco_2$.[136]

Patients with severe kyphoscoliosis are at significant risk for developing progressive respiratory insufficiency and cor pulmonale.[147, 148] While most patients with those complications have marked spinal deformity, the severity of respiratory insufficiency does not always correspond to the degree of deformity, and some patients with severe kyphoscoliosis survive into their seventh or eighth decade with

no significant cardiopulmonary disease.[149] Mechanical abnormalities of the thoracic cage that decrease chest wall compliance and lung volume undoubtedly increase the work of breathing. Inspiratory muscle function also is impaired in these
patients because of distortion of the thorax, decreased compliance of the abdominal compartment, and abnormalities of apposition of the diaphragm with the lower
rib cage.[150]

However, sleep studies in patients with kyphoscoliosis suggest that disordered
central respiratory drive, particularly when the patient is asleep, is a major
contributor to the development of hypercapnia and cor pulmonale. In several
small studies of patients with kyphoscoliosis, those with hypercapnia and cor pulmonale had severe fragmentation of sleep with frequent apneic and hypopneic episodes.[136, 151, 152] Disordered respiratory drive during sleep does not appear to be
due simply to chronic hypoxemia, hypercapnia, or cor pulmonale. Even if the
gas exchange and cardiac abnormalities are reversed with nocturnal ventilation,
sleep-disordered breathing still occurs if ventilatory support is discontinued temporarily.[136]

In some patients, the automatic control of ventilation fails although lungs and
chest bellows are normal. Patients with central alveolar hypoventilation have diminished or absent ventilatory responses to hypoxia or carbon dioxide inhalation,
but are capable of correcting their hypercapnia and hypoxia with voluntary hyperventilation.[153, 154] Central alveolar hypoventilation usually is associated with other
central nervous system disorders including ischemic brain stem infarcts, poliomyelitis, encephalitis, Parkinson's disease, syringomyelia, and Shy-Drager disease,
or after head trauma and certain neurosurgical procedures.

Patients with central alveolar hypoventilation can present with recurrent episodes of respiratory failure. Repeated hypoventilation, particularly when asleep,
will lead to hypoxemia, hypercapnia, cor pulmonale, and polycythemia. Common
presenting symptoms include chronic fatigue, morning headache, and daytime hy-
persomnolence, presumably as a consequence of sleep fragmentation and nocturnal hypoxemia and hypercapnia. Nocturnal ventilatory support of these patients
can ameliorate the symptoms and physiologic effects of central alveolar hypoventilation.[134, 155]

Ventilatory Strategies for Disorders of the Ventilatory Pump

Negative-Pressure Ventilators

Several types of negative-pressure ventilators have been used for chronic respiratory insufficiency, including the original Drinker or tank ventilator (the iron
lung), the chest shell (cuirass), and the pneumowrap (poncho).[137, 140, 143, 145]
These devices assist ventilation by intermittently applying subatmospheric pressure to the thorax and abdomen, expanding the chest wall and lungs. They differ

in ventilatory efficiency (the tidal volume delivered for a given pressure), size and portability of the device, and ease and comfort of fitting the device to each individual patient.[140, 156]

The efficiency of each ventilator is related directly to the surface area of the thoracoabdominal wall over which the pressure is distributed. For this reason, the tank ventilator is the most effective, but its size and the difficulty of patient access are obstacles to its routine use. A somewhat more portable unit weighing 45 kg is now available.[140] The pneumowrap, consisting of a nylon parka suspended over a rigid chest piece, is the next most efficient. It is readily portable, but can be uncomfortable because of the rigid chest piece and the tendency of the device to cause musculoskeletal pain in the shoulders or back. The cuirass, a rigid shell that fits firmly over the anterior chest and upper abdomen, is the least efficient ventilator. While quite portable, it can cause skin abrasion and musculoskeletal discomfort, and is difficult to fit to patients, particularly if they have thoracic cage deformities. Nonetheless, specially designed and fitted cuirasses have been used successfully in some patients with kyphoscoliosis.[137]

With all these devices, ventilation is initiated by setting the rate of the negative-pressure pump below the patient's spontaneous rate and then gradually increasing the magnitude of negative pressure until an adequate tidal volume is achieved. The pressure and rate then are adjusted to attain the desired minute ventilation and appropriate acid-base balance. These ventilators may not augment ventilation adequately in patients with significantly increased respiratory system impedance from severe chest wall deformity or pulmonary parenchymal disease. Another problem is that negative-pressure ventilation may induce or exacerbate upper airway obstruction, particularly during sleep, especially in patients with neuromuscular diseases that affect upper airway musculature.[156] Some patients require nasal CPAP or even a tracheostomy to resolve this problem, negating the noninvasive nature of these modes of ventilation.

Ventilators That Displace Abdominal Contents

The pneumobelt and rocking bed augment ventilation by generating passive motion of the diaphragm.[140, 157] The pneumobelt consists of an inflatable rubber bladder fitted over the abdomen with a cloth corset. Inflating the bladder assists exhalation by displacing the diaphragm upward. Inhalation is augmented during deflation of the bladder by the passive downward movement of the diaphragm and subsequent fall in intrathoracic pressure. To be effective, the corset must be fitted carefully to the patient and spontaneous respiratory efforts must be in synchrony with inflation and deflation of the bladder. In addition, the patient must be seated at an angle greater than 30 degrees, limiting its usefulness at night. It is not likely to be helpful to patients with expiratory flow limitation during tidal breathing.

The rocking bed tilts the patient forward and backward over an arc of 45 degrees; the resulting motion of the abdominal contents passively moves the diaphragm. Patients are unencumbered in the bed, and nursing care and respiratory therapy are administered easily. However, it is relatively inefficient, not portable, and poorly suited to patients with substantial impedance to lung inflation. In addition, some patients develop musculoskeletal complaints, become nauseated, or otherwise fail to tolerate the motion of the bed.

Neither the pneumobelt nor the rocking bed is effective for extremely obese or thin patients or for patients with kyphoscoliosis. The pneumobelt may be useful for supporting ventilatory efforts of patients with mild respiratory insufficiency during the day, but it is not well suited for those with severe airflow obstruction. The rocking bed, long used to support patients recovering from poliomyelitis,[157] recently has been used successfully to treat patients who developed bilateral diaphragmatic dysfunction as a complication of cardiac surgery.[158]

Electrophrenic Pacing of the Diaphragm

Diaphragm pacing has been employed in the last 25 years in selected patients with high cervical cord injury or central alveolar hypoventilation.[155, 159] Electrodes are placed directly on the phrenic nerve via a thoracotomy and are connected to an implanted radio frequency receiver. An external radio frequency transmitter provides power to the receiver, generating a series of direct current pulses to the phrenic nerve. The respiratory rate and amplitude of diaphragm contraction are controlled by adjusting the transmitter's rate and stimulus frequency respectively.[155, 159, 160]

Patients must have viable phrenic nerves, adequate diaphragm strength, and relatively normal lung mechanics and gas exchange. A center with specialized experience in adjusting diaphragm pacing must follow these patients closely. If the electrical current is too great or at too high a stimulus frequency, the phrenic nerve can be injured irreversibly. A new approach limits the risk of nerve fatigue; bilateral phrenic pacemakers are placed to pace both diaphragms simultaneously at low stimulus frequency (8.3 Hz).[160] Many patients still require a tracheostomy for back-up positive-pressure ventilation or for upper airway obstruction.[161] The need for thoracic surgery, problems with upper airway obstruction, and the specialized expertise required for adjusting the transmitter have limited the popularity of this mode of ventilation.

Positive-Pressure Ventilation Via the Mouth or Nose

There have been recent attempts to support respiratory efforts with positive pressure ventilation delivered through mouthpieces (mouth intermittent positive pressure ventilation, MIPPV).[131-133, 143] Positive pressure is delivered with pressure-preset, time-cycled ventilators, adjusting pressure to augment minute ventilation appropriately. Two to 3 breaths without exhaling provides a "sigh" that may limit or reverse atelectasis. Leakage through the nose is limited by having patients obstruct the nasopharynx with their soft palate. A lip seal designed to maintain the mouthpiece in place allows the use of MIPPV even when the patient is asleep.[131]

Alba and Bach used this technique in large series of patients with quadriplegia and neuromuscular disease.[131, 133] Their experience with MIPPV spans 3 decades, a fact that may explain why other institutions have not been able to duplicate their success.[143] Patients must be guided in how to tolerate the mouthpiece, how to handle oral secretions with the mouthpiece in place, and how to prevent air leaks with reflex movements of their upper airway. Therefore, the effectiveness of this mode of ventilation is dependent on the skill and experience of the staff working with the patient.

Experience with nasal CPAP as an effective therapy for sleep apnea[162] has led to the development of positive-pressure ventilation delivered through tight-fitting nasal masks (nasal intermittent positive pressure ventilation, NIPPV).[72, 132,–136, 142, 144] Initial studies used either standard pressure-cycled or volume-cycled ventilators. Recently, investigators have adapted a device designed to provide a higher inspiratory pressure than expiratory pressure during nasal CPAP for obstructive sleep apnea (Fig 10).[163, 164] The difference between inspiratory and expiratory applied pressure rep-

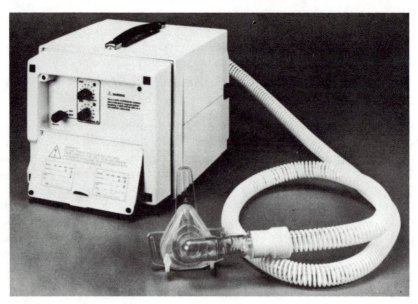

FIG 10.
Nasal BiPAP S Airway Management System (Respironics, Inc., Murrysville, Pa) consisting of a tight-fitting nasal mask and a pressure-cycled ventilator. This system can augment patient ventilation by cycling to a higher inspiratory positive airway pressure (IPAP) from a set baseline expiratory pressure (expiratory positive airway pressure, EPAP) in response to the patient's inspiratory efforts. The ventilator cycles down to the expiratory pressure when flow slows to a predetermined level that signals the end of the inspiration. The level of pressure support is determined by the clinician-set difference between expiratory and inspiratory pressure (the "pressure boost"). (Used by permission of Respironics, Inc.)

resents a "pressure boost" that acts to augment ventilation in a way similar to that of PSV. Recent adaptations of the machine permit the device to provide not only patient-initiated pressure increases but also a back-up ventilatory rate. In addition, the machine provides end-expiratory pressure (PEEP) that may help maintain alveolar recruitment.[164]

There are a number of case reports and patient series in which NIPPV was effective for patients with a variety of respiratory disorders.[72, 132, 134–136, 142, 144] An advantage of NIPPV or MIPPV, in comparison to negative-pressure ventilation, is that they prevent rather than precipitate upper airway obstruction. In a comparative study of NIPPV vs. negative-pressure ventilation in patients with neuromuscular disease, significant oxygen desaturation occurred during rapid eye movement sleep with negative-pressure ventilation because of upper airway obstruction.[135] On the other hand, in a study of long-term ventilation of eight patients with Duchenne's muscular dystrophy, all eight patients preferred negative-pressure ventilation to NIPPV or MIPPV.[143] Further development of noninvasive modes of ventilation should benefit patients with chronic respiratory insufficiency. As the experience with these modes expands, they may be applied increasingly to patients with acute respiratory failure, perhaps as a "bridge" from full ventilatory support to fully spontaneous breathing.[71, 73]

REMOVAL OF MECHANICAL VENTILATORY SUPPORT

Physiology

The vast majority of patients who require mechanical ventilation can resume spontaneous breathing once the illness that led to respiratory failure resolves. Ventilatory support can be withdrawn successfully by a number of methods. The choice of which method to use is not critical. Rather, the clinician's primary task is to determine when the patient can resume unsupported breathing. This decision is based on a judgment of the patient's medical condition, level of consciousness, ability to clear secretions, oxygenation status, and ventilatory capability. While a number of "weaning indices" have been developed, a trial of spontaneous breathing accompanied by clinical assessment remains the best indicator of a patient's overall ventilatory capability.[165–168] Newer modes of ventilation, particularly PSV, may facilitate this evaluation.

Approximately 10% of patients placed on ventilators require prolonged ventilatory assistance, resulting in increased morbidity and cost. Many factors contribute to ventilator dependence, including hemodynamic instability, lung disease, psychologic dependency, and unresolved medical illnesses. However, in most cases, a failure to wean occurs because the patient's ventilatory capability cannot meet the ventilatory demand imposed by the patient's minute ventilation and the work required per liter of gas flow.[38, 39, 41, 165] Physiologic studies of respiratory muscle function and ventilatory control mechanisms give us a greater understanding of the determinants of demand and capability, and guide our approach to these patients.

Minute ventilation is determined by the metabolic rate of production of CO_2, the fraction of ventilation that is wasted (dead space), and the ventilatory set point (or drive), indicated by the Pa_{CO_2} (Table 2). The other component of ventilatory demand—the work of breathing—is determined by resistive and elastic loads on

TABLE 2.

Physiologic Determinants of Weaning

I. Factors affecting ventilatory demand.
   A. CO_2 production.
      1. Fever.
      2. Shivering.
      3. Pain/agitation.
      4. Trauma.
      5. Sepsis.
      6. Overfeeding.
   B. Ventilatory dead space.
      1. Lung disease.
      2. Hypovolemia.
      3. Vascular occlusion.
      4. External apparatus.
   C. Central drive.
      1. Neurogenic.
      2. Psychogenic.
      3. Metabolic.
         a. Acidosis.
         b. Sepsis.
         c. Hypoxemia.
         d. Hypotension.
II. Factors affecting ventilatory capability
   A. Central drive.
      1. Sedatives.
      2. Central nervous system disorders.
      3. Resetting of drive for Pa_{CO_2}.
      4. Hypothyroidism.
      5. Metabolic alkalosis.
      6. Starvation.
   B. Muscle performance.
      1. Poor nutrition.
      2. Metabolic abnormalities.
      3. Hyperinflation.
      4. Corticosteroids.
      5. Hypercapnia.
      6. Respiratory impedance (Pi/Pi max).
      7. Respiratory muscle blood flow.

the respiratory muscles, including the elastic load caused by dynamic hyperinflation.[169, 170] Lung or chest wall diseases increase respiratory system impedance, but an additional mechanical burden is imposed by endotracheal tubes, ventilator circuits, exhalation valves, and PEEP devices.[171, 172]

A patient's ventilatory capability is determined by the integrity of central respiratory drive and the strength and endurance of the respiratory muscles. Primary failure of central respiratory drive appears to be an uncommon cause of prolonged ventilatory dependence.[173] Instead, patients failing attempts at spontaneous breathing frequently have evidence of respiratory muscle fatigue, inability of the muscles to sustain the required force output. We now understand that the response to a fatiguing load is complex, and may include a "downregulation" of central respiratory output that prevents depletion of cellular energy reserves and irreversible damage to respiratory muscles. Supporting this hypothesis are observations in patients who respond to a fatiguing load with a rapid onset of respiratory alternans and abrupt changes in respiratory rate and tidal volume, before actual muscle fatigue could develop.[173]

What defines a fatiguing load also has been established better. Normal subjects cannot sustain respiratory efforts in which the pressure generated by the inspiratory muscles exceeds a certain percentage of the maximal inspiratory pressure (Pi mus/Pi max).[64] The specific ratio of Pi mus/Pi max that is associated with fatigue depends on the inspiratory time fraction (Ti/T tot). The probability of fatigue is higher if the product of these two variables (the pressure time index) exceeds 0.15.[174] The use of this index is limited by the difficulty of measuring maximal inspiratory pressure in uncooperative critically ill patients. However, these studies of the pressure time index illustrate the value not only of decreasing the pressure required for tidal breathing, but also of increasing the maximal performance of the inspiratory muscles.

Ventilatory Strategies for Ventilator Dependence

Treating a patient with prolonged ventilator dependence requires attention to all the elements contributing to the imbalance between ventilatory demand and capability. Factors responsible for an elevated minute ventilation are minimized; secretion clearance is improved; and bronchospasm, pulmonary edema, and atelectasis are treated. Inspiratory muscle performance is optimized by avoiding catabolic states, correcting metabolic abnormalities, and limiting the use of corticosteroids, if possible. Lung hyperinflation also should be corrected to improve performance by placing the respiratory muscles on a more advantageous portion of their length-tension curve.[42]

Lemaire and colleagues demonstrated that hemodynamic instability and cardiac ischemia frequently are present in patients who fail weaning attempts.[127] The studies of Morganroth and colleagues in ventilator-dependent patients also emphasize the importance of addressing nonpulmonary medical problems when weaning patients.[168] Other ancillary strategies for patients on ventilatory support, such as inspiratory muscle training and the appropriate level and composition of nutritional support, are still being studied.[175]

There are few data to support the use of one ventilatory "weaning" mode over another. Patients probably perform enough breathing work to prevent atrophy of the respiratory muscles when triggering an assisted breath even on assist-control modes of ventilation.[169, 170] The best method of making the transition to unsupported breathing is not known, and may be less important than the efforts made to reverse underlying medical problems that contribute to respiratory failure. Nonetheless, many patients who have prolonged ventilator dependence may not tolerate an abrupt transition to spontaneous breathing, and instead will require partially supported ventilation until the muscles are reconditioned and respiratory efforts become better coordinated.

Monitoring during this transition is critically important. Simple indices using observed respiratory rate and tidal volume may guide this transition and help the clinician avoid a transition that is either so rapid that it precipitates fatigue, or so slow that it extends the period of mechanical ventilation unnecessarily.[167] During this process, some patients may benefit from biofeedback techniques that reduce anxiety, increase respiratory drive, and improve inspiratory muscle efficiency.[176]

Intermittent Spontaneous Breathing (T-Piece)

Weaning can be accomplished by alternating periods of full ventilator support with periods of independent breathing. The periods of independent breathing are lengthened progressively as tolerated by the patient. Although traditional, this approach may be an effective method to retrain and condition respiratory muscles by providing periods of stress leading to mild fatigue, punctuated by periods of rest and muscle recovery. Unfortunately, it is difficult to determine the appropriate duration of spontaneous breathing that provides an optimal stress. This mode of ventilation also requires careful supervision, since the patient is not attached to the ventilator with its monitoring systems and alarms. In addition, this mode does not compensate for the added resistance of the endotracheal tube and ventilatory circuit.

Continuous Positive Airway Pressure

During spontaneous breathing trials, CPAP restores the 600 to 1,200 mL of lung volume that is lost in the transition from the upright to the supine position. By increasing the end-expiratory lung volume from which spontaneous efforts are initiated, the problems of progressive atelectasis and secretion retention are prevented or at least limited. For this reason, it may be appropriate to apply a low level of applied PEEP in all intubated patients. As discussed in the section on airflow obstruction, CPAP also reduces the work of breathing of patients who have airflow obstruction and dynamic hyperinflation, facilitating the weaning process.[35, 36] Finally, when CPAP is applied by a mechanical ventilator, the patient is monitored by the ventilator alarm system. Early circuits that provided CPAP added a substantial resistive work load on to the patient.[172] Fortunately, the latest equipment employs either sensitive valving or bias flow mechanisms to provide more responsive systems that have less resistance.

Pressure-Support Ventilation

PSV was introduced as a mode of ventilation in 1981 in the Engstrom Erica and Siemens 900C ventilators and now is available on most ventilators with microprocessors.[177] During PSV, the clinician chooses the maximum level of pressure to be applied to the airway opening to support the patient's own breathing effort. Transpulmonary pressure is then the difference between the pressure support level and the pleural pressure. The patient retains control over the rate of respiration and the inspiratory time. When the machine senses an inspiratory effort, a rapid flow of gas (up to 3.3 L/sec^{-1}) enters the lungs until the pressure support level is reached. The gas flow necessary to maintain that pressure continues until flow rate falls to a set minimum (typically 25% of the peak flow), at which point flow is shut off. Pressure support of almost any amount can be applied up to levels that provide a significant proportion of ventilatory requirements. Several studies have confirmed that PSV effectively reduces the inspiratory work of breathing.[126, 178–181]

The most essential and unique role for PSV is compensating for the resistance imposed by the endotracheal tube. Even with an ideal ventilator circuit that maintains pressure at a constant level in the external circuit, the patient still must generate the pressure necessary to overcome endotracheal tube resistance unless a phasic bias pressure (provided by PSV) offsets this tube resistance during inspiration (Fig 11). In order to simulate the resistance of spontaneous breathing unimpeded by the endotracheal tube, PSV should be added, if possible, to all spontaneous breaths during CPAP or synchronized intermittent mandatory ventilation (SIMV). The level of pressure support needed to offset tube resistance is a function of tube caliber and flow rate and ranges from 4 to 12 cm H_2O.[182]

Higher levels of pressure support have been advocated as a method of providing varying levels of machine support to patients undergoing the gradual transition to spontaneous breathing.[177, 180] Unfortunately, there are significant disadvantages to PSV as a primary support mode. First, each PSV-aided breath must be initiated by the patient, a problem when a patient has unstable respiratory drive, especially if there is no back-up minute ventilation. Second, as with all pressure-preset modes of ventilation, the delivered tidal volume varies with changes in the impedance of the respiratory system. A pressure support level that provides an acceptable tidal volume and minute ventilation initially may become inadequate as secretions accumulate or bronchospasm increases. The development of autoPEEP can reduce the efficacy of PSV dramatically. Finally, the patient may adopt a strategy of tak-

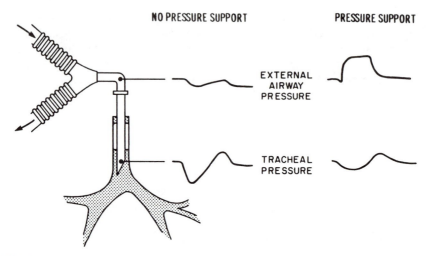

FIG 11.
Effect of endotracheal tube resistance on airway and tracheal pressures. The addition of pressure support attenuates the inspiratory effort required for a spontaneous breath, as reflected by the tracheal pressure configuration that demonstrates a decreased negative inspiratory pressure during pressure support. (From Marini JJ: *Crit Care Clin* 1990; 6:635–661. Used by permission.)

ing many small tidal breaths in order to maximize the percentage of work done by the ventilator. As a result, the transfer of work to the patient's own inspiratory muscles simply may be deferred until the latter stages of PSV withdrawal.

There are other problems with current configurations of PSV. The pressure profile often deviates from the optimal rectangular configuration if ventilation requirements or respiratory rates are very high. A delay in valve opening may cause flow delivery to lag behind the patient's demand, severely distorting the pressure waveform and limiting the effective ventilatory support. If there are leaks in the circuit or around the endotracheal cuff, pressure and flow may continue past the point when the patient begins exhalation, in effect creating a high level of CPAP equal to the set pressure.[183] To minimize this problem, most PSV circuits terminate flow after a certain arbitrary inspiratory time.

Synchronized Intermittent Mandatory Ventilation

During synchronized intermittent mandatory ventilation (SIMV), a clinician-selected number of volume-cycled breaths are interspersed each minute among unsupported (or PSV-supported) spontaneous breaths.[184, 185] Unless the patient's underlying respiratory rate is less than the set frequency, each machine cycle is initiated by the patient. However, unlike PSV, the set SIMV rate provides a back-up minute ventilation should the patient's inspiratory efforts fail. As would be expected, higher set levels of SIMV (greater number of machine cycles per minute) provide more machine support. However, the patient expends a similar effort, as estimated by the pleural pressure time product, for both the unsupported and supported breaths.[186] Apparently, dyspneic patients are unable to alter breathing effort quickly in response to intermittent unloading of the ventilatory work load. The patient's inspiratory efforts increase as the level of machine support is withdrawn in a manner similar to that during PSV.[186]

There are several problms with the use of SIMV. First, many SIMV circuits in older machines added a substantial resistance to spontaneous breathing. Second, if applied continuously, SIMV may stress the patient's respiratory muscles to the point of fatigue without allowing sufficient time for rest and full recovery. Finally, clinicians may reduce the SIMV rate so cautiously that the weaning process is perpetuated beyond the time when ventilatory support could have been discontinued safely.

Mandatory Minute Ventilation

Mandatory minute ventilation (MMV) guarantees a preset minimum level of ventilation, but provides only as much support as the spontaneously breathing patient requires to achieve it.[187] As during SIMV, the amount of ventilatory support can vary from full support to only a portion. However, unlike SIMV, the machine supplies only the support necessary to reach the minimum ventilatory target, receding to the background if the patient requires no aid. At intervals, the interrogating logic circuit of MMV examines the recent ventilation history, comparing it to the desired trajectory. If the pace of ventilation is too slow, MMV intervenes with either volume-cycled breaths or variable amounts of pressure support. Unfortunately, if the patient, in response to fatigue or respiratory loading, takes more breaths of smaller volume, he may reach the targeted minute ventilation (inactivating additional machine support) but without achieving an adequate alveolar ventilation.

MMV may be of considerable value as a method of providing a back-up mode of ventilation for patients on PSV, especially when they have unstable ventilatory drive or variable respiratory system impedance. Used in this way, it may allow patients to wean at the fastest rate compatible with the patient's ventilatory capability. However, it is difficult to determine what the appropriate minimum level of minute ventilation should be in each case. Set too low, MMV could perpetuate respiratory muscle fatigue.

Proportional Assist Ventilation

Recently, Younes and colleagues developed a form of ventilatory support in which the machine acts as if it were an "auxiliary muscle."[188] During proportional assist ventilation (PAV), the pressure assistance provided on each spontaneous breath is proportional to a variable combination of the inspired volume and the inspiratory flow rate. If the patient increases either the tidal volume or the inspiratory flow rate, the machine increases its support in proportion to a clinician-set gain. PAV is an intuitively attractive mode of ventilation, in that it attempts to use the patient's own neuromuscular control mechanisms to guide matching the patient's needs to the level of machine support. However, it assumes that the patient's ventilatory control centers are intact. The development of PAV is still in its earliest phase, and extensive clinical testing has not been performed yet.

REFERENCES

1. Petty TL: The modern evolution of mechanical ventilation. *Clin Chest Med* 1988; 9:1–10.

2. Matthay MA: New modes of mechanical ventilation for ARDS: How should they be evaluated? *Chest* 1989; 95:1175–1177.

3. Haake R, Schlichtig R, Ulstad DR, et al: Barotrauma: Pathophysiology, risk factors, and prevention. *Chest* 1987; 91:608–613.

4. Macklin MT, Macklin CC: Malignant interstitial emphysema of the lungs and mediastinum as an important occult complication in many respiratory diseases and other conditions: An interpretation of the clinical literature in the light of laboratory experiment. *Medicine* 1944; 23:281–352.

5. Maunder RJ, Pierson DJ, Hudson LD: Subcutaneous and mediastinal emphysema: Pathophysiology, diagnosis, and management. *Arch Intern Med* 1984; 144:1447–1453.

6. Pierson DJ: Alveolar rupture during mechanical ventilation: Role of PEEP, peak airway pressure, and distending volume. *Respir Care* 1988; 33:472–486.

7. Albelda SM, Gefter WB, Kelley MA, et al: Ventilator-induced subpleural air cysts: Clinical, radiologic, and pathologic significance. *Am Rev Respir Dis* 1983; 127:360–365.

8. Marini JJ, Culver BH: Systemic gas embolism complicating mechanical ventilation in the adult respiratory distress syndrome. *Ann Intern Med* 1989; 110:699–703.

9. Schaefer KE, McNulty WP, Carey C, et al: Mechanisms in development of interstitial emphysema and air embolism on decompression from depth. *J Appl Physiol* 1958; 13:15–29.

10. Borelli M, Kolobow T, Spatola R, et al: Severe acute respiratory failure managed with continuous positive airway pressure and partial extracorporeal carbon dioxide removal by an artificial membrane lung. *Am Rev Respir Dis* 1988; 138:1480–1487.

11. Dreyfuss D, Basset G, Soler P, et al: Intermittent positive-pressure hyperventilation with high inflation pressures produces microvascular injury in rats. *Am Rev Respir Dis* 1985; 132:880–884.

12. Dreyfuss D, Soler P, Basset G, et al: High inflation pressure pulmonary edema: Respective effects of high airway pressure, high tidal volume, and positive end-expiratory pressure. *Am Rev Respir Dis* 1988; 137:1159–1164.

13. Kolobow T, Moretti MP, Fumagalli R, et al: Severe impairment in lung function induced by high peak airway pressure during mechanical ventilation: An experimental study. *Am Rev Respir Dis* 1987; 135:312–315.

14. Parker JC, Hernandez LA, Longenecker GL, et al: Lung edema caused by high peak inspiratory pressures in dogs: Role of increased microvascular filtration pressure and permeability. *Am Rev Respir Dis* 1990; 142:321–328.

15. Tsuno K, Prato P, Kolobow T: Acute respiratory insufficiency induced by mechanical ventilation at peak airway pressure of 30 cm H_2O. An experimental study (abstract). *Am Rev Respir Dis* 1985; 131:A154.

16. Webb HH, Tierney DF: Experimental pulmonary edema due to intermittent positive pressure ventilation with high inflation pressures. Protection by positive end-expiratory pressure. *Am Rev Respir Dis* 1974; 110:556–565.

17. Pinsky MR: The effects of mechanical ventilation on the cardiovascular system. *Crit Care Clin* 1990; 6:663–678.

18. Robotham JL, Takata M: Cardiorespiratory interactions, Vincent J (ed): *Update in Intensive Care and Emergency Medicine,* vol 10. New York, Springer-Verlag, 1990, pp 291–304.

19. Zwillich CW, Pierson DJ, Creagh CE, et al: Complications of assisted ventilation: A prospective study of 354 consecutive episodes. *Am J Med* 1974; 57:161–170.

20. Stauffer JL, Olson DE, Petty TL: Complications and consequences of endotracheal intubation and tracheotomy. *Am J Med* 1981; 70:65–75.

21. Knodel AR, Beckman JF: Unexplained fevers in patients with nasotracheal intubation. *JAMA* 1982; 248:868–870.

22. Pingleton SK: Complications of acute respiratory failure. *Am Rev Respir Dis* 1988; 137:1463–1493.

23. Fagon J-Y, Chastre J, Domart Y, et al: Nosocomial pneumonia in patients receiving continuous mechanical ventilation. *Am Rev Respir Dis* 1989; 139:877–884.

24. Torres A, Aznar R, Gatell JM, et al: Incidence, risk, and prognosis factors of nosocomial pneumonia in mechanically ventilated patients. *Am Rev Respir Dis* 1990; 142:523–528.

25. Bell RC, Coalson JJ, Smith JD, et al: Multiple organ system failure and infection in adult respiratory distress syndrome. *Ann Intern Med* 1983; 99:293–298.

26. Montgomery AB, Stager MA, Carrico CJ, et al: Causes of mortality in patients with the adult respiratory distress syndrome. *Am Rev Respir Dis* 1985; 132:485–489.

27. Marini JJ: Paying the piper—the linkage of alveolar ventilation to alveolar pressure. *Intensive Care Med* 1990; 16:73–74.

28. Hickling KG: Ventilatory management of ARDS: Can it affect outcome? *Intensive Care Med* 1990; 16:219–226.

29. Bernasconi M, Ploysongsang Y, Gottfried SB, et al: Respiratory compliance and resistance in mechanically ventilated patients with acute respiratory failure. *Intensive Care Med* 1988; 14:547–553.

30. Broseghini C, Brandolese R, Poggi R, et al: Respiratory mechanics during the first day of mechanical ventilation in patients with pulmonary edema and chronic airway obstruction. *Am Rev Respir Dis* 1988; 138:355–361.

31. Don HF, Robson JC: The mechanics of the respiratory system during anesthesia. The effect of atropine and carbon dioxide. *Anesthesiology* 1965; 26:168–178.

32. Rossi A, Gottfried SB, Zocchi L, et al: Measurements of static compliance of the total respiratory system in patients with acute respiratory failure during mechanical ventilation: The effect of intrinsic positive end-expiratory pressure. *Am Rev Respir Dis* 1985; 131:672–677.

33. Marini JJ: Should PEEP be used in airflow obstruction? *Am Rev Respir Dis* 1989; 140:1–3.

34. Pepe PE, Marini JJ: Occult positive end-expiratory pressure in mechanically ventilated patients with airflow obstruction: The auto-PEEP effect. *Am Rev Respir Dis* 1982; 126:166–170.

35. Smith TC, Marini JJ: Impact of PEEP on lung mechanics and work of breathing in severe airflow obstruction. *J Appl Physiol* 1988; 65:1488–1499.

36. Petrof BJ, Legare M, Goldberg P, et al: Continuous positive airway pressure reduces work of breathing and dyspnea during weaning from mechanical ventilation in severe chronic obstructive pulmonary disease. *Am Rev Respir Dis* 1990; 141:281–289.

37. Stalcup SA, Mellins RB: Mechanical forces producing pulmonary edema in acute asthma. *N Engl J Med* 1977; 297:592–596.

38. Roussos S, Macklem PT: The respiratory muscles. *N Engl J Med* 1982; 307:786–797.

39. Macklem PT: Respiratory muscles: The vital pump. *Chest* 1980; 78:753–758.

40. Rochester DF: The diaphragm: Contractile properties and fatigue. *J Clin Invest* 1985; 75:1397–1402.

41. Grassino A, Macklem PT: Respiratory muscle fatigue and ventilatory failure. *Annu Rev Med* 1984; 35:625–647.

42. Macklem PT: Hyperinflation. *Am Rev Respir Dis* 1984; 129:1–2.

43. Juan G, Calverley P, Talamo C, et al: Effect of carbon dioxide on diaphragmatic function in human beings. *N Engl J Med* 1984; 310:874–879.

44. Cohen CA, Zagelbaum G, Gross D, et al: Clinical manifestations of inspiratory muscle fatigue. *Am J Med* 1982; 73:308–316.

45. Aubier M, Murciano D, Milic-Emili J, et al: Effects of O_2 administration on ventilation and blood gases in acute respiratory failure of patients with chronic obstructive lung disease. *Am Rev Respir Dis* 1980; 122:747–754.

46. Milic-Emili J: Recent advances in clinical assessment of control of breathing. *Lung* 1982; 160:1–17.

47. O'Quin R, Marini JJ: Pulmonary artery occlusion pressure: Clinical physiology, measurement, and interpretation. *Am Rev Respir Dis* 1983; 128:319–326.

48. Tuxen DV, Lane S: The effects of ventilatory pattern on hyperinflation, airway pressures, and circulation in mechanical ventilation of patients with severe airflow obstruction. *Am Rev Respir Dis* 1987; 136:872–879.

49. Marini JJ, Crooke PS, Truwit JD: Determinants and limits of pressure preset ventilation: A mathematical model of pressure control. *J Appl Physiol* 1989; 67:1081–1092.

50. Wasserfallen J-B, Schaller M-D, Feihl F, et al: Sudden asphyxic asthma: A distinct entity? *Am Rev Respir Dis* 1990; 142:108–111.

51. Braman SS, Kaemmerlen JT: Intensive care of status asthmaticus. *JAMA* 1990; 264:366–368.

52. Mountain RD, Sahn SA: Clinical features and outcome in patients with acute asthma presenting with hypercapnia. *Am Rev Respir Dis* 1988; 138:535–539.

53. Scoggin CH, Sahn SA, Petty TL: Status asthmaticus: A nine-year experience. *JAMA* 1977; 238:1158–1162.

54. Darioli R, Perret C: Mechanical controlled hypoventilation in severe acute asthma. *Am Rev Respir Dis* 1984; 129:385–387.

55. Connors AF, McCaffree RD, Gray BA: Effect of inspiratory flow rate on gas exchange during mechanical ventilation. *Am Rev Respir Dis* 1981; 124:537–543.

56. Qvist J, Andersen JB, Pemberton M, et al: High level PEEP in severe asthma. *N Engl J Med* 1982; 307:1347–1348.

57. Tenaillon A, Salmona JP, Burdon M: Continuous positive airway pressure in asthma. *Am Rev Respir Dis* 1983; 127:658.

58. Tuxen DV: Detrimental effects of positive end-expiratory pressure during controlled mechanical ventilation of patients with severe airflow obstruction. *Am Rev Respir Dis* 1989; 140:5–9.

59. Gluck EH, Onorato DJ, Castriotta R: Helium-oxygen mixtures in intubated patients with status asthmaticus and respiratory acidosis. *Chest* 1990; 98:693–698.

60. Bellemare F, Grassino A: Force reserve of the diaphragm in patients with chronic obstructive pulmonary disease. *J Appl Physiol* 1983; 55:8–15.

61. Oliven A, Kelsen SG, Deal EC, et al: Mechanisms underlying CO_2 retention during flow-resistive loading in patients with chronic obstructive pulmonary disease. *J Clin Invest* 1983; 71:1442–1449.

62. Pardy RL, Roussos C: Endurance of hyperventilation in chronic airflow obstruction. *Chest* 1983; 83:744–750.

63. Rochester DF, Braun NMT, Laine S: Diaphragmatic energy expenditure in chronic respiratory failure: The effect of assisted ventilation with body respirators. *Am J Med* 1977; 63:223–232.

64. Roussos C, Macklem PT: Diaphragmatic fatigue in man. *J Appl Physiol* 1977; 43:189–197.

65. Partridge BL, Abrams JH, Bazemore C, et al: Prolonged neurouscular blockade after long-term infusion of vecuronium bromide in the intensive care unit. *Crit Care Med* 1990; 18:1177–1179.

66. O'Donnell DE, Sanii R, Younes M: Improvement in exercise endurance in patients with chronic airflow limitation using continuous positive airway pressure. *Am Rev Respir Dis* 1988; 138:1510–1514.

67. Braun NMT, Marino WD: Effect of daily intermittent rest of respiratory muscles in patients with severe chronic airflow limitation (CAL). *Chest* 1984; 85(suppl 6):59–60S.

68. Corrado A, Bruscoli G, De Paola E, et al: Respiratory muscle insufficiency in acute respiratory failure of subjects with severe COPD: Treatment with intermittent negative pressure ventilation. *Eur Respir J* 1990; 3:644–648.

69. Cropp A, Dimarco AF: Effects of intermittent negative pressure ventilation on respiratory muscle function in patients with severe chronic obstructive pulmonary disease. *Am Rev Respir Dis* 1987; 135:1056–1061.

70. Zibrak JD, Hill NS, Federman EC, et al: Evaluation of intermittent long-term negative-pressure ventilation in patients with severe chronic obstructive pulmonary disease. *Am Rev Respir Dis* 1988; 138:1515–1518.

71. Brochard L, Isabey D, Piquet J, et al: Reversal of acute exacerbations of chronic obstructive lung disease by inspiratory assistance with a face mask. *N Engl J Med* 1990; 323:1523–1530.

72. Carroll N, Branthwaite MA: Control of nocturnal hypoventilation by nasal intermittent positive pressure ventilation. *Thorax* 1988; 43:349–353.

73. Marino W: Intermittent volume cycled mechanical ventilation via nasal mask in patients with respiratory failure due to COPD. *Chest* 1991; 99:681–684.

74. Ashbaugh DG, Bigelow DB, Petty TL: Acute respiratory distress in adults. *Lancet* 1967; 2:319–323.

75. Marini JJ: Lung mechanics in adult respiratory distress syndrome: Recent conceptual advances and implications for management. *Clin Chest Med* 1990; 11:1–18.

76. Gattinoni L, Pesenti A, Bombino M, et al: Relationships between lung computed tomographic density, gas exchange, and PEEP in acute respiratory failure. *Anesthesiology* 1988; 69:824–832.

77. Maunder RJ, Shuman WP, McHugh JW, et al: Preservation of normal lung regions in the adult respiratory distress syndrome. *JAMA* 1986; 255:2463–2465.

78. Dantzker DR, Brock CJ, Dehart P, et al: Ventilation-perfusion distributions in adult respiratory distress syndrome. *Am Rev Respir Dis* 1979; 120:1039.

79. Ralph DD, Robertson HT, Weaver LJ, et al: Distribution of ventilation and perfusion during positive end-expiratory pressure in the adult respiratory distress syndrome. *Am Rev Respir Dis* 1985; 131:54–60.

80. Benito S, Lemaire F: Pulmonary pressure-volume relationship in acute respiratory distress syndrome in adults: Role of positive end expiratory pressure. *J Crit Care* 1990; 5:27–34.

81. Gattinoni L, Pesenti A, Avalli L, et al: Pressure-volume curve of total respiratory system in acute respiratory failure: Computed tomographic scan study. *Am Rev Respir Dis* 1987; 136:730–736.

82. Holzapfel L, Robert D, Perrin F, et al: Static pressure-volume curves and effect of positive end-expiratory pressure on gas exchange in adult respiratory distress syndrome. *Crit Care Med* 1983; 11:591–597.

83. Matamis D, Lemaire F, Harf A, et al: Total respiratory pressure-volume curves in the adult respiratory distress syndrome. *Chest* 1984; 86:58–66.

84. Boros SJ, Matalon SV, Ewald R, et al: The effect of independent variations in inspiratory-expiratory ratio and end expiratory pressure during mechanical ventilation in hyaline membrane disease: The significance of mean airway pressure. *J Pediatr* 1977; 91:794–798.

85. Boros SJ: Variations in inspiratory:expiratory ratio and airway pressure wave form during mechanical ventilation: The significance of mean airway pressure. *J Pediatr* 1979; 94:114–117.

86. Cournand A, Motley HL, Werko L, et al: Physiologic studies of the effects of intermittent positive pressure breathing on cardiac output in man. *Am J Physiol* 1948; 52:162–174.

87. Jardin F, Farcot J-C, Boisante L, et al: Influence of positive end-expiratory pressure on left ventricular performance. *N Engl J Med* 1981; 304:387–392.

88. Hudson LD: Ventilatory management of patients with adult respiratory distress syndrome. *Semin Respir Med* 1981; 2:128–139.

89. Pesenti A, Marcolin R, Prato P, et al: Mean airway pressure vs. positive end-expiratory pressure during mechanical ventilation. *Crit Care Med* 1985; 13:34–37.

90. Albert RK, Leasa D, Sanderson M, et al: The prone position improves arterial oxygenation and reduces shunt in oleic-acid-induced acute lung injury. *Am Rev Respir Dis* 1987; 135:628–633.

91. Piehl MA, Brown RS: Use of extreme position changes in acute respiratory failure. *Crit Care Med* 1976; 4:13–14.

92. Coggeshall JW, Marini JJ, Newman JH: Improved oxygenation after muscle relaxation in adult respiratory distress syndrome. *Arch Intern Med* 1985; 145:1718–1720.

93. Al-Saady N, Bennett ED: Decelerating inspiratory flow waveform improves lung mechanics and gas exchange in patients on intermittent positive-pressure ventilation. *Intensive Care Med* 1985; 11:68–75.

94. Knelson JH, Howatt WF, DeMuth GR: Effect of respiratory pattern on alveolar gas exchange. *J Appl Physiol* 1970; 29:328–331.

95. Jansson L, Jonson B: A theoretical study of flow patterns of ventilators. *Scand J Respir Dis* 1972; 53:237–246.

96. Marcy TW, Burke WC, Adams AB, et al: Mean alveolar pressure is higher during ventilation with constant pressure than with constant flow or sinusoidal flow wave forms (abstract). *Am Rev Respir Dis* 1990; 141:A239.

97. Abraham E, Yoshihara G: Cardiorespiratory effects of pressure controlled ventilation in severe respiratory failure. *Chest* 1990; 98:1445–1449.

98. Marcy TW, Marini JJ: Inverse ratio ventilation: Rationale and implementation. *Chest* 1991; 100:494–504.

99. Cole AGH, Weller SF, Sykes MK: Inverse ratio ventilation compared with PEEP in adult respiratory failure. *Intensive Care Med* 1984; 10:227–232.

100. Abraham E, Yoshihara G: Cardiorespiratory effects of pressure controlled inverse ratio ventilation in severe respiratory failure. *Chest* 1989; 96:1356–1359.

101. Lachman B, Danzmann E, Haendley B, et al: Ventilator settings and gas exchange in respiratory distress syndrome, in Prakash O (ed): *Applied Physiology in Clinical Respiratory Care.* The Hague, Martinus Nijhoff Publishers, 1982, pp 141–176.

102. Lain DC, DiBenedetto R, Morris SL, et al: Pressure control inverse ratio ventilation as a method to reduce peak inspiratory pressure and provide adequate ventilation and oxygenation. *Chest* 1989; 95:1081–1088.

103. Tharratt RS, Allen RP, Alberston TE: Pressure controlled inverse ratio ventilation in severe adult respiratory failure. *Chest* 1988; 94:755–762.

104. Reynolds EOR: Effect of alterations in mechanical ventilator settings on pulmonary gas exchange in hyaline membrane disease. *Arch Dis Child* 1971; 46:152–159.

105. Fuleihan SF, Wilson RS, Pontoppidan H: Effect of mechanical ventilation with end-inspiratory pause on blood-gas exchange. *Anesth Analg* 1976; 55:122–130.

106. Sykes MK, Lumley J: The effect of varying inspiratory:expiratory ratios on gas exchange during anesthesia for open-heart surgery. *Br J Anaesth* 1969; 41:374–380.

107. Gurevitch MJ, Van Dyke J, Young ES, et al: Improved oxygenation and lower peak airway pressure in severe adult respiratory distress syndrome: Treatment with inverse ratio ventilation. *Chest* 1986; 89:211–213.

108. Downs JB, Stock MC: Airway pressure release ventilation: A new concept in ventilatory support. *Crit Care Med* 1987; 15:459–461.

109. Zapol WM, Snider MT: Membrane lungs for acute respiratory failure. *Am Rev Respir Dis* 1980; 121:907–909.

110. Zapol WM, Snider MT, Hill JD, et al: Extracorporeal membrane oxygenation in severe acute respiratory failure: A randomized prospective study. *JAMA* 1979; 242:2193–2196.

111. Keszler M, Subramanian KNS, Smith YA, et al: Pulmonary management during extracorporeal membrane oxygenation. *Crit Care Med* 1989; 17:495–500.

112. Gattinoni L, Pesenti A, Mascheroni D, et al: Low-frequency positive-pressure ventilation with extracorporeal CO_2 removal in severe acute respiratory failure. *JAMA* 1986; 256:881–886.

113. Sinard JM, Bartlett RH: Extracorporeal life support in critical care medicine. *J Crit Care* 1990; 5:265–278.

114. Mortensen JD, Berry G: Conceptual and design features of a practical, clinically effective intravenous mechanical blood/carbon dioxide exchange device (IVOX). *Int J Artif Organs* 1989; 12:384–389.

115. Bove AA, Santamore WP: Ventricular interdependence. *Prog Cardiovasc Dis* 1981; 23:356–388.

116. Butler J: The heart is in good hands. *Circulation* 1983; 67:1163–1168.

117. Buda AJ, Pinsky MR, Ingels NB, et al: Effect of intrathoracic pressure on left ventricular performance. *N Engl J Med* 1979; 301:453–459.

118. Pinsky MR, Summer WR: Cardiac augmentation by phasic high intrathoracic pressure support in man. *Chest* 1983; 84:370–375.

119. Pinsky MR, Matuschak GM, Itzkoff JM: Respiratory augmentation of left ventricular function during spontaneous ventilation in severe left ventricular failure by grunting: An auto-EPAP effect. *Chest* 1984; 86:267–269.

120. Robotham JL: Ventilator-assisted myocardial performance (editorial). *Chest* 1983; 84:366–367.

121. Aubier M, Trippenbach T, Roussos CH: Respiratory muscle fatigue during cardiogenic shock. *J Appl Physiol* 1981; 51:499–508.

122. Field S, Kelly SM, Macklem PT: The oxygen cost of breathing in patients with cardiorespiratory disease. *Am Rev Respir Dis* 1982; 126:9–13.

123. Mathru M, Rao TLK, El-Etr A, et al: Hemodynamic response to changes in ventilatory patterns in patients with normal and poor left ventricular reserve. *Crit Care Med* 1982; 10:423–426.

124. Rasanen J, Nikki P, Heikkila J: Acute myocardial infarction complicated by respiratory failure. The effects of mechanical ventilation. *Chest* 1984; 85:21–28.

125. Rasanen J, Vaisanen IT, Heikkila J, et al: Acute myocardial infarction complicated by left ventricular dysfunction and respiratory failure: The effects of continuous positive airway pressure. *Chest* 1985; 87:158–162.

126. Prakash O, Meij S: Cardiopulmonary response to inspiratory pressure support during spontaneous ventilation vs conventional ventilation. *Chest* 1985; 88:403–408.

127. Lemaire F, Teboul J-L, Cinotti L, et al: Acute left ventircular dysfunction during unsuccessful weaning from mechanical ventilation. *Anesthesiology* 1988; 69:171–179.

128. Permutt S: Circulatory effects of weaning from mechanical ventilation: The importance of transdiaphragmatic pressure. *Anesthesiology* 1988; 69:157–160.

129. O'Donohue WJ, Baker JP, Bell GM, et al: Respiratory failure in neuromuscular disease. *JAMA* 1976; 235:733–735.

130. Shackford SR, Virgilio RW, Peters RM: Selective use of ventilator therapy in flail chest injury. *J Thorac Cardiovasc Surg* 1981; 81:194–201.

131. Bach JR, Alba AS, Bohatiuk G, et al: Mouth intermittent positive pressure ventilation in the management of postpolio respiratory insufficiency. *Chest* 1987; 91:859–864.

132. Bach JR, Alba A, Mosher R, et al: Intermittent positive pressure ventilation via nasal access in the management of respiratory insufficiency. *Chest* 1987; 92:168–170.

133. Bach JR, Alba AS: Noninvasive options for ventilatory support of the traumatic high level quadriplegic patient. *Chest* 1990; 98:613–619.

134. DiMarco AF, Connors AF, Altose MD: Management of chronic alveolar hypoventilation with nasal positive pressure breathing. *Chest* 1987; 92:952–954.

135. Ellis E, Bye PTP, Bruderer JW, et al: Treatment of respiratory failure during sleep in patients with neuromuscular disease: Positive-pressure ventilation through a nose mask. *Am Rev Respir Dis* 1987; 135:148–152.

136. Ellis ER, Grunstein RR, Chan S, et al: Noninvasive ventilatory support during sleep improves respiratory failure in kyphoscoliosis. *Chest* 1988; 94:811–815.

137. Fulkerson WJ, Wilkins JK, Esbenshade AM, et al: Life threatening hypoventilation in kyphoscoliosis: Successful treatment with a molded body brace-ventilator. *Am Rev Respir Dis* 1984; 129:185–187.

138. Garay SM, Turino GM, Goldring RM: Sustained reversal of chronic hypercapnia in patients with alveolar hypoventilation syndromes: Long-term maintenance with noninvasive nocturnal mechanical ventilation. *Am J Med* 1981; 70:269–274.

139. Goldstein RS, Molotiu N, Skrastins R, et al: Reversal of sleep-induced hypoventilation and chronic respiratory failure by nocturnal negative pressure ventilation in patients with restrictive ventilatory impairment. *Am Rev Respir Dis* 1987; 135:1049–1055.

140. Hill NS: Clinical applications of body ventilators. *Chest* 1986; 90:897–905.

141. Hoeppner VH, Cockcroft DW, Dosman JA, et al: Nighttime ventilation improves respiratory failure in secondary kyphoscoliosis. *Am Rev Respir Dis* 1984; 129:240–243.

142. Kerby GR, Mayer LS, Pingleton SK: Nocturnal positive pressure ventilation via nasal mask. *Am Rev Respir Dis* 1987; 135:738–740.

143. Mohr CH, Hill NS: Long-term follow-up of nocturnal ventilatory assistance in patients with respiratory failure due to Duchenne-type muscular dystrophy. *Chest* 1990; 97:91–96.

144. Segall D: Noninvasive nasal mask-assisted ventilation in respiratory failure of Duchenne muscular dystrophy. *Chest* 1990; 93:1298–1300.

145. Splaingard ML, Frates RC, Jefferson LS, et al: Home negative pressure ventilation: Report of 20 years of experience in patients with neuromuscular disease. *Arch Phys Med Rehabil* 1985; 66:239–242.

146. Braun NMT, Arora NS, Rochester DF: Respiratory muscle and pulmonary function in polymyositis and other proximal myopathies. *Thorax* 1983; 38:616–623.

147. Bergofsky EH: Respiratory failure in disorders of the thoracic cage. *Am Rev Respir Dis* 1979; 119:643–669.

148. Libby DM, Briscoe WA, Boyce B, et al: Acute respiratory failure in scoliosis or kyphosis. *Am J Med* 1982; 73:532–538.

149. Rom WN, Miller A: Unsuspected longevity in patients with severe kyphoscoliosis. *Thorax* 1978; 33:106–110.

150. Lisboa C, Moreno R, Fava M, et al: Inspiratory muscle function in patients with severe kyphoscoliosis. *Am Rev Respir Dis* 1985; 132:48–52.

151. Guilleminault C, Kurland G, Winkle R, et al: Severe kyphoscoliosis, breathing and sleep: The "Quasimodo" syndrome during sleep. *Chest* 1981; 79:626–630.

152. Mezon BL, West P, Israels J, et al: Sleep breathing abnormalities in kyphoscoliosis. *Am Rev Respir Dis* 1980; 122:617–621.

153. Mellins RB, Balfour HH, Turino GM, et al: Failure of automatic control of ventilation (Ondine's cures). *Medicine (Baltimore)* 1970; 49:487–504.

154. Reichel J: Primary alveolar hypoventilation. *Clin Chest Med* 1980; 1:119–124.

155. Glenn WWL, Sairenji H: Diaphragm pacing in the treatment of chronic ventilatory insufficiency, in Roussos C, Macklem P (eds): *The Thorax.* New York, Marcel Dekker, 1985, pp 1407–1440.

156. Simonds AK, Branthwaite MA: Efficiency of negative pressure ventilatory equipment (abstract). *Thorax* 1985; 40:213.

157. Plum F, Whedon GD: The rapid rocking bed: Its effect on the ventilation of poliomyelitis patients with respiratory paralysis. *N Engl J Med* 1951; 245:235–241.

158. Abd AG, Braun NMT, Baskin MI, et al: Diaphragmatic dysfunction after open heart surgery: Treatment with a rocking bed. *Ann Intern Med* 1989; 111:881–886.

159. Marcy TW, Loke JSO: Diaphragm pacing for ventilatory insufficiency. *J Intensive Care Med* 1987; 2:345–353.

160. Glenn WWL, Hogan JF, Loke JSO, et al: Ventilatory support by pacing of the conditioned diaphragm in quadriplegia. *N Engl J Med* 1984; 310:1150–1155.

161. Hyland RH, Hutcheon MA, Perl A: Upper airway occlusion induced by diaphragm pacing for primary alveolar hypoventilation: Implications for the pathogenesis of obstructive sleep apnea. *Am Rev Respir Dis* 1981; 124:180–185.

162. Sullivan CE, Issa FG, Berthon-Jones M, et al: Reversal of obstructive sleep apnoea by continuous positive airway pressure applied through the nares. *Lancet* 1981; 1:862–865.

163. Sanders MH, Kern N: Obstructive sleep apnea treated by independently adjusted inspiratory and expiratory positive airway pressures via nasal mask: Physiologic and clinical implications. *Chest* 1990; 98:317–324.

164. Strumpf DA, Carlisle CC, Millman RP, et al: An evaluation of the Respironics BiPAP bi-level CPAP device for delivery of assisted ventilation. *Respir Care* 1990; 35:415–422.

165. Marini JJ: The physiologic determinants of ventilator dependence. *Respir Care* 1986; 31:271–282.

166. Milic-Emili J: Is weaning an art or a science? *Am Rev Respir Dis* 1986; 134:1107–1108.

167. Yang K, Tobin MJ: A prospective study of predicting outcome of trials of weaning from mechanical ventilation. *N Engl J Med* 1991; 324:1445–1450.

168. Morganroth ML, Morganroth JL, Nett LM, et al: Criteria for weaning from prolonged mechanical ventilation. *Arch Intern Med* 1984; 144:1012–1016.

169. Marini JJ, Capps JS, Culver BH: The inspiratory work of breathing during assisted mechanical ventilation. *Chest* 1985; 87:612–618.

170. Marini JJ, Rodriquez RM, Lamb V: The inspiratory workload of patient-initiated mechanical ventilation. *Am Rev Respir Dis* 1986; 134:902–909.

171. Marini JJ, Culver BH, Kirk W: Flow resistance of exhalation valves and positive end-expiratory pressures devices used in mechanical ventilation. *Am Rev Respir Dis* 1985; 131:850.

172. Banner MJ, Lampotang S, Boysen P, et al: Flow resistance of expiratory positive-pressure valve systems. *Chest* 1986; 90:212–217.

173. Tobin MJ, Perez W, Guenther SM: Does ribcage-abdominal paradox signify respiratory muscle fatigue? *J Appl Physiol* 1987; 63:851–860.

174. Bellemare F, Grassino A: Evaluation of human diaphragm fatigue. *J Appl Physiol* 1982; 53:1196–1206.

175. McMahon MM, Benotti PN, Bistrian BR: A clinical application of exercise physiology and nutritional support for the mechanically ventilated patient. *JPEN J Parenter Enteral Nutr* 1990; 14:538–532.

176. Holliday JE, Hyers TM: The reduction of weaning time from mechanical ventilation using tidal volume and relaxation biofeedback. *Am Rev Respir Dis* 1990; 141:1214–1220.

177. MacIntyre NR: Respiratory function during pressure support ventilation. *Chest* 1986; 89:677–683.

178. Brochard L, Pluskwa F, Lemaire F: Improved efficacy of spontaneous breathing with inspiratory pressure support. *Am Rev Respir Dis* 1987; 136:411–415.

179. Brochard L, Harf A, Lorino H, et al: Pressure support prevents diaphragmatic fatigue during weaning from mechanical ventilation. *Am Rev Respir Dis* 1989; 139:513–521.

180. MacIntyre NR, Leatherman NE: Ventilatory muscle loads and the frequency-tidal volume pattern during inspiratory pressure-assisted (pressure-supported) ventilation. *Am Rev Respir Dis* 1990; 141:327–331.

181. Viale JP, Annat GJ, Bouffard YM, et al: Oxygen cost of breathing in postoperative patients: Pressure support ventilation versus continuous positive airway pressure. *Chest* 1988; 93:506–509.

182. Fiastro JF, Habib MP, Quan SF: Pressure support compensation for inspiratory work due to endotracheal tubes and demand continuous positive airway pressure. *Chest* 1988; 93:499–505.

183. Black JW, Grover BS: A hazard of pressure support ventilation. *Chest* 1988; 93:333–335.

184. Weisman IM, Rinaldo JE, Rogers RM, et al: State of the art: Intermittent mandatory ventilation. *Am Rev Respir Dis* 1983; 127:641–647.

185. Downs JB, Klein EF Jr, Desautels D, et al: Intermittent mandatory ventilation: A new approach to weaning patients from mechanical ventilation. *Chest* 1973; 64:331–335.

186. Marini JJ, Smith TC, Lamb VJ: External work output and force generation during synchronized intermittent ventilation. *Am Rev Respir Dis* 1988; 138:1169–1179.

187. Hewlett A, Platt A, Terry V: Mandatory minute ventilation. *Anaesthesia* 1977; 32:163–169.

188. Younes M, Bilan D, Jung D, et al: An apparatus for altering the mechanical load of the respiratory system. *J Appl Physiol* 1987; 62:2491–2499.

CHAPTER 4

Nutritional Support of the Critically Ill

Diana S. Dark, M.D.

Associate Professor of Medicine, Division of Pulmonary Disease and Critical Care Medicine, University of Kansas Medical Center School of Medicine, Kansas City, Kansas

Susan K. Pingleton, M.D.

Professor of Medicine, Division of Pulmonary Disease and Critical Care Medicine, University of Kansas Medical Center School of Medicine, Kansas City, Kansas

Nutritional support of the intensive care unit (ICU) patient is accepted as the standard of care in most institutions. There have been dramatic changes in nutritional support in the last 50 years. In 1940, the only common intravenous nutrition used was 5% dextrose administered in 2 to 3 L of solution per day as a means of replenishing water needs rather than as a form of nutrition. By 1950, investigators in both the United States and Europe were exploring the possibility of using protein hydrolysates intravenously as an additional means of supplementing nutrition. Administering intravenous fat proved to be much more difficult. Since the formulation of an acceptable form of intravenous fat in Sweden in the early 1960s,[1] quickly followed by use in this country,[2] total parenteral nutrition (TPN) has become commonplace in many ICUs. The use of nutritional support is still controversial, however, and can present special challenges to the ICU team. The critically ill patient and his nutritional needs can change very quickly. In addition, the critically ill patient may have multiorgan involvement and increased susceptibility to a variety of complications, including those related to nutritional support, some of which may be life-threatening.

It now has been more than 20 years since the publication of Dudrick's landmark article announcing the successful use of TPN in supporting the growth and development of animals.[2] Even though TPN is readily accessible now, the prevalence of "malnutrition" in the hospitalized patient is said to approach 50%.[3-5] The incidence of malnutrition in the critically ill population may be even higher due to the nature of the underlying disease. ICU patients with respiratory failure who are receiving mechanical ventilation appear to be at particular risk of malnutrition. Driver and LeBrun found that 88% of mechanically ventilated patients received inadequate nutritional support.[6] Pollack and associates evaluated the prevalence of protein calorie malnutrition (PCM) in a pediatric ICU. Although patients with chronic illness and malignancy were excluded from the study, all were critically ill, requiring ICU monitoring. Nineteen percent had acute malnutrition, and 18% had chronic PCM based on anthropometric techniques.[7] Recent studies have shown that malnutrition among hospitalized medical patients, even now, generally remains undetected and largely untreated. Lack of physician awareness due to inadequate training seemed, in Roubenoff's study,[8] to be the key; this was found to be easily correctable, however, with minimal education. Nutritional education appears inadequate and needs to be addressed at the medical school level and throughout training.

NUTRITIONAL ASSESSMENT

Nutritional assessment of hospitalized patients can be difficult; assessing critically ill patients is even more so. The primary goal of nutritional assessment is identifying patients with *clinically relevant* malnutrition, i.e., the state of altered nutritional status associated with adverse clinical events.[9]

The ideal markers for nutritional assessment are somewhat controversial. Commonly used parameters for malnutrition include patient weight, anthropometric determinations, and various biochemical markers such as serum levels of albumin, transferrin, cholesterol, prealbumin, and retinol-binding protein. Weight is notoriously unreliable in the ICU due to rapid and frequent fluid shifts. Anthropometric measurements such as triceps skin fold and the midarm muscle circumference, used in many epidemiologic studies, may not be applicable to the critically ill patient. Since the status of visceral proteins (albumin, transferrin, retinol-binding protein) depends on the concentration of serum transport proteins synthesized by the liver, it is assumed that a fall in the serum concentration of these proteins is due to a nutrition-related decrease in protein synthesis. However, the plasma level of any protein is the result of a balance between synthesis and catabolism. In the presence of either abnormal losses or liver disease, the abnormal plasma level may not be due to malnutrition but rather to an underlying disease. These measurements also are variably affected by fluid balance, blood or blood product transfusion, and acute illness, rendering them inaccurate, at best, in critically ill patients. Because albumin has a half-life of 20 days[10] and transferrin has a half-life of 9 days,[11] they are not good indicators of an acute negative protein balance. Steadily rising values, on the other hand, reflect nutritional improvement. Somatic indices such as creatinine-height index and 3-methylhistidine are used also, but are dependent on renal function and generally are not reliable with a creatinine clearance less than 20 mL/min.[12] This leaves the clinician with the problem of sorting through the available data and applying them to each individual critically ill patient in order to assess his nutritional status adequately.

In the great majority of cases, routine laboratory measurements of visceral proteins and serum cholesterol along with anthropometric measurements are used to estimate nutritional status, however inaccurate. It is important to emphasize the role of the history and physical examination in nutritional assessment. Baker and associates compared the ability of the clinician to discern malnutrition by history and physical examination to the use of anthropometry, biochemical and whole-body composition studies.[13] Two independent investigators agreed in 81% of instances in classifying patients as normal, moderately malnourished, or severely malnourished. This classification correlated with patient morbidity and mortality as well as with objective parameters derived from anthropometry and body composition studies. A "prognostic nutritional index" based on several parameters, including serum albumin and total lymphocyte count, has been proposed and is used by some,[14] but is probably more accurate in the assessment of stable patients scheduled to undergo elective surgery than in critically ill patients.[15] A clinical technique called subjective global assessment, which utilizes features of the history and physical examination, also has been proposed for nutritional assessment.[16] While many parameters are utilized, a definitive test of nutritional status has not been developed yet. However, it is clear that general clinical assessment is a reproducible and valid technique for evaluating nutritional status. A carefully obtained history and physical examination often are sufficient for nutritional assessment.

CONSEQUENCES OF MALNUTRITION IN CRITICALLY ILL PATIENTS

Malnutrition is a condition in which nutritional deficiency or potential alteration in the dietary or nutritional requirements may lead to an abnormality in body mass or composition. Abnormalities produced by malnutrition can affect critically ill patients in a number of ways, including altering their immune function, respiratory muscle function, and ventilatory drive. The first report of the adverse effects of reduction in body weight was reported by Studley in 1936.[17] In this study, acute weight loss was associated with increased postoperative mortality; this finding, however, was not substantiated by later studies.[18]

Malnutrition has been shown to alter immune function. PCM is the most frequent cause of acquired immunodeficiency in humans.[19] Polymorphonuclear leukocytes are normal in number; chemotaxis, opsonic function, and phagocytic function usually remain normal or are mildly depressed, but intracellular killing decreases.[20] Thymus, spleen, and lymph nodes become markedly atrophic, and lymphocytes may decrease. While immunoglobulins remain normal or slightly increased, antibody response may be depressed.[20]

Lung defense mechanisms are altered by effects on the antioxidant defense system and surfactant production and by changes in immunologic competence.[21-23] Although death from starvation frequently is accompanied by pneumonia, it is unclear whether this is an immune deficit or a defect in the respiratory system predisposing the patient to infection. Rosenbaum et al. have demonstrated a marked decrease in "sighing" in hospitalized patients with malnutrition.[24] Studies of patients with chest wall weakness due to muscle disease or submaximal paralyzing doses of curare have demonstrated a decrease in functional residual capacity.[25, 26] This reported decrease may predispose the patient to atelectasis and infection, providing one possible mechanism for the increased respiratory morbidity associated with starvation.

Respiratory muscle function is altered by malnutrition.[27, 28] Respiratory muscle strength is related to muscle size and fuel supply, both of which are decreased in nutritional depletion. Diaphragm weight and maximal inspiratory mouth pressures have been shown to be decreased in malnutrition.[29] Ventilatory drive is affected as well. Zwillich et al. suggested that the interaction of nutrition and ventilatory drive seems to be a direct function of the influence of nutrition on metabolic rate.[30] In general, conditions that reduce metabolic rate, such as starvation,[31-33] reduce ventilatory drive. Doekel et al. demonstrated a parallel fall in metabolic rate and hypoxic ventilatory response that returned toward normal with refeeding.[34] Studies of hospitalized patients receiving TPN demonstrated a marked effect of protein intake on the ventilatory response to CO_2.[35] This effect could be detrimental, however, in patients with limited pulmonary reserve by leading to an unnecessary increase in respiratory effort.

The link between undernutrition and cardiac wasting has been established within the past 40 to 50 years. The position that the heart was spared during starvation was advocated by many in the early 1900s and widely held to be true until the mid-1940s. Keys and his associates refuted this belief in their study of 32 young men who voluntarily lost 25% of their body weight over 6 months.[36] They showed that undernutrition was associated with a decrease in heart rate, arterial and venous pressures, stroke volume, cardiac output, and cardiac index. Additionally, metabolic rate and oxygen consumption, as well as arterial and venous oxygen content, were decreased. There were multiple electrocardiographic changes demonstrated as well, including sinus bradycardia, increased QT interval, and diffusely decreased voltage.

Deficiency of a specific vitamin, trace element, or inorganic ion, despite adequate caloric intake, can lead to cardiac dysfunction. Thiamine deficiency, for example, is associated with high-output heart failure. Selenium deficiency is associated with Keshan's disease, a juvenile cardiomyopathy seen in some regions in China. This deficiency also is related to the development of fatal cardiomyopathy in patients receiving long-term TPN.[37, 38]

Starvation also results in reduced levels of the main anabolic hormone, insulin. This promotes the mobilization of adipose tissue as free fatty acids, providing the fuel required for peripheral tissues as well as the substrate for ketone production by the liver. Despite the increased output of free fatty acids in early fasting, there is catabolism of muscle protein that supplies amino acids. These amino acids are deaminated in the liver and kidneys; the carbon skeletons of the deaminated keto acids are converted to glucose, while the nitrogen moiety is excreted as urea and ammonia.[39] Muscle breakdown provides substrate for gluconeogenesis, which supplies the brain with glucose, its main fuel, at a time of deprivation.[40] In injury and sepsis, counterregulatory hormones that oppose the action of insulin, namely glucagon, cortisol, and catecholamines, commonly are elevated and lead to hyperglycemia as well as accelerated nitrogen loss.[41, 42] Starvation superimposed on critical illness promotes glucose intolerance and leads to mobilization of fat stores. In starved critical illness, there is a continuous, rapid breakdown of muscle protein, resulting in a more rapid loss of vital tissue when compared to starvation alone.

NUTRITIONAL NEEDS OF CRITICALLY ILL PATIENTS

ICUs are available even in many small community hospitals. Charts and formulas applying to most procedures and practices are readily available and accessible for nursing and paramedical personnel. What is not as easily defined and readily accessible are dictates for nutritional supplementation. However, guidelines are available, as is the expertise of the hospital dietitian to help direct the physician's nutrition orders. Standardized nutritional regimens also are available in most institutions and, because of cost and time savings, physicians are encouraged to utilize these products. Caution must be used, however, as these standardized regimens will fail to meet some patients' needs and will exceed the needs of others.

First, the optimal caloric needs of the patient must be determined. This may be done in several ways. Levels of energy expenditure can be estimated, calculated with formulas or nomograms, or determined by using measurements of energy expenditure. Accepted rules for estimating daily energy requirements are 20 to 30 kcal/kg for minimally ill patients, 30 to 40 kcal/kg for moderately stressed patients, and 40 to 50 kcal/kg for critically ill patients.[43, 44] Resting energy expenditure probably is estimated better using formulas based on age, sex, and body size, adjusting this value for the patient's physical activity and severity of illness. There are more than 190 equations utilizing variables such as weight, height, and age to predict energy needs. The formula used most frequently for estimating resting energy expenditure is the Harris-Benedict equation, developed from oxygen consumption measurements and established standard basal metabolic rates for both men and women[45]:

$$Male: BMR (kcal/24 hr) = 66.5 + 13.8W + 5.0H - 6.8A$$
$$Female: BMR (kcal/24 hr) = 655 + 9.6W + 1.9H - 4.7A$$

where BMR equals basic metabolic rate, W equals weight (kg), H equals height (cm), and A equals age (years). A "stress factor," or percent increase in energy requirements, based on the severity of the patient's illness then is added. The stress factor guidelines have been determined, to a large degree, by indirect calorimetry studies done primarily in the surgical patient population.[46] Stress factors are based on estimated metabolic needs over and above basal needs and will vary with body temperature, degree of physical activity and agitation, extent of injury, etc.[47]

While estimates for burned and traumatized patients may be fairly reliable, few good studies are available for determining the stress factors needed in medical ICU patients. Because caloric requirements can be affected by many factors, estimates and predictive equations may not be accurate for severely ill patients; many actually prefer to measure the energy expenditure of these patients using indirect calorimetry. Caloric expenditure can be determined indirectly by measuring the rate of oxygen consumption, with each liter representing approximately 4 to 5 kcal.[43, 48, 49] Stand-alone metabolic measurement carts can be used to measure oxygen consumption in both mechanically ventilated and spontaneously breathing patients, but they are expensive ($40,000 and above) and require some technical expertise. Although they have limitations, accurate information usually can be obtained reliably when they are used regularly.[49] Energy expenditure also can be measured using a pulmonary artery catheter by determining oxygen consumption from the measured thermodilution cardiac output and the O_2 content differences between arterial and mixed venous blood.[50] Caloric needs determined by this method have been shown to correlate with the caloric needs estimated by the Harris and Benedict method without modification unless sepsis is present.[51]

Once energy needs are established, the proportions of protein, carbohydrate, and fat are determined. It is estimated that a 70- to 80-kg person has 10 to 13 kg of protein, approximately half of which is intracellular.[52] The average person stores approximately 20,000 kcal as protein, 1,000 as carbohydrates, and over 140,000 as fats.[39, 53] It takes only a few days of inadequate nutrition to begin depleting these stores. In the presence of prolonged or severe trauma or sepsis, the demand for amino acids will exceed the supply from endogenous protein sources. The response of body protein to injury is characterized by a mobilization of amino acids from skeletal muscle and connective tissue to more active tissues involved in host defense and recovery.[54] Studies by Anderson and associates[55] showed that the nitrogen requirement for balance in stable adults is only 0.4 g/kg/day. Daily protein turnover (synthesis and breakdown) is 200 to 300 g.[15, 52] During semistarvation, the anabolic rate markedly decreases, with only a marginal change in catabolic rate.[56] Schiller and Blakemore have shown a rapid loss of nitrogen (protein) in patients with serious trauma.[57] With severe illness or trauma, protein requirements may increase to 1.5 to 2.0 g/kg/day.[58, 59]

One of the goals of nutritional supplementation is providing adequate calories and protein to meet endogenous requirements, avoiding loss of body protein, and preventing alterations in respiratory muscle function, as detailed above. In general, large protein intakes (>2 g/kg/day) can maintain positive nitrogen balance with only minimal caloric intake.[60] However, a positive *energy* balance is important for other reasons. Nonprotein energy spares utilization of protein for energy. Several standard amino acid solutions are available in variable concentrations for use in critically ill patients who do not have significant renal or hepatic disease.

There is some controversy surrounding the proportions of nutritional supplementation given to carbohydrates vs. fats. The respiratory quotient is the ratio of carbon dioxide production to oxygen consumption during substrate utilization. Proteins yield 4 kcal/g using about 1 L of oxygen, and therefore have a respiratory quotient of 0.8. Metabolism of carbohydrates yields approximately 4 kcal/g with a respiratory quotient of 1.0. Fats yield 9 kcal/g with a respiratory quotient of 0.7. When excess energy is delivered to the patient, it is stored as fat by lipogenesis; this is accompanied by a high respiratory quotient (~8.0) and, therefore, the production of a large amount of CO_2. Carbohydrates traditionally have been considered a more efficient source of energy in acute illness, since they are the source of energy on which most cells normally function.[61] However, this may not be true in seriously ill patients because of a decreased ability to utilize carbohydrates.[62] Wiener et al. suggested that fat may be a preferable source of energy in critically ill patients.[63]

Definite guidelines have yet to be established for appropriate proportions of carbohydrates and fats. In practice, once the necessary amino acids are provided, the remaining nonprotein calories usually are delivered in equal proportions ±20%. A minimum of 150 g/day of glucose probably is needed to provide an optimal energy substrate for certain areas and to obtain a maximal protein-sparing effect.[63] Some fat is needed as well to avoid fatty acid deficiency, but this can be done with minimal fat administration, as little as 1% to 5% of the daily caloric intake.

ELECTROLYTES

The importance of fluid and electrolyte replacement for adequate tissue perfusion and ionic equilibrium is self-evident. Malnutrition and refeeding may be associated with major changes in electrolyte balance.[62] With malnutrition there is loss of the intracellular ions potassium, magnesium, and phosphorus, and a gain in sodium and water. Hence, on refeeding, it is necessary to supply additional electrolytes, especially potassium, magnesium, and phosphorus to reverse intracellular ion loss. "Refeeding edema," from sodium and water retention, often occurs, particularly during refeeding with carbohydrate.[40, 64] In malnourished patients, particularly the elderly and those with cardiopulmonary disease, refeeding has to be undertaken very carefully because of the risk of pulmonary edema.

MICRONUTRIENTS

Although provided in small or minute amounts, micronutrients are essential for utilization of protein, carbohydrates, and fats. The two main groups are vitamins and trace elements.

Vitamins, enzyme cofactors in many metabolic pathways, play a crucial role in normal food substrate utilization as well as in host defense. Phagocytosis and, to a lesser degree, bactericidal function appear to be affected adversely by PCM and especially by folic acid deficiency.[65]

Multivitamins usually are given daily. With normal kidney function, daily administration of a standard multivitamin supplement is sufficient, since excessive vitamins will be excreted. Recommended dietary allowances for most vitamins are readily accessible but may not apply to the elderly and critically ill patient populations. Nor have the optimal dose and frequency of administration been studied in detail in patients receiving TPN.

Trace element preparations are essential in TPN to maintain good nutritional status. Recommended dietary allowances for each element are available (Table 1). Seven trace elements have been proven to be essential to humans: iron, zinc, copper, chromium, selenium, iodine, and cobalt; manganese, molybdenum, and vanadium may be important also.[66-69] Selenium and vitamin E have interrelated actions as antioxidants; deficiency of one can be corrected partially by giving the other. Selenium deficiency is associated with depression of humoral immune responsiveness, with a delay in appearance of antibody and lower titers of antibody. While fluoride imparts caries resistance to the enamel of teeth, there are no other known biologic needs for this element.

Other trace elements are believed to be essential for man based on studies on experimental animals or on their presence in human enzyme systems. Phillips and Garnys[70] carried out balance studies for zinc, copper, manganese, chromium, selenium, and molybdenum in three critically ill patients in an ICU. Their need for zinc was great; the need for copper and manganese was less. There were small negative chromium and selenium balances. Studies of molybdenum, iron, cobalt, and iodine balances were attempted but were difficult to interpret. It was clear that requirements for each trace element varied from patient to patient, influenced by the presence of gastrointestinal fluid loss and renal function. This study demonstrates that trace element requirements in critically ill patients will be difficult to determine.

Most trace element solutions are administered as multiple-ingredient formulations which, while avoiding deficiency states, may not be ideal. Additional zinc,

TABLE 1.
Daily Electrolyte, Trace Element, Vitamin, and
Mineral Requirements

	Dosage	
Component	Enteral	Parenteral
Electrolytes		
Sodium	—	90–150 mEq
Potassium	—	60–90 mEq
Trace elements		
Chromium	5–200 μg	10–15 μg
Manganese	2.5–5.0 mg	0.15–0.80 mg
Copper	2–3 mg	0.5–1.5 mg
Zinc	15 mg	2.5–4.0 mg
Iron	10 mg	2.5 mg
Iodine	150 μg	2.5 mg
Fluoride	1.5–4.0 mg	—
Selenium	0.05–0.20 mg	20–40 μg
Molybdenum	0.15–0.50 mg	20–120 μg
Vitamins		
Ascorbic acid	60 mg	100 mg
Retinol (A)	1,000 μg	3,300 IU
Vitamin D	5.0 μg	200 IU
Thiamine (B_1)	1.4 mg	3.0 mg
Riboflavin (B_2)	1.7 mg	3.6 mg
Pyridoxine (B_6)	2.2 mg	4.0 mg
Niacin	19 mg	40 mg
Pantothenic acid	4–7 mg	15 mg
Vitamin E	10.0 mg	10 IU
Biotin	100–200 μg	60 μg
Folic acid	400 μg	400 μg
Cobalamin (B_{12})	3.0 μg	5.0 μg
Vitamin K	70–140 μg	10 mg
Minerals		
Calcium	800 mg	0.20–0.30 mEq/kg
Phosphorus	800 mg	300–400 mg/kg
Magnesium	350 mg	0.34–0.45 mEq/kg
Sulfur	2–3 g	—

for example, may be needed by patients in an acute catabolic state or with substantial losses of gastrointestinal fluids. Intravenous administration of trace elements presents a risk of toxic effects, since the regulatory absorptive mechanism of the intestinal mucosa is bypassed. Renal excretion will minimize danger from modest excesses of zinc and chromium, but when there is renal dysfunction, caution is necessary to ensure against excess dosage. Copper and manganese are excreted primarily via the biliary tract. Therefore, in patients with obstruction of the biliary tract it is essential to avoid the possibility of excess retention of these elements by decreasing intake or omitting them from TPN.[71] Alternatively, blood levels of these elements can be monitored, but the tests are not generally available. In considering the effects of an excess or deficiency of any ingested trace mineral, direct actions of the mineral on the organism must be distinguished from its effects on the metabolism of other metals that potentially may affect the entire organism. Copper, manganese, and zinc all are known to interact with each other and with many other trace elements such as cadmium, molybdenum, iron, silver, mercury, selenium, arsenic, and chromium. Studying the actions and interactions of the trace elements, therefore, is very difficult.

METHODS OF DELIVERING NUTRITION

There are several methods for delivering nutritional supplementation to critically ill patients. The simplest and most straightforward is by the oral route. Many critically ill patients are able to eat and can meet their energy and protein needs with careful nutritional supervision. If the patient becomes increasingly catabolic, as with sepsis, diet supplementation may become necessary. If possible, oral intake should be supplemented with high-energy, high-nitrogen feedings. Between-meal and bedtime snacks may be adequate.

Critically ill patients frequently are unable to eat or must be kept without oral intake, necessitating an alternative method of feeding. The opinion of the authors parallels that of Heimburger: "If the gut works, use it."[72] There is increasing evidence that the route by which nutrients are administered is of major biologic importance. For example, when the same nutrient mix is administered, enterally fed animals are more resistant to an infectious challenge than are parenterally fed animals.[73, 74] While the reason is not clear, nutrients appear to preserve the structure[75] and function[76] of the intestine better when administered enterally than parenterally.

The rationale for enteral feeding is based on the physiologic effects of digestion, absorption, and hormone-substrate. In addition to the well-accepted primary roles of digestion and absorption of nutrients, the gastrointestinal tract has important defense mechanisms. The intestinal mucosa functions as a major local defense barrier to prevent bacteria colonizing the gut from invading systemic organs and tissues. Thus, the normal intestine protects the host from intraluminal bacteria and their toxins. The structural maintenance of normal intestinal epithelial cells prevents transepithelial migration. A variety of immunologic mechanisms complement this barrier function. The intestinal wall contains immunologically active cells such as lymphocytes and macrophages and the mesentery is filled with regional lymph nodes. Intraluminal secretory IgA prevents the adherence of bacteria to mucosal cells and is the principal component of the gut mucosal defense system. Kupffer cells of the liver and spleen provide a back-up barrier to trap and detoxify bacteria and their toxic products if the epithelium and regional lymph nodes are penetrated. Thus, the gut can be described as a metabolically active, immunologically important and bacteriologically decisive organ in critical illness.

After insult to the intestinal epithelium, indigenous bacteria colonizing the gastrointestinal tract pass through the epithelial mucosa to infect the mesenteric lymph nodes and systemic organs. This microbial migration has been termed bacterial translocation.[77] Three major mechanisms promote bacterial translocation: altered permeability of the intestinal mucosa as caused by hemorrhagic shock, sepsis, or endotoxemia; decreased host defense mechanisms such as immunosuppression; and increased bacterial numbers within the intestine from bacterial overgrowth or intestinal stasis. Parenteral nutrition has been shown, in animals, to promote bacterial translocation from the gut by increasing the cecal bacterial count and impairing intestinal defense.[78] There is some evidence, again in animals, that diets lacking bulk or fiber may not maximally support intestinal antibacterial barrier function.[79, 80] Much of the data evaluating bacterial translocation have been gathered in animals, but, because the factors that facilitate translocation often are present in critically ill patients, they may be vulnerable to the invasion of enteral bacteria as well. The clinical significance of these observations remains uncertain in humans.

Further justification for enteral feeding includes its safety, convenience, and economy. Enteral feeding also may help maintain gut mucosal integrity and decrease the incidence of stress-induced hemorrhagic gastritis.[81] Enteral feeding by tube is indicated for all patients who require involuntary nutritional support when there is no contraindication or any suspicion that enteral nutrient absorption will be ineffective. There are fewer complications with enteral nutrition than with central line placement, including the risk of infection associated with a central line. Enteral feeding is not possible when there is intestinal obstruction, vomiting, or ileus. Relative contraindications for enteral feeding include enterocutaneous fistula, severe diarrhea, inflammatory bowel disease, or other conditions requiring temporary bowel rest. Many effects of critical illness on the gastrointestinal tract may affect the decision to feed enterally. Despite an otherwise healthy gastrointestinal tract, enteral nutrition is often impossible in the critically ill patient because of malabsorption and ileus. Alterations in gastrointestinal enzymes and the structure of villi impede the absorption of nutrients from the gastrointestinal tract of the critically ill.[82] Ileus may be due to many causes; each may act alone or in combination. Abdominal surgery is the most frequent cause of ileus in the critically ill patient. The etiology of postoperative ileus is still not well understood, but is probably multifactorial.[82]

The various segments of the gastrointestinal tract are not equally susceptible to paralytic ileus. The small bowel is rather resistant; when it does occur, the ileus usually is of shorter duration than is ileus of the colon or delay in gastric function.[83-85] Since the small bowel is the major site of nutrient absorption, bypassing the stomach and feeding into the small bowel has been used widely,[86] although not without some risk.[87] Paralytic ileus is an important and common finding in critically ill patients and usually is a result of many ongoing physiologic changes.

In addition to oral supplementation, enteral feeding solutions can be delivered via a nasogastric, nasoduodenal, or, less commonly, oral-gastric tube. A tube enterostomy also can be placed either in the stomach or jejunum. For critically ill patients, nasoenteric tubes are preferred for short-term enteral nutrition. There are a number of inexpensive (<$20), soft, small-bore tubes available that are composed of nonreactive materials such as Silastic or polyurethane; many have weighted tips that will enable them to pass into the small bowel with peristalsis. The risk of aspiration may be less if the feedings are delivered into the duodenum or proximal jejunum.

Tube enterostomy is preferred for long-term enteral feeding. It generally is placed into the stomach either surgically or with endoscopic guidance (percutaneous endoscopic gastrostomy).[88-90] Jejunal extensions can be placed through gastrostomies if there is a risk of aspiration, although this entails a much longer procedure and additional expense. Jejunostomy also is used as a feeding route for critically ill patients at risk for aspiration. A combined gastrostomy-jejunal feeding tube has been developed that allows simultaneous gastric decompression and jejunal feeding.[91]

Many solutions are available for enteral administration (Table 2). When selecting an enteral formulation, several dietary characteristics should be considered: (1) nutrient completeness within reasonable fluid limitation, (2) digestibility and absorbability, (3) residue content, (4) lactose content, (5) osmolarity, (6) viscosity, (7) stability, (8) preparation requirements, (9) versatility, and (10) cost.[86] In most instances, hospitals will have available a variety of solutions from which to choose.

There are several classifications of enteral feedings. The most straightforward, based on nutrient composition, will be used here: (1) polymeric, (2) oligomeric, and (3) modular.[92, 93] Polymeric formulas contain 100% of the recommended daily allowance for vitamins and minerals when a total daily prescription of, on average, 2 L is administered. These formulas are semiisotonic or hypertonic solutions, most of which have a relatively high carbohydrate/fat ratio, contain intact or almost intact protein, are low in residue and sodium, and usually are lactose-free. Lactose-containing solutions are given rarely to critically ill patients because of gastrointestinal intolerance. The nitrogen source is a natural protein (egg, soy, or lactalbumin) that may be intact or partially hydrolyzed. These diets require the ability to digest protein, carbohydrate, and fat. Because polymeric diets are composed of high–molecular weight compounds, their osmolarity is low. These formulations are fairly palatable and can be used for oral feedings as well as tube feedings. A polymeric formula is the initial choice for nutritional supplementation, is relatively inexpensive, and is adequate for the great majority of patients.[82]

Oligomeric diets usually are hyperosmolar and composed of elemental or nearly elemental nutrients that require minimal digestion. They are absorbed almost com-

TABLE 2.
Enteral Diets*

Product	kcal/mL	Protein (g/dL)	Fat (g/dL)	CHO (g/dL)	Osmolality	Volume to Meet RDA
Isotein HN	1.2	6.8	3.4	15.6	300	1,770
Precision NH	1.05	4.4	0.1	21.6	525	2,850
Precision Isotonic	1.0	2.9	3.0	14.4	300	1,560
Precision LR	1.1	2.6	0.2	24.8	530	1,710
Isocal	1.06	3.4	4.4	13.3	300	1,890
Sustacal	1.01	6.1	2.3	14.0	620	1,060
Enrich	1.1	4.0	3.7	16.0	480	1,391
Ensure	1.06	3.7	3.7	14.5	470	1,887
Ensure HN	1.06	4.4	3.6	14.1	470	1,321
Osmolite	1.06	3.7	3.9	14.5	300	1,887
Osmolite HN	1.06	4.4	3.7	14.1	300	1,321
Travasorb HN	1.0	4.5	1.6	17.5	560	2,000
Travasorb	1.0	3.0	1.6	18.5	560	2,000
Magnacal	2.0	7.0	8.0	25.0	590	1,000
Isocal HCN	2.0	7.5	10.2	20.0	690	1,000
Sustacal HC	1.5	6.1	5.8	19.0	700	1,180
Ensure Plus	1.5	5.5	5.3	20.0	690	1,420
Ensure Plus HN	1.5	6.3	5.0	20.0	650	947
Tolerex	1.0	2.1	0.15	22.6	550	2,000
Vivonex T.E.N.	1.0	3.8	0.3	20.6	630	2,000
Critcare HN	1.06	3.8	0.5	22.0	650	1,890
Vital HN	1.0	4.2	1.1	18.5	500	1,500

*CHO = carbohydrate; RDA = recommended daily allowance.

pletely and leave little residue in the colon. Oligomeric diets contain either crystalline amino acids (elemental) or oligopeptides and amino acids. The carbohydrate sources are oligosaccharides and disaccharides. The formulas contain variable amounts of fat (1% to 30%) and all essential minerals and vitamins.[82] Oligomeric diets require digestion of both carbohydrate and fat; therefore, some pancreatic enzyme activity is necessary. Because the diets are hyperosmolar, osmotic diarrhea may occur if they are delivered too rapidly. These formulas are significantly more expensive but may be useful, particularly when administered during periods of digestive or absorptive insufficiency, as during the transition stage of gut recovery following peritonitis, prolonged ileus, or major surgery.[94]

There may be rare patients with unusual dietary requirements who cannot use a standard diet and require dietary supplementation using a modular diet. A module consists of single or multiple nutrients that can be combined to produce a nutritionally complete diet. Complete modular feeding is expensive, complicated, and requires some expertise, and, fortunately, is needed rarely.[95]

Specialized formulas are available for specific illnesses. Specialized formulas for hepatic encephalopathy contain high quantities of branched chain amino acids and low quantities of aromatic amino acids and methionine designed to correct the and low quantities of aromatic amino acids and methionine designed to correct the abnormal plasma ratio of these amino acids.[96] These formulas are expensive and should be restricted to those patients with hepatic encephalopathy. Specialized formulas for renal failure contain crystalline essential amino acids as the major nitrogen source; the solutions were developed with the intent of decreasing urea production by recycling nitrogen into the synthesis of nonessential amino acids. Renal failure formulations are lactose-free, contain few or no electrolytes, and are hyperosmolar.

Enteral feeding preparations that are relatively low in carbohydrate and high in fat concentration are commercially available and advocated by some for use in respiratory failure. Although proper nutrition can facilitate weaning from mechanical ventilation,[91] excessive calories are stored as fat; CO_2 yielded by this process (respiratory quotient $\sim$ 8.0) greatly increases ventilatory demands.[97, 98] The importance of this is somewhat controversial; there is some question as to whether the total carbohydrate load or the total caloric load is more important in producing excessive CO_2.

Regardless of the choice of enteral feeding solution and the type of feeding tube used, once enteral feeding is begun, proper administration must be maintained. There are few indications, if any, for bolus feeding of enteral nutrition. Continuous infusion, although it requires the use of an infusion pump, generally is better tolerated[99] and may decrease the risk of aspiration.[82, 100] There may be, in addition, better nutrient utilization, although further study is needed.[100]

PARENTERAL NUTRITION

Although parenteral nutrition is more costly and is associated with more serious complications than is enteral feeding, one should not hesitate to use it in critically ill patients with inadequate gastrointestinal tract function. Parenteral nutrition can be delivered to a critically ill patient either peripherally or centrally. Peripheral and central parenteral solutions are similar, but the volume and concentration of nutrients that can be given through a smaller peripheral vein are somewhat limited. Recently, the use of lipid-based, low-osmolality, three-in-one solutions for peripheral administration has increased.[101] The University of Southern California group has nearly 15 years of experience with such solutions and advocates their use. Their solution combines 500 mL of 10% lipid solution, 350 mL of 8.5% amino acid solution, 100 mL of $D_{50}W$ per liter, and distilled water added to make 1 L. Each liter of this solution provides 720 nonprotein calories and 31 g of protein with a calorie:nitrogen of 144:1. Three liters of this solution often is adequate to meet the patient's nutritional needs. Vitamins and trace elements usually are added to 1 L daily; electrolytes are added as needed. This solution is significantly less concentrated (900 mOsm/L) than standard TPN solutions ($\sim$1,500 mOsm/L) and is well tolerated peripherally. This avoids the risks associated with central venous line placement but does require additional pharmacist preparation time, since there are no commercially available lipid-based solutions in this country. Peripheral nutrition is not optimal for long-term maintenance of patients with markedly elevated nutritional needs, but it is well suited for short-term maintenance or for supplementation of patients with limited oral intake. Adequate peripheral intravenous access may limit the use of peripheral parenteral hyperalimentation. The usual recommended duration for three-in-one solution administration is 10 days.[101]

If peripheral hyperalimentation is not possible or adequate to meet patients' nutritional needs, TPN can be infused centrally. Central TPN is administered as dextrose and amino acid solution either mixed with lipid or with lipid infused separately. Vitamins and trace elements are added to the dextrose/amino acid mixture, because a separate rapid infusion could result in the urinary loss of some vitamins.[102] The solution is hyperosmolar (>1,000 mOsm/L) and must be infused through a central vein, usually a subclavian or internal jugular vein.

Crystalline amino acid solutions contain amino acids precipitated as chloride or hydrochloride salts; their amino acid contents are adapted to meet metabolic requirements of specific diseases. Unless designed specifically for patients in renal failure, amino acid solutions contain both essential and nonessential amino acids. Premixed dextrose/amino acid solutions are available, usually 50% dextrose or 70% dextrose premixed with 8.5% amino acid solution. If fluid restriction is necessary (congestive heart failure, renal failure), higher concentrations of amino acids can be used. Ten percent and even 15% amino acid solutions are available.

Some medical conditions require alterations in standard TPN. Specialty parenteral solutions for hepatic failure and renal failure are available and similar in composition to enteral formulations mentioned. Liberal administration of intravenous lipid solutions is not recommended for patients with multiple organ failure or severe hepatic dysfunction,[15, 103] because long-chain triglycerides require hepatic metabolism.[104, 105] Recently published data,[106] however, suggest that the cautious use of a feeding protocol relatively rich in lipids and poor in carbohydrates could have some direct beneficial effect in patients with hepatic encephalopathy. Such a diet also may potentiate favorable effects of hepatic solutions poor in aromatic and rich in branched-chain amino acids. This remains a controversial area.

Specialized parenteral formulas for renal failure are available; they are designed to minimize elevations of blood urea nitrogen and the accumulation of toxic waste products, potassium, and fluid. It is difficult to meet protein needs with these formulations in an extremely catabolic patient. Because of this, and because of the high cost of these formulas, we reserve their use for patients with acute renal failure when attempting to avoid or delay dialysis rather than giving them to those already on dialysis.[82]

There are data to suggest that the use of increased amounts of branched chain amino acids may be advantageous for critically ill patients. Preparations rich in branched chain amino acids are more efficient in achieving positive nitrogen balance in patients with severe physiologic stress (e.g., major trauma, sepsis, or burns)[107–112] but, with no proven effect on clinical outcome[109–114] yet a significant increase in expense, there is no clear indication for their use other than in hepatic encephalopathy as previously discussed.[91]

Glutamine is a nonessential amino acid that is undergoing intensive study to determine its role in nutritional supplementation of critically ill patients. Animal studies document decreased bacterial translocation with the use of glutamine-enriched TPN compared to standard formulas. This is associated with normalization of S-IgA levels and a decrease in bacterial adherence to enterocytes, suggesting that glutamine-supplemented TPN may enhance gut immune function. Additional studies have shown that both glutamine-enriched enteral and parenteral formulas accelerate intestinal glutamine uptake.[115, 116] Thus, in various stress states (shock, sepsis, trauma) associated with bacterial translocation, the provision of diets that are glutamine-supplemented may reduce the incidence of bacterial translocation, promote "bowel rescue," and possibly improve overall survival.[117] Although these data suggest that glutamine-supplemented diets may have significant impact in some clinical settings, it should be emphasized that additional carefully designed studies are necessary before the use of glutamine-enriched enteral or parenteral solutions in critically ill patients can be advocated.

MONITORING NUTRITIONAL SUPPORT

Ongoing assessment of the dynamic changes in the patient's underlying condition, as well as nutritional status, is important in monitoring nutritional support. Fluids, electrolytes, and acid-base balance should be monitored until stable.[118] Carefully maintained intake and output charts are needed to monitor changes in fluid balance; patient weight also must be monitored regularly. Although weight changes may reflect fluid balance rather than nutritional status, stable weight indicates adequate nutritional support if fluid balance is stable. Anthropometric measurements probably are not accurate in critically ill patients and are not followed routinely.

Changing serum concentrations of proteins such as albumin and transferrin may not reflect nutritional status. Because albumin has a long half-life[10] and transferrin has a half-life of 9 days,[11] they are not good indicators of short-term protein balance; rather, they must be monitored on a long-term basis.

Changing energy requirements can be calculated utilizing the Harris-Benedict equation and adding the estimated *changing* stress factor for the patient. This calculation involves several potential sources of error. Although height is stable, weight probably is not accurate. Clinical impressions of stress estimates may underestimate or, more likely, overestimate actual stress, leading to inappropriate nutritional support. Energy requirements of the critically ill patient can be assessed utilizing indirect calorimetry; this may be more accurate than the Harris-Benedict method.[119, 120] However, technical difficulties and expense limit the routine use of indirect calorimetry, especially in critically ill patients receiving supplemental oxygen and/or mechanical ventilatory support.

Urine urea nitrogen excretion is used commonly to monitor nutritional support but is dependent on renal function. Nitrogen balance over a short period may reflect only the "temporary" gain on the labile protein pool. Over longer periods, the extent of gain in tissue nitrogen can be studied more appropriately by estimating total body nitrogen.[121, 122] However, few institutions are equipped with the nuclear medicine facilities necessary for this study, rendering it clinically inapplicable.

With these limitations in mind, we monitor routine laboratory measurements of visceral proteins and 24-hour urine urea nitrogen excretion. Other measurements such as serum cholesterol and long-term body weight are followed also. It is clear, in our opinion, that the ideal method for following the response to nutritional supplementation and evaluating its adequacy has not been developed yet.

COMPLICATIONS OF NUTRITIONAL SUPPORT

Enteral Nutrition

Although regarded as relatively safe, complications do occur with enteral feeding. They are generally one of three types: mechanical, gastrointestinal, or metabolic.

Mechanical problems include knotting or clogging of the tube and improper tube placement. Proper tube placement can be assisted by endoscopic visualization or fluoroscopic guidance, if necessary, and should always be confirmed by either endoscopy or x-ray. Clogging of the tube, if caught early, often can be corrected by flushing the tube; occasionally, the tube must be replaced. Other mechanical problems such as epistaxis, nasopharyngeal erosions, sinusitis, otitis, gagging, esophageal reflux, esophagitis, tracheoesophageal fistula, and rupture of esophageal varices are uncommon, especially with the advent of small-bore, pliable tubes.[93, 123–126] Nasoenteral tubes are not recommended for patients with known or suspected cribriform plate fracture because of the risk of inadvertent tube placement into the cranial vault.[93]

Gastrointestinal complications of enteral nutrition are numerous. Nausea and vomiting occur commonly.[126–128] Contributing factors include a rapid infusion rate, large infusion volume, lactose intolerance, fat intolerance, hyperosmolality, and delayed gastric emptying. Most of these can be avoided by careful management and formula selection. Delayed gastric emptying, common in critically ill patients, can be difficult to manage. Metoclopramide may be beneficial if no intestinal obstruction is present; in addition, metoclopramide may facilitate the transpyloric passage of a feeding tube.[129]

Diarrhea is the most common and often the most difficult gastrointestinal complication to manage in enterally fed patients. Although the etiology often is multifactorial (infectious, dietary, drug-induced), following simple guidelines may help to avoid diarrhea. Many enteral solutions are hypertonic and cause osmotic diarrhea. Inappropriate volume and infusion rate also are important causes[130]; continuous infusion of the solution may decrease this risk. Bacterial contamination of the enteral solution has been reported as a potential cause of diarrhea; this has been eradicated largely by routine changing of containers and tubing.[131, 132]

Drugs that can induce diarrhea include antibiotics, magnesium-containing antacids, and other drugs such as quinidine. Hypoalbuminemia is related to an increased incidence of diarrhea in hospitalized patients.[133] The treatment of diarrhea depends on the cause. Eliminating causative drugs and decreasing the concentration and/or infusion rate of the enteral solution may be helpful. If bacterial overgrowth of the small intestine is suspected, a trial of broad-spectrum antibiotics is indicated. Bulking agents have been tried periodically with some success. Some commercially available enteral formulas include dietary fiber which may decrease stool volume.

Although there are significantly fewer metabolic complications of enteral alimentation than parenteral hyperalimentation, they do occur, especially in critically ill patients. Metabolic complications associated with enteral alimentation include nutrient intolerance and fluid and electrolyte imbalance. Careful monitoring, especially when starting enteral feeding, will identify these abnormalities quickly. Some patients, particularly those with preexisting glucose intolerance, will exhibit hyperglycemia. Its treatment is straightforward. The hyperglycemia may be corrected, at least partially, by the use of a commercially available specialty formula specifically designed for diabetics. Other fluid and electrolyte imbalances will be identified as the patient is monitored closely and treated accordingly.

Aspiration has been reported to occur in up to 40% of patients who are fed enterally. Although gross aspiration can occur, it usually can be prevented by proper positioning of the patient and frequent checks for increased residual gastric volume of the enteral solution. Microaspiration, often undetected, has been demonstrated in mechanically ventilated patients receiving enteral alimentation and has been associated with the development of nosocomial respiratory infection.[134] This can occur early in the patient's hospital course and may contribute to increased morbidity and mortality.

Parenteral Nutrition

Peripheral parenteral hyperalimentation generally is regarded as safe with relatively few complications, although, since lipids are the primary calorie source, complications related to lipid intolerance can occur. Patients must be monitored closely for hypertriglyceridemia, especially if there is preexisting hyperlipidemia.

Diabetics tolerate the lipid-based three-in-one solution extremely well with a low incidence of hyperalimentation-induced hyperglycemia. Peripheral administration over long periods of time may lead to problems with access. The sclerosing effect of the hypertonic solution can cause superficial phlebitis. However, complications associated with central line placement and maintenance are avoided. In some studies, lipid-based TPN was associated with elevated circulating free fatty levels.[135] The consequences of this in acute myocardial ischemia are controversial,[136] but there is some evidence that arrhythmias may be precipitated and that the area of ischemic damage may be extended in patients with acute myocardial infarctions.[137, 138] Glucose-based TPN administered centrally is preferable for fluid-restricted patients and for those with poor peripheral venous access, disorders of lipid metabolism, or acute myocardial ischemia.[101] It is the authors' experience that the lipid-based, peripherally administered solutions work extremely well for short periods, i.e., 10 days or less, either as a stand-alone method of nutritional support or as a supplement to oral or nasoenteral feedings.

Centrally administered total parenteral nutrition has numerous potential complications and, therefore, requires very close supervision and monitoring. Complications from catheter insertion have been reported to occur in 1% to 15% of patients.[139–141] The majority of studies emphasize the relation between the operator's experience with the procedure and morbidity. Pneumothorax is the most common major complication following percutaneous central vein catheterization (~5%) and usually is due to improper technique. It is more likely to occur on the left side because the left pleural dome is higher. Several other anatomic factors can increase the risk, even with good technique; these are cachexia, barrel chest, kyphosis, and morbid obesity. Other risk factors include mechanical ventilation and positive end-expiratory pressure. Late development of a pneumothorax[142] may be suggested by the onset of scapular or supraclavicular pain. A high index of suspicion will help identify this complication.

Catheter misdirection usually is not serious if recognized early. It most often involves the subclavian catheter traveling up the ipsilateral internal jugular vein. This occurs more commonly on the right side because of the abrupt descent of the superior vena cava from its junction with the subclavian vein.[143] It is suggested by ipsilateral neck, auricular, or mandibular pain during catheter manipulation. More dangerous misdirection is placement of the catheter tip in the hepatic vein or in the cardiac chambers. The use of shorter catheters usually prevents this problem. The most serious form of misdirection is perforation of the great veins or heart and entry of the guidewire or catheter into the pericardium or mediastinum. This can occur with the overaggressive or improper use of flexible guidewires or with the use of stiff catheters. Accidental puncture of a subclavian or carotid artery is not rare and often only requires prolonged pressure over the puncture site. However, significant bleeding can occur, especially in patients with coagulation abnormalities. Mediastinal hematoma, airway obstruction, and pericardial tamponade are life-threatening but rare sequelae of inadvertent great vessel puncture.[144] Inadvertent injury to the thoracic duct resulting in a chylothorax can occur. Obviously, this occurs more commonly with left-sided cannulation.

Infectious complications, both bacterial and fungal, occur fairly frequently (3% to 7%) with parenteral feeding.[145, 146] Strict adherence to a protocol that ensures sterility during insertion, manipulation, and dressing changes is important for prevention. Reserving the central line exclusively for TPN administration is also important.[146] There is some evidence of a greater incidence of sepsis with the use of triple-lumen catheters than with single-lumen catheters.[147, 148]

Due to the high insulin level that develops in response to hypertonic glucose infusion, serum concentrations of components of lean tissue (potassium, magnesium, phosphorus, and nitrogen) or glycogen (potassium) may fall dramatically. Adequate amounts of these components must be supplied continually. A rapid fall in potassium can lead to cardiac arrhythmias and even sudden death; close monitoring of potassium, however, usually is routine. Magnesium and phosphorus may not be monitored so closely, yet a fall in blood concentration can develop precipitously.[143] A rapid fall in the magnesium level can result in either cardiac arrhythmias or dysfunction of calcium metabolism.[149] Acute reductions in plasma phosphate concentration have been associated with numerous abnormalities of the erythrocyte,[150] leukocyte,[151] neurologic system,[152] and cardiovascular system,[153] and with respiratory muscle dysfunction.[154] Disorders of calcium metabolism have been documented during TPN administration, mandating monitoring of serum calcium.[155]

Hyperglycemia often occurs, even when nondiabetic critically ill patients initially are given parenteral nutrition. There are several reasons for this: persistent gluconeogenesis, blunted insulin response, decreased tissue sensitivity to insulin, impaired peripheral utilization of glucose or phosphate, or chromium deficiency, which further diminishes tissue sensitivity to insulin. Blood sugars in excess of 220 mg/dL have been shown to impair phagocyte function[156] and should be treated. When insulin is required with TPN, it should be added to the solution and administered continuously. It is somewhat less effective than parenteral dosing, but controls blood sugar better than intermittent subcutaneous dosing.[143]

Hypoglycemia results from either a decreased or an uneven infusion rate of the TPN solution or, rarely, from excessive insulin administration. Because parenteral feeding eventually induces relative hyperinsulinemia in most patients, it must be discontinued gradually (over 72 to 96 hours) to avoid rebound hypoglycemia.[93] For the same reason, a peripheral infusion of 20% dextrose should be started immediately if the central infusion of TPN is interrupted.

Hyperlipidemia can occur with TPN administration. Usually, triglyceride levels peak 4 hours after intravenous infusion and are back to baseline in 6 to 8 hours, but their clearance may be impaired in patients with liver disease or multiple-organ failure.[157–159] Excessive or rapid infusion of lipids can result in transient hyperlipidemia. Pulmonary function has been shown to be worsened by intravenous lipid infusions in some patients, but its clinical significance is unknown.[160]

Abnormal liver function tests and fatty liver infiltration often develop with parenteral nutrition, but only rarely with enteral feedings.[161] Most cases are self-limited and require only a lowered caloric intake. Intravenous lipid infusions have been associated with liver function abnormalities, mandating close monitoring of liver function tests.[162]

Multiple acid-base abnormalities can occur with administration of TPN. Acetate, as sodium or potassium acetate, can be added to the solution for additional buffering. Many acid-base abnormalities are exacerbated by other aspects of the patient's underlying illness or other therapeutic modalities and, when caught early, can be remedied easily.

The administration of nutritional support is not without morbidity, even with careful supervision. There are no prospective, randomized, controlled trials of critically ill patients to assess outcome following nutritional support. It is unlikely, with current practices, that these trials ever will be done in the United States. Skeie et al. have examined the effects of long-term parenteral nutrition in patients with cystic fibrosis and demonstrated a marked increase in maximal work load during exercise testing.[163] This was thought to be due to a reduction in anaerobic metabolism after institution of TPN. Although these data are preliminary and are from cystic fibrosis patients rather than critically ill patients, they demonstrate definite benefit from the administration of TPN.

In summary, nutritional support of the critically ill patient remains a complex and challenging therapeutic modality of intensive care medicine. Providing adequate nutrition requires a multidisciplinary approach utilizing support services such as dietetics and pharmacy as well as nursing. Patients receiving nutritional support of any kind require close monitoring and frequent adjustments of their therapy. Nutritional support continues to be controversial and demands continued study of many aspects.

REFERENCES

1. Schuberth O, Wretlind A: Intravenous infusion of fat emulsions, phosphatides and emulsifying agents. Clinical and experimental studies. *Acta Chir Scand* 1961; 278(suppl 1):1–21.

2. Dudrick SJ, Wilmore DW, Vars HM, et al: Long-term parenteral nutrition with growth, development and positive nitrogen balance. *Surgery* 1968; 64:134–142.

3. Bistrian BR, Blackburn GL, Vitale J, et al: Prevalence of malnutrition in general medical patients. *JAMA* 1976; 235:1567–1570.

4. Bistrian BR, Blackburn GL, Hallowell E, et al: Protein status of general surgical patients. *JAMA* 1974; 230:858–860.

5. Willcutts HE: Nutritional assessment of 1000 surgical patients in an affluent suburban community hospital. *JPEN J Parenter Enteral Nutr* 1977; 1:25A.

6. Driver AG, LeBrun M: Iatrogenic malnutrition in patients receiving ventilatory support. *JAMA* 1980; 244:2195–2196.

7. Pollack MM, Wiley JS, Kanter R, et al: Malnutrition in critically ill infants and children. *JPEN J Parenter Enteral Nutr* 1982; 6:20–24.

8. Roubenoff R, Roubenoff RA, Preto J, et al: Malnutrition among hospitalized patients. *Arch Intern Med* 1987; 147:1462–1465.

9. Mullen JL, Gertner MH, Buzby GP, et al: Implications of malnutrition in the surgical patient. *Arch Surg* 1979; 114:121–125.

10. Burritt MF, Anderson CF: Laboratory assessment of nutritional status. *Hum Pathol* 1984; 15:130–133.

11. Roza AM, Tuitt D, Shizgal HM: Transferrin—a poor measure of nutritional status. *JPEN J Parenter Enteral Nutr* 1984; 8:523–528.

12. Kosanovich JM, Dumler F, Horst M, et al: Use of urea kinetics in the nutritional care of the acutely ill patient. *JPEN J Parenter Enteral Nutr* 1985; 9:165–169.

13. Baker JP, Detsky AS, Wesson DE, et al: Nutritional assessment. A comparison of clinical judgement and objective measurements. *N Engl J Med* 1982; 306:969–972.

14. Dempsey DT, Buzby GP, Mullen JL: Nutritional assessment in the seriously ill patient. *J Am Coll Nutr* 1983; 2:15–23.

15. Silberman H: *Parenteral and Enteral Nutrition,* ed 2. Norwalk, Conn, Appleton & Lange, 1989.

16. Detsky AS, McLaughlin JR, Baker JP, et al: What is subjective global assessment of nutritional status? *JPEN J Parenter Enteral Nutr* 1987; 11:8–13.

17. Studley HO: Percentage of weight loss. A basic indicator of surgical risk in patients with chronic peptic ulcer. *JAMA* 1936; 106:458.

18. Ryan JA, Taft DA: Preoperative nutritional assessment does not predict morbidity and mortality in abdominal operations. *Surg Forum* 1980; 31:96–98.

19. Chandra RK: Malnutrition, in Chandra RK (ed): *Primary and Secondary Immunodeficiency Disorders.* New York, Churchill Livingstone, 1983, p 187.

20. Shizgal HM: Nutrition and immune function. *Surg Annu* 1981; 12:15–29.

21. Brown LAS, Bliss AS, Longmore WJ: Effect of nutritional status on the lung surfactant system: Food deprivation and caloric restriction. *Exp Lung Res* 1984; 6:133–147.

22. Chandra RK, Newberne PM: *Nutrition, Immunity and Infection: Mechanisms of Interaction.* New York, Plenum Press, 1977.

23. Halliwell B, Gutteridge JMC: Oxygen toxicity, oxygen radicals, transition metals and disease. *Biochem J* 1984; 219:1–14.

24. Rosenbaum SH, Askanazi J, Hyman AI, et al: Respiratory patterns in profound nutritional depletion. *Anesthesiology* 1979; 51(suppl 1):366.

25. De Troyer A, Bastenier-Geens J: Effects of neuromuscular blockade on respiratory mechanics in conscious man. *J Appl Physiol* 1979; 47:1162–1168.

26. Gibson GJ, Pride NB, Newsom Davis J: Pulmonary mechanics in patients with respiratory muscle weakness. *Am Rev Respir Dis* 1978; 118:373.

27. Arora NS, Rochester DF: Effect of body weight and muscularity on human diaphragm muscle mass, thickness, and area. *J Appl Physiol* 1982; 52:64–70.

28. Thurlbeck WM: Diaphragm and body weight in emphysema. *Thorax* 1978; 33:483–487.

29. Arora NS, Rochester DF: Respiratory muscle strength and maximal voluntary ventilation in undernourished patients. *Am Rev Respir Dis* 1982; 126:5–8.

30. Zwillich CW, Sahn SA, Weil JV: Effects of hypermetabolism on ventilation and chemosensitivity. *J Clin Invest* 1977; 60:900–906.

31. Benedict FC, Miles WR, Roth P, et al: *Human Vitality and Efficiency Under Prolonged Restricted Diet.* Carnegie Institute, Washington Publications No 280, 1919.

32. Keys A, Brozek J, Henschel A, et al: *Biology of Human Starvation.* Minneapolis, University of Minnesota Press, 1950.

33. Wilhelmj CM: The specific dynamic action of food. *Physiol Rev* 1935; 15:202–220.

34. Doekel RC Jr, Zwillich CW, Scoggin CH: Clinical semi-starvation: Depression of hypoxic ventilatory response. *N Engl J Med* 1976; 295:358–361.

35. Askanazi J, Rosenbaum SH, Hyman AI, et al: Effects of parenteral nutrition on ventilatory drive. *Anesthesiology* 1980; 53(suppl 1):185.

36. Keys A, Henschel A, Taylor HL: The size and function of the human heart at rest in semi-starvation and in subsequent rehabilitation. *Am J Physiol* 1947; 50:153–169.

37. Johnson RA, Baker SS, Fallon JT, et al: An occidental case of cardiomyopathy and selenium deficiency. *N Engl J Med* 1981; 304:1210–1212.

38. Van Rij AM, Thomson CD, McKenzie J, et al: Selenium deficiency in total parenteral nutrition. *Am J Clin Nutr* 1979; 32:2076–2085.

39. Cahill GF Jr: Starvation in man. *N Engl J Med* 1970; 282:668–675.

40. Lemoyne M, Jeejeebhoy KN: Total parenteral nutrition in the critically ill patient. *Chest* 1986; 89:568–575.

41. Baracos V, Rodeman HP, Dinarello CA, et al: Stimulation of muscle protein degradation and prostaglandin E$_2$ release by leukocytic pyrogen (interleukin-1). *N Engl J Med* 1983; 308:553–558.

42. Shamoon H, Hendler R, Sherwin RS: Synergistic interactions among antiinsulin hormones in the pathogenesis of stress hyperglycemia in humans. *J Clin Endocrinol Metab* 1981; 52:1235–1241.

43. Bartlett RH: Assessment and management of nutrition in critical illness, in Bone RC (ed): *Critical Care: A Comprehensive Approach*, ed 1. Park Ridge, Ill, American College of Chest Physicians, 1984, pp 60–81.

44. Jeejeebhoy KN: Total parenteral nutrition. *Ann R Coll Phys Surg Can* 1976; 9:287–300.

45. Harris JA, Benedict FG: *A Biometric Study of Basal Metabolism in Man*. Washington, DC, Carnegie Institute of Washington, Publication 297, 1919.

46. Kinney JM, Duke JH Jr, Long CL, et al: Tissue fuel and weight loss after injury. *J Clin Pathol* 1970; 23(suppl 1):65–69.

47. Long CL, Schaffel N, Geiger JW, et al: Metabolic response to injury and illness: Estimation of energy and protein needs from indirect calorimetry and nitrogen balance. *JPEN J Parenter Enteral Nutr* 1979; 3:452–456.

48. Feurer ID, Crosby LO, Mullen JL: Measured and predicted resting energy expenditure in clinically stable patients. *Clin Nutr* 1984; 3:27–34.

49. Damask MC, Schwarz Y, Weissman C: Energy measurements and requirements of critically ill patients. *Crit Care Clin* 1987; 3:71–96.

50. Liggett SB, St John RE, Lefrak SS: Determination of resting energy expenditure utilizing the thermodilution pulmonary artery catheter. *Chest* 1987; 91:562–566.

51. Liggett SB, Renfro AD: Energy expenditures of mechanically ventilated nonsurgical patients. *Chest* 1990; 98:682–686.

52. Moore FD: Surgical care and metabolic management of the postoperative patient, in Winters RW, Green HL (eds): *Nutritional Support of the Seriously Ill Patient*. Bristol-Myers Nutrition Symposia Series, vol 1. New York, Academic Press, 1983, pp 5–12.

53. Blackburn GL, Flatt JP, Hensle TW: Peripheral amino acid infusions, in Fischer JE (ed): *Total Parenteral Nutrition*. Boston, Little, Brown & Co, 1976, pp 363–394.

54. Blackburn GL: Protein metabolism and nutritional support. *J Trauma* 1981; 21(suppl):707–711.

55. Anderson GH, Patel DG, Jeejeebhoy KN: Design and evaluation by nitrogen balance and blood aminograms of an amino acid mixture for total parenteral nutrition of adults with gastrointestinal disease. *J Clin Invest* 1974; 53:904–912.

56. Wilmore DM, Black PR, Muhlbacher FM: Injured man: Trauma and sepsis, in Winters RW, Greene H (eds): *Nutritional Support of the Seriously Ill Patient*. Bristol-Myers Nutrition Symposia Series, vol 1. New York, Academic Press, 1983, pp 34–52.

57. Schiller WR, Long CL, Blakemore WS: Creatinine and nitrogen excretion in seriously ill and injured patients. *Surg Gynecol Obstet* 1979; 149:561–566.

58. Long CL, Jeevanandam M, Kim BM, et al: Whole body protein synthesis and catabolism in septic man. *Am J Clin Nutr* 1977; 30:1340–1344.

59. Herrmann VM, Clarke D, Wilmore DW, et al: Protein metabolism: Effect of disease and altered intake on the stable ^{15}N curve. *Surg Forum* 1980; 31:92–94.

60. Elwyn DH: Protein metabolism and requirements in the critically ill patient. *Crit Care Clin* 1987; 3:57–69.

61. Fischer JE: Nutritional support in the seriously ill patient. *Curr Probl Surg* 1980; 17:465–532.

62. Wolfe RR: Carbohydrate metabolism in the critically ill patient: Implications for nutritional support. *Crit Care Clin* 1987; 3:11–23.

63. Wiener M, Rothkopf MM, Rothkopf G, et al: Fat metabolism in injury and stress. *Crit Care Clin* 1987; 3:25–56.

64. MacFie J, Smith RC, Hill GL: Glucose or fat as a nonprotein energy source? A controlled clinical trial in gastroenterological patients requiring intravenous nutrition. *Gastroenterology* 1981; 80:103–107.

65. Youinou PY, Garre MA, Menez JF, et al: Folic acid deficiency and neutrophil dysfunction. *Am J Med* 1982; 73:652–657.

66. Cotzias GC: Role and importance of trace substance in environmental health, in Hemphill DD (ed): *Proceedings of the First Annual Conference on Trace Substances and Environmental Health*. Columbia, Mo, University of Missouri Press, 1967, pp 5–19.

67. Doisy EA Jr: Micronutrient control in biosynthesis of clotting protein and cholesterol, in Hemphill DD (ed): *Trace Substances in Environmental Health*. Columbia, Mo, Curators of the University of Missouri, 1972, pp 193–199.

68. Abumrad NN, Scneider AJ, Steel D, et al: Amino acid intolerance during prolonged total parenteral nutrition (TPN) reversed by molybdenum (abstract). *Am J Clin Nutr* 1981; 34:618.

69. Golden MHN, Golden BE: Trace elements: Potential importance in human nutrition with particular reference to zinc and vanadium. *Br Med Bull* 1981; 37:31–36.

70. Phillips GD, Garnys VP: Parenteral administration of trace elements to critically ill patients. *Anaesth Intensive Care* 1981; 9:221–225.

71. Shils ME, Burke AW, Greene HL, et al: Guidelines for essential trace element preparations for parenteral use. *JAMA* 1979; 241:2051–2054.

72. Heimburger DC: Enteral feeding. *Ala J Med Sci* 1982; 19:387–391.

73. Kudsk KA, Stone JM, Carpenter G, et al: Enteral and parenteral feeding influences mortality after hemoglobin-*E. coli* peritonitis in normal rats. *J Trauma* 1983; 23:605–609.

74. Kudsk KA, Stone JM, Carpenter G, et al: Effects of enteral versus parenteral feeding on body composition of malnourished animals. *J Trauma* 1982; 22:904–906.

75. Johnson LR, Copeland EM, Dudrick SJ, et al: Structural and hormonal alterations in the gastrointestinal tract of parenterally fed rats. *Gastroenterology* 1975; 68:1177–1183.

76. Levine GM, Deren JJ, Steiger E, et al: Role of oral intake in maintenance of gut mass and disaccharidase activity. *Gastroenterology* 1974; 67:975–982.

77. Berg RD: Translocation of indigenous bacteria from the intestinal tract, in Hentges DJ (ed): *Human Intestinal Microflora in Health and Disease*. New York, Academic Press, 1983.

78. Alverdy JC, Aoys E, Moss GS: Total parenteral nutrition promotes bacterial translocation from the gut. *Surgery* 1988; 104:185–190.

79. Spaeth G, Specian RD, Berg RD, et al: Bulk prevents bacterial translocation induced by the oral administration of total parenteral nutrition solution. *JPEN J Parenter Enteral Nutr* 1990; 14:442–447.

80. Alverdy JC, Aoys E, Moss GS: Effect of commercially available chemically defined liquid diets on the intestinal microflora and bacterial translocation from the gut. *JPEN J Parenter Enteral Nutr* 1990; 14:1–6.

81. Pingleton SK, Hadzima SK: Enteral alimentation and gastrointestinal bleeding in mechanically ventilated patients. *Crit Care Med* 1983; 11:13–16.

82. Koruda MJ, Guenter P, Rombeau JL: Enteral nutrition in the critically ill. *Crit Care Clin* 1987; 3:133–153.

83. Rothnie NG, Kemp Harper RA, Catchpole BN: Early postoperative gastrointestinal activity. *Lancet* 1963; 2:64–67.

84. Wilson JP: Postoperative motility of the large intestine in man. *Gut* 1975; 16:689–692.

85. Woods JH, Erickson LW, Condon RE, et al: Postoperative ileus: A colonic problem. *Surgery* 1978; 84:527.

86. Ryan JA, Page CP: Intrajejunal feeding: Development and current status. JPEN J Parenter Enteral Nutr 1984; 8:187–198.

87. Hayashi JT, Wolfe BM, Calvert CC: Limited efficacy of early postoperative jejunal feeding. *Am J Surg* 1985; 150:52–57.

88. Ponsky JL, Gauderer MWL, Stellato TA, et al: Percutaneous approaches to enteral alimentation. *Am J Surg* 1985; 149:102–105.

89. Dye KR, Pattison CP, Dye NV: Percutaneous endoscopic gastrostomy: Technical modifications for improved results. *South Med J* 1986; 79:24–27.

90. Ponsky JL, Aszodi A: Percutaneous endoscopic jejunostomy. *Am J Gastroenterol* 1984; 79:113–116.

91. Rombeau JL, Twomey PL, McLean GK, et al: Experience with a new gastrostomy-jejunal feeding tube. *Surgery* 1983; 93:574–578.

92. Rolandelli RH, Rombeau JL: Liquid defined formula diets. *Curr Ther Gastro Liv Disease* vol 2. 1984–85.

93. Berger R, Adams L: Nutritional support in the critical care setting. *Chest* 1989; 96:139–150, 372–380.

94. Randall HT: Enteral nutrition: Tube feeding in acute and chronic illness. *JPEN J Parenter Enteral Nutr* 1984; 8:113–136.

95. Macburney MM, Jacobs DO, Apelgren KN, et al: Modular feeding, in Rombeau JL, Caldwell MD (eds): *Enteral and Tube Feeding*. Philadelphia, WB Saunders Co, 1984, pp 199–211.

96. Heimburger DC, Weinsier RL: Guidelines for evaluating and categorizing enteral feeding formulas according to therapeutic equivalence. *JPEN J Parenter Enteral Nutr* 1985; 9:61–67.

97. Askanazi J, Elwyn DH, Silverberg PA, et al: Respiratory distress secondary to a high carbohydrate load: A case report. *Surgery* 1980; 87:596–598.

98. Dark DS, Pingleton SK, Kerby GR: Hypercapnia during weaning: A complication of nutritional support. *Chest* 1985; 88:141–142.

99. Hiebert JM, Brown A, Anderson RG, et al: Comparison of continuous vs. intermittent tube feedings in adult burn patients. *JPEN J Parenter Enteral Nutr* 1981; 5:73–75.

100. Orr G, Wade J, Bothe A, et al: Alternatives to total parenteral nutrition in the critically ill patient. *Crit Care Med* 1980; 8:29–34.

101. Silberman H: Total parenteral nutrition by peripheral vein: Current status of fat emulsions. *Nutr Intelligence* 1986; 2:145–149.

102. Messing B, Beliah M, Girard-Pipau F, et al: Technical hazards of using nutritive mixtures in bags for cyclical intravenous nutrition: A comparison with standard intravenous nutrition in 48 gastroenterological patients. *Gut* 1982; 23:297–303.

103. Shields HM: Nutritional therapy, in Campbell JW, Frisse M (eds): *Manual of Medical Therapeutics, ed 24*. Boston, Little, Brown & Co, 1983, pp 211–224.

104. Hallberg D: Therapy with fat emulsion. *Acta Anaesthesiol Scand* 1974; 55(suppl 1):1336.

105. Meng HC: Fat emulsions in parenteral nutrition, in Fischer JE (ed): *Total Parenteral Nutrition*. Boston, Little, Brown & Co, 1976, pp 305–334.

106. Glynn MJ, Powell-Tuck J, Reaveley DA, et al: High lipid parenteral nutrition improves portasystemic encephalopathy. *JPEN J Parenter Enteral Nutr* 1988; 12:457–461.

107. Freund H, Hoover HC Jr, Atamian S: Infusion of the branched chain amino acids in postoperative patients. *Ann Surg* 1979; 190:18–23.

108. Mizock BA: Branched-chain amino acids in sepsis and hepatic failure. *Arch Intern Med* 1985; 145:1284–1288.

109. Bower RH, Kern KA, Fischer JE: Use of a branched chain amino acid enriched solution in patients under metabolic stress. *Am J Surg* 1985; 149:266–270.

110. Cerra FB, Mazuski J, Teasley K, et al: Nitrogen retention in critically ill patients is proportional to the branched chain amino acid load. *Crit Care Med* 1983; 11:775–778.

111. Cerra FB, Upson D, Angelico R, et al: Branched chains support postoperative protein synthesis. *Surgery* 1982; 92:192–199.

112. Takala J, Klossner J, Irjala J, et al: Branched-chain amino acids in surgically stressed patients, in Johnston ID (ed): *Advances in Clinical Nutrition*. Boston, MTP Press, 1983, pp 77–82.

113. Cerra FB, Mazuski JE, Chute E, et al: Branched chain metabolic support: A prospective randomized double-blind trial in surgical stress. *Ann Surg* 1984; 199:286–291.

114. Echenique MM, Bistrian BR, Moldawer LL, et al: Improvement in amino acid use in the critically ill patient with parenteral formulas enriched with branched chain amino acids. *Surg Gynecol Obstet* 1984; 159:233–241.

115. Klimberg VS, Souba WW, Sitren H, et al: Glutamine-enriched total parenteral nutrition supports gut metabolism. *Surg Forum* 1989; 40:175–177.

116. Salloum RM, Souba WW, Klimberg VS, et al: Glutamine is superior to glutamate in supporting gut metabolism, stimulating intestinal glutaminase activity, and preventing bacterial translocation. *Surg Forum* 1989; 40:6.

117. Souba WW, Herskowitz K, Austgen TR, et al: Glutamine nutrition: Theoretical considerations and therapeutic impact. *JPEN J Parenter Enteral Nutr* 1990; 14(suppl 1):237s–243s.

118. Lakshman K, Blackburn GL: Monitoring nutritional status in the critically ill adult. *J Clin Monit* 1986; 2:114–120.

119. Cortes V, Nelson LD: Errors in estimating energy expenditure in critically ill surgical patients. *Arch Surg* 1989; 124:287–290.

120. Makk LJK, McClave SA, Creech PW, et al: Clinical application of the metabolic cart to the delivery of total parenteral nutrition. *Crit Care Med* 1990; 18:1320–1327.

121. McNeill KG, Harrison JE, Mernagh JR, et al: Changes in body protein, body potassium and lean body mass during total parenteral nutrition. *JPEN J Parenter Enteral Nutr* 1982; 6:106–108.

122. McNeill KG, Mernagh JR, Jeejeebhoy KN, et al: In vivo measurements of body protein based on the determination of nitrogen by prompt gamma analysis. *Am J Clin Nutr* 1979; 32:1955–1961.

123. Hendry PJ, Akyurekli Y, McIntyre R, et al: Bronchopleural complications of nasogastric feeding tubes. *Crit Care Med* 1986; 14:892–894.

124. Aronchick J, Epstein DM, Gefter WB, et al: Pneumothorax as a complication of placement of a nasoenteric tube. *JAMA* 1984; 252:3287–3288.

125. Lind LJ, Wallace DH: Submucosal passage of a nasogastric tube complicating attempted intubation during anesthesia. *Anesthesiology* 1978; 49:145–147.

126. Cataldi-Betcher EL, Seltzer MH, Slocum BA, et al: Complications occurring during enteral nutritional support: A prospective study. *JPEN J Parenter Enteral Nutr* 1983; 7:546–552.

127. Dark DS, Pingleton SK: Gastrointestinal complications of enteral alimentation in respiratory failure patients (abstract). *Chest* 1984; 86:

128. Dark DS, Pingleton SK: Nonhemorrhagic gastrointestinal complications in acute respiratory failure. *Crit Care Med* 1989; 17:755–758.

129. Whatley K, Turner WW, Dey M, et al: When does metoclopramide facilitate transpyloric intubation? *JPEN J Parenter Enteral Nutr* 1984; 8:679–681.

130. Keohane PP, Attrill H, Love M, et al: Relation between osmolality of diet and gastrointestinal side effects in enteral nutrition. *BMJ* 1984; 288:678–680.

131. Hostetler C, Lipman TO, Geraghty M, et al: Bacterial safety of reconstituted continuous drip tube feeding. *JPEN J Parenter Enteral Nutr* 1982; 6:232–235.

132. Schroeder P, Fisher D, Volz M, et al: Microbial contamination of enteral feeding solutions in a community. *JPEN J Parenter Enteral Nutr* 1983; 7:364–367.

133. Brinson RR, Kolts BE: Hypoalbuminemia as an indicator of diarrheal incidence in critically ill patients. *Crit Care Med* 1987; 15:506–509.

134. Pingleton SK, Hinthorn DR, Liu C: Enteral nutrition in patients receiving mechanical ventilation. *Am J Med* 1986; 80:827–832.

135. Jeejeebhoy KN, Anderson GH, Nakhooda AF, et al: Metabolic studies in total parenteral nutrition with lipid in man. Comparison with glucose. *J Clin Invest* 1976; 57:125–136.

136. Jones JW, Tibb D, McDonald LK, et al: 10% Soybean oil emulsion as a myocardial energy substrate after ischemic arrest. *Surg Forum* 1977; 28:284–285.

137. Free fatty acids and arrhythmias after acute myocardial infarction (editorial). *Lancet* 1975; 1:313.

138. Opie LH, Tansey M, Kennelly BM: Proposed metabolic vicious circle in patients with large myocardial infarcts and high plasma-free-fatty-acid concentrations. *Lancet* 1977; 2:890–892.

139. Ryan JA, Able RM, Abbott WM, et al: Catheter complications in total parenteral nutrition: A prospective study of 200 consecutive patients. *N Engl J Med* 1974; 290:757–761.

140. Bernard RW, Stahl WM: Subclavian vein catheterizations. *Ann Surg* 1971; 173:184–190.

141. Eisenhauer ED, Derveloy RJ, Hastings PR: Prospective evaluation of central venous pressure (CVP) catheters in a large city-county hospital. *Ann Surg* 1982; 196:560–564.

142. Sivak SL: Late appearance of pneumothorax after subclavian venipuncture. *Am J Med* 1986; 80:323–324.

143. Benotti PN, Bistrian BR: Practical aspects and complications of total parenteral nutrition. *Crit Care Clin* 1987; 3:115–131.

144. Hunt LB, Olshansky B, Hiratzka LF: Cardiac tamponade caused by pulmonary artery perforation after central venous catheterization. *JPEN J Parenter Enteral Nutr* 1984; 8:711–713.

145. Snydman DR, Murray SA, Kornfeld SJ, et al: Total parenteral nutrition-related infections: Prospective epidemiologic study using semiquantitative methods. *Am J Med* 1982; 73:695–699.

146. Saunders RA, Sheldon GF: Septic complications of total parenteral nutrition: A five year experience. *Am J Surg* 1976; 132:214–220.

147. Pemberton LB, Lyman B, Lander V, et al: Sepsis from triple- vs single-lumen catheters during total parenteral nutrition in surgical or critically ill patients. *Arch Surg* 1986; 121:591–594.

148. Lee RB, Buckner M, Sharp KW: Do multi-lumen catheters increase central venous catheter sepsis compared to single-lumen catheters? *J Trauma* 1988; 28:1472–1475.

149. Ryzen E, Wagers PW, Singer FR, et al: Magnesium deficiency in a medical ICU population. *Crit Care Med* 1985; 13:19–21.

150. Klock JC, Williams HE, Mentzer WC: Hemolytic anemia and somatic cell dysfunction in severe hypophosphatemia. *Arch Intern Med* 1974; 134:360–364.

151. Craddock PR, Yawata Y, Van Santen L, et al: Acquired phagocyte dysfunction: A complication of the hypophosphatemia of parenteral hyperalimentation. *N Engl J Med* 1974; 290:1403–1407.

152. Silvis SE, Paragas PD: Paresthesias, weakness, seizures and hypophosphatemia in patients receiving hyperalimentation. *Gastroenterology* 1972; 62:513–520.

153. O'Connor LR, Wheeler WS, Bethune JE: Effect of hypophosphatemia on myocardial performance in man. *N Engl J Med* 1977; 297:901–903.

154. Aubier M, Murciano D, Lecocguic Y, et al: Effect of hypophosphatemia on diaphragmatic contractility in patients with acute respiratory failure. *N Engl J Med* 1985; 313:420–424.

155. Weissman C, Askanazi J, Hyman AI, et al: Hypercalcemia and hypercalciuria in a critically ill patient. *Crit Care Med* 1983; 11:576–578.

156. Rossini AA: Why control blood glucose levels? *Arch Surg* 1976; 111:229–233.

157. Askanazi J, Carpentier YA, Elwyn DH, et al: Influence of total parenteral nutrition on fuel utilization in injury and sepsis. *Ann Surg* 1980; 191:40–46.

158. Silberman H: Parenteral nutrition: The lipid system, in Silberman H, Eisenberg D (eds): *Parenteral and Enteral Nutrition,* ed 2. Norwalk, Conn, Appleton & Lange, 1989, pp 265–292.

159. Wretlind A: Current status of Intralipid and other fat emulsions, in Meng HC, Wilmore DW (eds): *Fat Emulsions in Parenteral Nutrition.* Chicago, American Medical Association, 1976, pp 109–122.

160. Greene HL, Hazlett D, Demaree R: Relationship between Intralipid-induced hyperlipidemia and pulmonary function. *Am J Clin Nutr* 1976; 29:127–135.

161. Bower RH, Talamini MA, Sax HC, et al: Postoperative enteral vs parenteral nutrition: A randomized controlled trial. *Arch Surg* 1986; 121:1040–1045.

162. Jacobson S, Ericsson JLE, Obel AL: Histopathological and ultrastructural changes in the human liver during complete intravenous nutrition for 7 months. *Acta Chir Scand* 1971; 137:335–349.

163. Skeie B, Askanazi J, Rothkopf MM, et al: Improved exercise tolerance with long-term parenteral nutrition in cystic fibrosis. *Crit Care Med* 1987; 15:960–962.

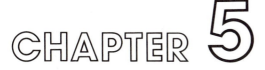

CHAPTER 5

Viral Infections of the Respiratory Tract

Frederick L. Ruben, M.D.

Professor of Medicine, University of Pittsburgh School of Medicine, Montefiore University Hospital, Pittsburgh, Pennsylvania

Respiratory infections are the most common short-term illness in the American population.[1] Viruses play a major role as pathogens in these illnesses, as shown by many population-based studies of respiratory illness. The populations of children studied have included those in prepaid health plans,[2, 3] those receiving hospital-based care[4] and those from rural communities.[5] Other studies have focused on an entire community,[6] civilian adults,[7] a military base,[8] or special groups such as adults with chronic obstructive pulmonary disease (COPD)[9] or asthma.[10] Given the high frequency of these viral respiratory illnesses, much effort has been devoted to defining the clinical picture of illness from differing viruses, developing diagnostic methods, and providing means for treatment and prevention. This review will discuss the major respiratory viruses from a clinical viewpoint and will emphasize the most current approaches to diagnosis and treatment.

INFLUENZA VIRUSES

Influenza A and B viruses regularly cause epidemics of respiratory illness leading to loss of productivity, physician visits, hospitalizations, and deaths. These viruses frequently change the antigenic structure of their surface antigens, the hemagglutinin (HA) and neuraminidase, circumventing prior immunity and making the population again susceptible to infection.[11] The molecular basis for this interpandemic variation has been shown to be minor changes in amino acid sequences at one of several epitopes.[12] A remarkable finding is the evidence for genetic reassortment between human and avian influenza A viruses to create strains responsible for the 1957 (Asian) and 1968 (Hong Kong) pandemics.[13]

When influenza viruses infect humans, upper airways typically are the site involved. Viral HA attaches to respiratory epithelial cells, and HA must be cleaved, presumably by proteases,[14] before entering the cell. Viral multiplication leads to epithelial cell destruction sparing the basal layer,[15] and virions budding from the dying cell surface are released to infect other cells by the enzymatic action of their neuraminidase. The infection leads to loss of host defenses, particularly mucociliary clearance,[16] but also abnormalities in airflow both acutely[17] and for weeks thereafter.[18] Upper airway infection causes pharyngitis, otitis, and sinusitis. Virus also can infect the lungs, causing primary viral pneumonia.[19] In fatal cases, virus has been found in extrapulmonary sites including liver, spleen, heart, and brain.[20, 21] A strong association exists between influenza and bacterial pneumonia[22] because of the loss of host defenses induced by the virus.[23]

Both humoral and cell-mediated immunity are important in defense against influenza viruses. Humoral antibodies reduce the likelihood of infection and illness,[24] while cell-mediated immunity probably plays a prime role in elimination of the virus and recovery.[25]

Influenza A and B viruses tend to cause relatively minor upper respiratory tract illnesses in infants and children.[2, 3] Up to 4% of bronchiolitis and 6% of croup in infants was caused by influenza in one study.[5] By contrast, in adults, up to 60% of lower respiratory infection was caused by influenza viruses.[6] Influenza has been associated with attacks of asthma[10] and exacerbations of COPD.[9] Elderly and debilitated persons of any age are prone to complications from influenza, including pneumonia.[26, 27] A number of reports describe severe influenza pneumonia during pregnancy.[28, 29]

The clinical features of influenza are characteristic in adolescents and young adults.[30] They show an abrupt onset of symptoms including headache, chills, and dry cough, followed by fever, malaise, and myalgias. Then weakness, loss of appetite, and the need for bed rest ensues, with illness lasting up to a week. In contrast, children may have fever alone, or they may show convulsions, vomiting, irritability, and photophobia.[31] In the elderly, the only symptoms may be fever, headache, and cough before pneumonia presents.[31] Radiographically, patchy localized infiltrates or diffuse bilateral infiltrates can occur.[22] Bacterial superimposed infection may be present. Hypoxemia may be profound[32] and may necessitate ventilatory support.[33] Patients surviving severe viral pneumonia may develop pulmonary fibrosis.[33]

Our ability to diagnose influenza is improving. An important feature is the reported occurrence of influenza in a community, usually by surveillance conducted by local or regional public health laboratories. Until the presence of a local outbreak has been documented, the diagnosis of influenza should rest on virologic proof. Once documented, patients presenting with classic features of influenza described above are diagnosed easily. However, influenza A cannot be distinguished from influenza B on clinical grounds, so the physician must know the identity of the viruses that have been recovered by the local authorities. In children and older adults, because of the lack of typical features, diagnosing influenza is more difficult. Virologic or serologic proof is needed, as is early diagnosis if treatment is being considered. One always must be concerned about bacterial superinfection in any patient at high risk (see below) for complications of influenza. Appropriate gram stains and bacterial cultures should guide antibacterial therapy.

Identifying influenza by culture requires an appropriate specimen. Throat swabs, nasal washings or aspirates, and, in cases with pneumonia, either sputum or secretions collected at endoscopy are used. Virus is grown in the allantoic fluid of embryonated eggs or in cell culture. Such cultures require 3 to 4 days and are useful for surveillance. Techniques for rapid diagnosis now exist.

The immunofluorescence of nasopharyngeal cells for influenza virus when first developed gave inconsistent results. Improved results came with monoclonal antisera for use in immunofluorescence, which showed 69% sensitivity and 86% accuracy.[34] Monoclonal antibodies also have been used to confirm cell culture at 48 hours of growth,[35] as well as to detect isotype-specific antibodies to influenza in sera.[36] An immunoperoxidase technique using monoclonal antibodies compared favorably with a time-resolved fluoroimmunoassay in cell culture at 48 hours.[37] Using a 24-hour fluorescence focus assay, chamber slides and shell vials showed comparably good responses, with 75% to 84% sensitivity and 96% to 100% specificity.[38] A fluorometric assay for viral neuraminidase at 24 hours showed 92% sensitivity and 96% specificity.[39] Detecting IgM class anti-influenza antibody by hemadsorption immunoadsorbent assay was 36% positive in patients at first physician contact, suggesting its usefulness as an adjunct to other methods.[40] Centrifugation of cell cultures has been shown to enhance virus isolation with low levels of virus.[41, 42] A limitation of any of the above techniques is that they have not been adopted yet by clinical laboratories.

An enzyme-linked immunosorbent assay (ELISA) using monoclonal secondary antibodies to detect influenza A viral core antigens (matrix and nucleoproteins) showed 50% sensitivity in naturally acquired influenza and 57% sensitivity in experimental infection.[43] The ELISA correlated directly with the titer of live virus in nasal washes. There is a commercially available kit, Directigen Flu A, which also uses the ELISA; however, there are no published data on its efficacy. Based on the published ELISA study,[43] the kit would be more useful in the rapid diagnosis of children since they shed higher titers of virus.

In the near future, rapid diagnostic tests should become more widely available. A new technique, the polymerase chain reaction (PCR), is being applied to rapid diagnosis by detecting viral RNA. For the present, a physician must rely on clinical judgment for the diagnosis of influenza and, when needed, on confirmation by cell culture or seroconversion.

The antiviral drug amantadine has been available since the 1960s for influenza A viruses.[44] Studies of the therapeutic efficacy of amantadine and its derivative, rimantadine, against naturally occurring influenza A showed significantly positive results.[45] Both drugs show efficacy against all influenza A strains, and numerous studies confirm therapeutic efficacy.[46–48] The drugs shorten symptom duration and decrease symptom severity. Amantadine accelerates the resolution of airway dysfunction.[49] A serious limitation of published studies is that neither drug has been studied in high-risk populations such as the elderly or been shown to reduce the incidence of complications such as pneumonia, despite working well in low-risk groups. Amantadine dosage must be adjusted for reduced renal function,[50] whereas the unlicensed drug rimantadine (which is metabolized in the liver) does not require dosage adjustment.[51] The safety profile of both drugs is excellent, with the most common side effects being minor gastrointestinal and central nervous system effects including nervousness, light-headedness, difficulty in concentrating, insomnia, and loss of appetite.[52] Side effects are dose-related and a 100-mg-per-day adult dose greatly diminished the incidence.[53]

A recent study[54] noted the development of rimantadine-resistant influenza A strains in a family study giving drug therapeutically to index cases and prophylactically to other family members. Rimantadine-resistant strains of influenza A were recovered from 8 index patients and 5 treated contacts in 61 drug-treatment families. The drug was ineffective in protecting household members as well. A reasonable conclusion from this study is that the drug should not be used simultaneously in home settings as both treatment and postexposure prophylaxis.

There is no current, well-studied antiviral agent for influenza B. However, ribavirin, a licensed antiviral for respiratory syncytial virus (RSV), is effective in vitro against influenza B.[55] A randomized, controlled trial[56] of aerosolized ribavirin showed efficacy against influenza A, as did a nonrandomized study.[57] A controlled study with 11 treated students showed aerosolized ribavirin to be effective against influenza B; however, treatment required up to 17 hr/day to deliver the dosage of drug. There are additional case reports of aerosolized ribavirin[58, 59] and a report of intravenous use in influenza myocarditis.[60]

Both influenzas A and B are preventable with the use of current inactivated whole- or split-virus vaccines.[61] High-risk groups who should receive vaccine annually include those 65 years or older; those with chronic cardiac or pulmonary disorders, including children with asthma; residents of nursing homes and other chronic care facilities; adults and children with chronic diseases (e.g., diabetes, renal dysfunction, immunosuppression); and children (up to 19 years) on long-term aspirin therapy and at risk for Reye's syndrome.

Live virus vaccines hold the promise of efficacy and the convenience of avoiding injections, making them feasible for use in schoolchildren, who are major spreaders of influenza.[62] Amantadine is an adjunct to vaccines for prophylaxis, and a replacement if a patient is allergic to eggs and cannot be immunized. Amantadine has been of use in prophylactically controlling influenza in nursing homes,[63] and rimatadine also has been safe and effective in this setting.[64]

RESPIRATORY SYNCYTIAL VIRUS

Since recognition in the 1950s,[65, 66] RSV has been shown to be the most important respiratory pathogen for infants and children. Although RSV long was considered to be a single broad serotype, it now is proved to have two subgroups, A and B.[67] These may circulate concurrently.[68] Subgroup A has proven to be the dominant clinical subgroup,[69] while B is associated with fewer bronchiolitis illnesses.[70]

RSV was the predominant cause of pneumonia in infants and caused sharp epidemics in winter and spring.[2] Epidemics last an average of 5 months.[4] In a recent study, RSV caused 65% of bronchiolitis and 24% of croup.[3] It was the most common infectious agent in hospitalized children, with 17% being culture-positive.[5] RSV also is a cause of respiratory illness in 20% of adults,[6] including patients with COPD[9] and asthma,[10] and the elderly (see later).

RSV is transmitted best by direct contact and fomites, with little spread by aerosol.[71] It infects respiratory epithelial cells, causing inclusions, cell membrane fusion between cells (forming syncytia), and necrosis of bronchial epithelium.[72] First infections are more severe and have higher attacks rates (98%) than second (75%) and third infections (65%).[73] Reinfection is related inversely to the level of neutralizing antibody.[74] Prolonged virus shedding in immunocompromised children suggests a role for cell-mediated immunity in eradicating the virus.[75]

The clinical features of RSV are those of croup, bronchitis, bronchiolitis, and pneumonia in children up to 5 years of age. Radiographic lung findings may be normal, or they may include overinflation, subsegmental atelectasis, peribronchial cuffing, or alveolar consolidation.[76] With bronchiolitis and pneumonia, hypoxemia may be present and persist for weeks.[77] Children with congenital heart disease or immunocompromised status[78] are prone to severe RSV illness, but fatal pneumonia also has been reported in a normal child.[79]

Nosocomial RSV infections have been a problem for infants,[80] with fomites playing a major role.[81] Glove and gown precautions may reduce nosocomial spread,[82] although cohorting at admission may be more useful.[83]

RSV can cause lower respiratory illness in the elderly,[84, 85] in healthy adults,[86-88] and in immunocompromised adults.[89, 90] In the latter group, case fatality rates can be high, and nosocomial spread has been demonstrated.[91]

Laboratory diagnosis of RSV now includes cell culture, serology, and rapid antigen detection. For any virus identification, the specimen must be adequate, and nasal washes are superior to throat or nasopharyngeal swabs,[92, 93] probably because of the yield of cells. In cell culture, the use of several cell types in combination maximized virus recovery.[94] Monoclonal antibodies are available for confirmation of cell cultures.[95]

Rapid diagnosis of RSV has come of age using direct fluorescent antibodies, enzyme immunoassay, or centrifugation culture with shell vials.[96] Enzyme immunoassay, while having 86% sensitivity and 91% to 95% specificity, has false-positive results up to 16% of the time,[97, 98] but it is also more simple than fluorescent antibodies.[99] In general, a combination of rapid diagnostic techniques with cell culture for a back-up seems appropriate.[96] At present, there are a variety of commercially available antigen detection kits.[100] Serology for RSV has improved greatly, with ELISA adding greater sensitivity and simplicity than traditional complement fixation or plaque reduction.[101]

Chemotherapy for RSV became available with U.S. Food and Drug Administration approval of ribavirin in aerosolized form for treating hospitalized children who do not require assisted ventilation. After in vitro studies showed efficacy, ribavirin, a synthetic nucleoside, was shown to be effective as an aerosol in an animal model.[102] Two randomized, double-blind studies in infants with RSV lower respiratory disease,[103, 104] and another in young adult volunteers[105] each showed decreased viral shedding and illness severity scores in ribavirin aerosol–treated groups, without any toxicity. Ribavirin also was effective in infants with underlying cardiopulmonary disease.

The American Academy of Pediatrics has made recommendations on the use of aerosolized ribavirin, emphasizing treatment for high-risk infants, those who are severely ill, or those with lower respiratory tract disease at risk for a complicated course.[107] Some have been critical of the lack of data on efficacy in children, and have suggested additional controlled studies.[108] Another concern is the safety of incidental exposure to aerosolized drug for health care personnel. Although absorption by these personnel has been low or absent,[109] risk should be made known to such persons. There are reports of ribavirin aerosol for treating adults with severe RSV pneumonia.[90, 110] In addition, techniques for the use of ribavirin aerosol in infants on ventilators are published now.[111]

The prevention of RSV with killed vaccines proved ineffective and disease was enhanced in vaccinees.[112] Live Ts mutant RSV vaccine showed no efficacy.[113] Live attenuated virus vaccine given parenterally induced low antibody levels, but showed no efficacy.[114] Future directions for vaccine could include subunit synthetic vaccines or live vaccines given topically.

PARAINFLUENZA VIRUSES

Like RSV, the parainfluenza viruses are important causes of lower respiratory tract disease. They were identified first in the 1950s from children with croup.[115] There are four antigenic types numbered 1 through 4, each known to cause upper or lower respiratory tract disease. Parainfluenza viruses caused 22% of respiratory tract illness with physician consultation.[1] They were second to RSV as a cause of pneumonia and bronchiolitis in infants, and were the leading cause of croup.[2] Parainfluenza type 3 disease occurs year-round, while other types show a seasonal pattern in the fall, winter, or spring. A recent study in children under 1 year of age found parainfluenza viruses to cause 45% of croup, 33% of pneumonia, and 14% of bronchiolitis.[3] In adults, parainfluenza viruses are associated with exacerbations of COPD,[9] wheezing episodes in asthmatics,[10] and pneumonia in Marine Corps recruits.[116]

Little has been documented on the mechanism of spread of parainfluenza viruses, but the respiratory route or via the hands seems likely. In one general practice, all age groups were infected, including the elderly.[117] Reinfections in children have been well documented.[118] The second illness was milder, and protection against reinfection was related to the level of serum-neutralizing antibody. Secretory IgA may be a more reliable indication of resistance to reinfection.[119] In a long-term study of patients with chronic bronchitis and emphysema, an epidemic of parainfluenza type 3 occurred with 8 of 29 infected patients demonstrating persistent infection up to 5 months.[120] This occurred despite the presence of local IgA. Persistent infection also was demonstrated in healthy young adults residing in social isolation at an Antarctic station.[121, 122]

Parainfluenza type 3 caused an epidemic in renal transplant recipients who experienced mild upper respiratory tract infection.[123] There was an increased frequency of acute rejection episodes in those infected compared with uninfected controls, although patient and graft survival at 6 months were not different in either group. Giant cell pneumonia caused by parainfluenza type 3 was documented serologically in a leukemic child, who survived the illness.[124]

The clinical diagnosis of parainfluenza infection is similar to that of RSV.[76] Croup, tracheobronchitis, bronchiolitis, and pneumonia each can occur.Wheezing is more common with parainfluenza type 3. It is necessary to recover the virus in cell culture or to show a serologic response to confirm the etiology.

Prevention of parainfluenza viruses with vaccines is in the developmental stage.[125, 126] At the present time, treatment is supportive, and infants should be observed closely for signs of respiratory failure that would necessitate ventilatory support.

ADENOVIRUSES

Since their initial isolation from adenoids and tonsils of children[127] and subsequent recovery from military recruits with respiratory illnesses,[128] there have been 42 different adenovirus serotypes found in humans. Primarily regarded as respiratory agents, adenoviruses cause a wide range of systemic disorders ranging from rashes to gastroenteritis. They were recovered from 3.9% of illnesses with physician consultation.[1] Another study found adenoviruses to be responsible for 2.8%

of pneumonia in children, most being types 1 and 2, while type 3 was common in croup.[2] A recent study found adenoviruses in 9% of croup cases in infants and in 2% of bronchiolitis.[3] Adenoviruses cause similar infection rates in urban and rural children.[5] Of the adenoviruses recovered in a community study, one third were from lower respiratory illnesses and two thirds were from the upper tract.[6] Although adenoviruses were recovered from adults with COPD, they were not associated significantly with illness.[9]

Adenovirus types 1, 2, and 5 cause endemic respiratory disease, but were found as latent infectious agents in up to 90% of tonsils removed at surgery,[129] with nearly half of all infections being without symptoms. Types 1, 2, 3, 5, and 7 accounted for 95% of all symptomatic illness.[130]

Adenoviral pneumonia in children usually will present with fever, coryza, tachypnea, and increasing cough. There also may be sore throat, conjunctivitis, and abdominal pain, with severe cases showing meningitis, hepatitis, myocarditis, and other extrapulmonic features.[131] Radiographic features are not specific. Lung pathology may show intranuclear inclusions and hyaline membranes.[132] Long-term complications include fibrosis.[133]

In military recruits, adenoviral pneumonia commonly presented with pharyngitis, rales and rhonchi, and rhinitis with fever. Cough was ubiquitous.[134] The pneumonia could be fatal.[135] In children with type 7 pneumonia, extrapulmonary features included coma.[136] Fatal adenoviral pneumonia was reported in a 60-year-old woman whose autopsy showed interstitial fibrosis and bronchiolitis obliterans.[137]

Adenoviruses can cause an overwhelming illness with high fatality in immunocompromised patients,[138] and also has been fatal in patients undergoing bone marrow transplantation.[129] The presence of severe graft vs. host disease was a significant risk factor for infection, although a source of virus was not identified.

The diagnosis of adenoviruses requires recovery of the virus in cell culture using specimens including nasopharynx, conjunctiva, or stool. At present, immune electron microscopy, counterimmunoelectrophoresis, radioimmunoassay, and ELISA are available for diagnosis.[140] DNA probes and monoclonal antibodies are used also, as is in situ detection of nucleic acid sequences of rapid diagnosis.[141]

There is no specific treatment for adenoviral infection. Nosocomial outbreaks have been reported,[142] and infection control measures should be started when an index case is identified.[143]

Prevention of adenoviral disease with vaccines has been highly successful in the military. Both live and inactivated vaccines given orally and parenterally to naval recruits were followed with no reactions and with the reduction of acute respiratory disease by about half.[144, 145] Large field trials continued to show benefit, and vaccine serotypes were not replaced by other serotypes in the vaccinees.[146] Cost-benefit analysis of the immunization also was highly favorable.[147] The use of live oral vaccines in civilians (including children), although it probably would be effective, has not been undertaken.

RHINOVIRUSES

With over 100 serotypes thus far identified that infect humans, it is no surprise that rhinoviruses cause a heavy disease burden. Although there is some seasonal variation, rhinoviruses cause respiratory disease throughout the year.[148] In a family study, rhinoviruses caused 11.9% of all reported respiratory illnesses.[149] Rhinovirus colds usually are mild, though they tend to be prolonged.[150] During a study of an isolated group of adults in the Antarctic, rhinovirus colds did not spread easily.[151] Transmission of rhinoviruses may occur via hands and self-inoculation;[152] hand-to-hand transmission between adults has been shown experimentally.[153] The virus survives on environmental surfaces and can be picked up by the fingers and infect the individual by autoinoculation.[154] Aerosol transmission also can occur.[155]

The common cold syndrome from rhinoviruses is experienced universally. Studies of lower airway function during rhinovirus infection showed that smokers experienced pulmonary function changes where nonsmokers did not.[156] These changes were reversible. Others have shown increased frequency dependence of compliance during rhinovirus infection of normal volunteers,[157] as well as changes in leukocyte functions.[158] Persons with chronic bronchitis were more susceptible to rhinovirus challenge than were nonbronchitic controls.[159] In hospitalized infants and children, a study showed evidence for cough, fever, respiratory distress, and focal radiologic changes on chest x-ray in association with rhinoviruses.[160] Rhinoviruses also are associated with acute otitis media.[161] Experimental challenge studies with rhinovirus in asthmatics showed no significant changes,[162] while a more recent study has demonstrated late-occurring asthmatic reactions (a 15% decrease in forced expiratory volume of the first second occurring 6 hours after challenge).[163] How rhinoviruses produce their symptoms is now known; however, inflammatory mediators and possibly kinins may play a role.[164]

Many studies have looked at means for treating or preventing rhinovirus colds. The use of aspirin for treatment has been shown to increase virus shedding to a highly significant degree,[165] while others have shown that aspirin or acetaminophen prolonged shedding and reduced the antibody response as well.[166] Atropine nasal spray produced nasal dryness and systemic side effects that offset any therapeutic benefit.[167] Antihistamine sprays showed no significant effects on nasal symptoms or mucus production.[168] Intranasal interferon-α2 as treatment led to decreased quantity and duration of viral shedding, but the effects were judged to be only modest at best.[169] Others used interferon-α2 as a preventative and showed protection that was significant,[170, 171] but the irritation of prolonged use, manifest as nasal mucosal bleeding, offset the value.[171] Interferon-β serine, a less toxic interferon, showed no prophylactic benefit.[172] Virucidal paper handkerchiefs or tissues for prophylaxis against rhinovirus colds have shown mixed results, with at best a modest reduction in incidence.[173, 174]

With the elucidation of the structure of rhinovirus type 14 using x-ray crystallography has come an appreciation for the viral immunogenic regions and receptor binding sites.[175] This opened possibilities for antiviral compounds tailored for attachment sites,[176] as well as for site-specific antibodies.[177] In addition, there are now highly sensitive molecular DNA probes for viral detection.[178] Animal studies show monoclonal antibodies that block receptor sites and thereby modify infection.[179] The future for rhinovirus control looks bright.

CORONAVIRUSES

Unrelated to other respiratory viruses, the coronaviruses are responsible for up to 15% of acute upper respiratory tract illnesses in children,[180] although they involve all age groups as well.[181] In a study of insurance company employees, 4% of all colds and 8% of winter and spring colds were related serologically to coronaviruses 229E and OC43, with reinfections occurring commonly.[182] These agents can cause pneumonia in infants[183] or military recruits,[184] and exacerbations of chronic bronchitis,[185] and may cause neurologic or cardiac diseases as well.[186] Using an ELISA for detecting antibody rises, these agents were found to cause disease throughout the year.[187] There are no human coronavirus vaccines to date; however, volunteers given prophylactic intranasal interferon-α2b had shorter illness duration and reduced severity of colds after challenge with coronavirus 229E.[188]

NONRESPIRATORY VIRUSES

Thus far, discussion has been about primary viral agents of the respiratory tract. Other viral agents also can cause minor to severe respiratory disease. The herpesvirus group (herpes simplex [HSV], varicella-zoster [VZV], cytomegalovirus [CMV]) is the most important nonrespiratory group of viruses affecting the respiratory tract.

Varicella-Zoster Virus

The first report of pneumonia as a manifestation of chickenpox came in 1942.[189] A subsequent report noted that varicella pneumonia was not rare, describing adults 19 to 71 years of age whose rash was followed in 2 to 5 days by severe respiratory distress associated with cough, chest pain, dyspnea, and tachypnea, as well as cyanosis and hemoptysis.[190] The clinical course was variable, but could be fatal.[190]

Intranuclear inclusion bodies were described in sputum cells.[191] A prominent radiographic feature was extensive, bilateral, nodular consolidation that became calcified nodules.[192] VZV has been cultured from the lungs.[193] Pulmonary infarction may accompany varicella pneumonia as a complication.[194] Immunocompromised children are at risk for VZV pneumonia.[195, 196] Population-based studies suggest that pneumonia occurs in children under 5 years of age and in persons 15 years and older with primary infections.[197] Varicella complicating pregnancy increases the risk of pneumonia for the mother, with mortality reaching 45%.[198, 199] A small series of normal adults with varicella pneumonia were treated successfully with the intravenous nucleoside antiviral drug, acyclovir.[200] In summary, varicella pneumonia is more common in adults with primary infection, in immunocompromised patients at any age, and in pregnancy. The rash of VZV is very characteristic, and respiratory symptoms should suggest pneumonia. Viral cultures and chest film can confirm the diagnosis. Intravenous acyclovir may be considered for therapy.

Herpes Simplex Viruses (Types 1 and 2)

HSVs are an infrequent cause of lower respiratory tract disease in humans. In a study of over 400 adult volunteers given challenges with live respiratory viruses, HSV was recovered from respiratory secretions in 5% and there was no relationship to the occurrence of illness.[201] HSVs have been recovered from the lungs of adults with burns,[202] renal failure,[203] cancer,[204] and organ transplantation.[205] A review of 20 cases of HSV pneumonia showed that skin or mucous membrane lesions preceded the onset in 17.[206] Pneumonia was diffuse or focal, resulting from viral hematogenous or contiguous spread, respectively, based upon viral typing and strain determination using restriction endonuclease analysis. HSV was found in the respiratory secretions of 30% of consecutive patients with adult respiratory distress syndrome.[207] The same authors later used acyclovir as prophylaxis for HSV in similar patients, but it did not improve the outcome.[203] Neonatal HSV pneumonia presents as respiratory distress, with the chest radiograph showing prominent hila and central interstitial infiltration.[208] Fatal cases in childhood have been reported.[209] Herpetic tracheobronchitis has been described, with findings of exudative, necrotizing disease by bronchoscopy in a group of elderly patients. Cytology, histopathology, and viral cultures all supported the viral diagnosis, and therapy with acyclovir was deemed beneficial.[210] Criteria for HSV of the lower respiratory tract have been suggested and include cytologic or histologic findings followed by viral confirmation.[211] In summary, HSV infrequently causes lower respiratory disease in neonates, and does so in selected older age groups usually with underlying diseases. Cytologic or virologic proof is needed for accurate diagnosis. Acyclovir may be considered for treatment because of the efficacy of the antiviral drug for actively replicating HSV.

Cytomegalovirus

CMV is a viral agent that causes primary pneumonia (in the absence of involvement of other organs) or pneumonia as part of disseminated infection.[212] Interstitial CMV pneumonia is seen with congenital CMV infection in neonates.[213] CMV caused less than 1% of community-acquired pneumonia in a study of 443 cases.[214] Usually, with reactivation of latent infection, CMV causes opportunistic pneumonia in patients with acquired immunodeficiency syndrome[215] and other immunocompromised states.[216, 217] CMV pneumonia may be asymptomatic and detected only by chest x-ray, or symptomatic, in which case the onset is insidious.[212] Chest films show bilateral, diffuse reticular or nodular patterns.[218] The natural course varies from being self-limited with full recovery to progressive with death. Diagnosis requires clinical suspicion, viral confirmation, and lung histopathology. Trials using the antiviral drug DHPG showed viral elimination but low survival.[219, 220] Ganciclovir also has been used to treat CMV pneumonia, showing both antiviral effect and some clinical benefit.[221] Prophylactic intravenous hyperimmune globulin has been shown to reduce the severity of CMV disease,[222] as has prophylaxis with acyclovir.[223] In summary, CMV pneumonia has become more common with the increasing immunocompromised population. Open lung biopsy is the current standard procedure for diagnosis. Although the antivirals DHPG and ganciclovir are used for treating CMV pneumonia, prophylaxis with hyperimmune globulin or acyclovir may be more effective in reducing disease.

Measles Virus

Although measles typically is recognized for its morbilliform rash, measles virus can cause giant cell pneumonia with or without accompanying rash.[224] Measles pneumonia also may follow apparent recovery from measles.[225] Of children hospitalized with measles, up to 50% may have clinical or radiologic evidence for pneumonia.[226, 227] Measles also predisposes to bacterial suprainfection from a variety of bacterial types,[228] although the proportion of bacterial or viral causes is unknown.[229] Underlying cardiac or pulmonary disorders[228, 230] and malignancies or immunodeficiencies predispose children and adults to fatal pneumonia during measles. Pulmonary infiltrates can develop in persons who received killed measles vaccine in the 1960s and later were exposed to natural measles, developing the atypical measles syndrome.[232, 233] Pulmonary function in these patients revealed hypoxemia and decreased lung volumes, with gradual resolution over 12 weeks.[234] Measles is diagnosed by recognizing the rash, and is confirmed by virus culture, antigen detection in the nasopharyngeal secretions, or detection of specific IgM class antibodies. There is no antiviral therapy, but bacterial suprainfections should be treated with appropriate antibiotics.

REFERENCES

1. Monto AS, Ullman BM: Acute respiratory illness in an American community. The Tecumseh study. *JAMA* 1974; 227:164–169.

2. Foy HM, Coony MK, Maletzky AJ, et al: Incidence and etiology of pneumonia, croup, and bronchiolitis in preschool children belonging to a prepaid medical care group over a four-year period. *Am J Epidemiol* 1973; 97:80–92.

3. Wright AL, Taussig LM, Ray CG, et al: The Tucson children's respiratory study. II. Lower respiratory tract illness in the first year of life. *Am J Epidemiol* 1989; 129:1232–1246.

4. Kim HW, Arrobio JO, Brandt CD, et al: Epidemiology of respiratory syncytial virus infection in Washington, DC. *Am J Epidemiol* 1973; 98:216–225.

5. Belshe RB, VanVoris LP, Mufson MA: Impact of viral respiratory disease on infants and young children in a rural and urban area of southern West Virginia. *Am J Epidemiol* 1983; 117:467–474.

6. Monto AS, Cavallaro JJ: The Tecumseh study of respiratory illness. *Am J Epidemiol* 1971; 94:280–289.

7. Mufson MA, Webb PA, Kennedy H, et al: Etiology of upper-respiratory-tract illnesses among civilian adults. *JAMA* 1966; 195:1–7.

8. Meiklejohn G: Viral respiratory disease at Lowry Air Force Base in Denver, 1952–1982. *J Infect Dis* 1983; 148:775–784.

9. Smith CB, Golden CA, Kanner RE, et al: Association of viral and *Mycoplasma pneumoniae* infections with acute respiratory illness in patients with chronic obstructive pulmonary disease. *Am Rev Respir Dis* 1980; 121:225–232.

10. Hudgel DW, Langston L, Selner JC, et al: Viral and bacterial infections in adults with chronic asthma. *Am Rev Respir Dis* 1979; 120:393–397.

11. Palese P, Young JF: Variation of influenza A, B and C viruses. *Science* 1982; 21:1468–1474.

12. Webster RG, Laver WG, Air GM, et al: Molecular mechanisms of variation in influenza viruses. *Nature* 1982; 296:115–121.

13. Kawaoka Y, Krauss S, Webster RG: Avian-to-human transmission of the PB1 gene of influenza A viruses in the 1957 and 1968 pandemics. *J Virol* 1989; 63:4603–4608.

14. Barbey-Moral CL, Oeltmann TN, Edwards KM, et al: Role of respiratory tract proteases in infectivity of influenza A virus. *J Infect Dis* 1987; 155:667–672.

15. Walsh JJ, Dietlein LF, Low FN, et al: Bronchotracheal response in human influenza. *Arch intern Med* 1961; 108:98–110.

16. Camner P, Jarstrand C, Philipson K: Tracheobronchial clearance in patients with influenza. *Am Rev Respir Dis* 1973; 108:131–135.

17. Little JW, Hall WJ, Douglas RG, et al: Airway hyperreactivity and peripheral airway dysfunction in influenza A infection. *Am Rev Respir Dis* 1978; 118:295–303.

18. Hall WJ, Douglas RG, Hyde RW, et al: Pulmonary mechanics after uncomplicated influenza A infection. *Am Rev Respir Dis* 1976; 113:141–147.

19. Soto PJ, Brown GO, Wyatt JP: Asian influenzal pneumonitis. *Am J Med* 1959; 27:18–25.

20. Oseasohn R, Adelson L, Kaji M: Clinicopathologic study of thirty-three fatal cases of Asian influenza. *N Engl J Med* 1959; 11:509–518.

21. Frankova V, Jiasek A, Tumova B: Type A influenza: Postmortem virus isolations from different organs in human lethal cases. *Arch Virol* 1977; 53:265–268.

22. Bisno AL, Griffin JP, Van Epps KA, et al: Pneumonia and Hong Kong influenza: A prospective study of the 1968–1969 epidemic. *Am J Med Sci* 1971; 261:251–263.

23. Couch RB: The effects of influenza on host defenses. *J Infect Dis* 1981; 144:284–291.

24. Hobson D, Curry RL, Beare AS, et al: The role of serum hemagglutination-inhibiting antibody in protection against challenge infection with influenza A2 and B viruses. *J Hyg Cambridge* 1972; 70:767–777.

25. Ada GL, Jones PD: The immune response to influenza virus infection, in Kendal A, Patriarca P (eds): *Options for the Control of Influenza*. New York, Alan R Liss Inc, 1986, pp 107–124.

26. Barker WH, Mullooly JP: Impact of epidemic A influenza in a defined adult population. *Am J Epidemiol* 1980; 112:798–811.

27. Goodman RA, Orenstein WA, Munro TF, et al: Impact of influenza A in a nursing home. *JAMA* 1982; 247:1451–1453.

28. Kost BA, Cefalo RC, Baker VV: Fatal influenza pneumonia in pregnancy. *Am J Perinatol* 1986; 3:179–182.

29. McKinney WP, Volkert P, Kaufman J: Fatal swine influenza pneumonia during late pregnancy. *Arch Intern Med* 1990; 150:213–215.

30. Stuart-Harris C, Schild GC: *Influenza*. Littleton, Mass, Publishing Sciences Group, Inc, 1976.

31. Bennett NM: Diagnosis of influenza. *Med J Aust* 1973; 1(suppl):19–22.

32. Noble RL, Lillington GA, Kempson RL: Fatal diffuse influenza pneumonia: Premortem diagnosis by lung biopsy. *Chest* 1973; 63:644–646.

33. Winterbauer RH, Ludwig WR, Hammar SP: Clinical course, management, and long-term sequelae of respiratory failure due to influenza viral pneumonia. *Johns Hopkins Med J* 1977; 141:148–155.

34. Shalit I, McKee PA, Beauchamp H, et al: Comparison of polyclonal antiserum versus monoclonal antibodies for the rapid diagnosis of influenza A virus infections by immunofluorescence in clinical specimens. *J Clin Microbiol* 1985; 22:877–879.

35. Walls HH, Harmon MW, Slagle JJ, et al: Characterization and evaluation of monoclonal antibodies developed for typing influenza A and influenza B viruses. *J Clin Microbiol* 1986; 23:240–245.

36. Harmon MW, Phillips DJ, Reimer CB, et al: Isotype-specific enzyme immunoassay for influenza antibody with monoclonal antibodies to human immunoglobuline. *J Clin Microbiol* 1986; 24:913–916.

37. Waris M, Ziegler T, Kiviverta M, et al: Rapid detection of respiratory syncytial virus and influenza A virus in cell cultures by immunoperoxidase staining with monoclonal antibodies. *J Clin Microbiol* 1990; 28:1159–1162.

38. Stokes CE, Bernstein JM, Kyger SA, et al: Rapid diagnosis of influenza A and B by 24-h fluorescent focus assays. *J Clin Microbiol* 1988; 26:1263–1266.

39. Pachucki CT, Creticos C: Early detection of influenza virus by using a fluorometric assay of infected tissue culture. *J Clin Microbiol* 1988; 26:2664–2666.

40. Vikerfors T, Lindegren G, Grandien M, et al: Diagnosis of influenza A virus infections by detection of specific immunoglobulins M, A, and G in serum. *J Clin Microbiol* 1989; 27:453–458.

41. Seno M, Kanamoto Y, Takav S, et al: Enhancing effect of centrifugation on isolation of influenza virus from clinical specimens. *J Clin Microbiol* 1990; 28:1669–1670.

42. Mills RD, Cain KJ, Woods GL: Detection of influenza virus by centrifugal inoculation of MDCK cells and staining with monoclonal antibodies. *J Clin Microbiol* 1989; 27:2505–2508.

43. Coonrod JD, Karathanasis P, Betts RF, et al: Enzyme-linked immunosorbent assay of core antigens for clinical diagnosis of influenza. *J Med Virol* 1988; 25:399–409.

44. Davies WL, Grunert RR, Haff RR, et al: Antiviral activity of 1-adamantanamine (amantadine). *Science* 1964; 144:862–863.

45. Wingfield WL, Pollock D, Grunert RR: Therapeutic efficacy of amantadine HCL and rimantadine HCL in naturally occurring influenza A2 respiratory illness in man. *N Engl J Med* 1969; 281:579–584.

46. Younkin SW, Betts RF, Roth FK, et al: Reduction in fever and symptoms in young adults with influenza A/Brazil/78 H1N1 infection after treatment with aspirin or amantadine. *Antimicrob Agents Chemother* 1983; 23:577–582.

47. Sears SD, Clements ML: Protective efficacy of low-dose amantadine in adults challenged with wild-type influenza A virus. *Antimicrob Agents Chemother* 1987; 31:1470–1473.

48. Hayden FG, Monto AS: Oral rimantadine hydrochloride therapy of influenza A virus H3N2 subtype infection in adults. *Antimicrob Agents Chemother* 1986; 29:339–341.

49. Little JW, Hall WJ, Douglas RG, et al: Amantadine effect on peripheral airways abnormalities. *Ann Intern Med* 1976; 85:177–182.

50. Aoki FY, Sitar DS: Amantadine kinetics in healthy elderly men: Implications for influenza prevention. *Clin Pharmacol Ther* 1985; 37:137–144.

51. Hayden FG, Minocha A, Spyker DA, et al: Comparative single-dose pharmacokinetics of amantadine hydrochloride in young and elderly adults. *Antimicrob Agents Chemother* 1985; 28:216–221.

52. Douglas RG: Prophylaxis and treatment of influenza. *N Engl J Med* 1990; 322:443–450.

53. Hayden FG, Gwaltney JM, Van de Castel RL, et al: Comparative toxicity of amantadine hydrochloride and rimantadine hydrochloride in healthy adults. *Antimicrob Agents Chemother* 1981; 19:226–233.

54. Hayden FG, Belshe RB, Clover RD, et al: Emergence and apparent transmission of rimantadine resistant influenza virus in families. *N Engl J Med* 1989; 321:1696–1702.

55. Togo Y: In vitro effect of virazole against influenza viruses. *Antimicrob Agents Chemother* 1973; 4:641–642.

56. Wilson SZ, Gilbert BE, Quarles JM, et al: Treatment of influenza A(H1N1) virus infection with ribavirin aerosol. *Antimicrob Agents Chemother* 1984; 26:200–203.

57. McClung HW, Knight V, Gilbert BE, et al: Ribavirus aerosol treatment of influenza B virus infection. *JAMA* 1983; 249:2671–2674.

58. Knight V, McClung HW, Wilson SZ, et al: Ribavirin small-particle aerosol treatment of influenza. *Lancet* 1981; 2:945–949.

59. Kirshon B, Faro S, Zurawin RK, et al: Favorable outcome after treatment with amantadine and ribavirin in a pregnancy complicated by influenza pneumonia. *J Reprod Med* 1988; 33:399–401.

60. Ray CG, Icenogle TB, Minnich LL, et al: The use of intravenous ribavirin to treat influenza virus-associated acute myocarditis. *J Infect Dis* 1989; 159:829–836.

61. Recommendations of the Immunization Practices Advisory Committee: Prevention and control of influenza. *MMWR* 1990; 39:1–15.

62. Ruben FL: Now and future influenza vaccines, in Schaffner W (ed): *Infectious Disease Clinics of North America*. Philadelphia, WB Saunders Co, 1990, pp 1–10.

63. Arden NH, Patriarca PA, Fasano MB, et al: The roles of vaccination and amantadine prophylaxis in controlling an outbreak of influenza A(H3N2) in a nursing home. *Arch Intern Med* 1988; 148:865–868.

64. Patriarca PA, Kater NA, Kendal AP, et al: Safety of prolonged administration of rimantadine hydrochloride in prophylaxis of influenza A virus infections in nursing homes. *Antimicrob Agents Chemother* 1984; 26:101–103.

65. Morris JA, Blount RE, Savage RE: Recovery of a cytopathogenic agent from chimpanzees with coryza. *Proc Soc Exp Biol Med* 1956; 92:544–549.

66. Chanock R, Roizman B, Myers R: Recovery from infants with respiratory illness of a virus related to chimpanzee coryza agent (CCA): I. Isolation, properties and characterization. *Am J Hyg* 1957; 66:281–290.

67. Mufson MA, Orvell C, Rafnar B, et al: Two distinct subtypes of human respiratory syncytial virus. *J Gen Virol* 1985; 66:2111–2124.

68. Hendry RM, Talis AL, Godfrey E, et al: Concurrent circulation of antigenically distinct strains of respiratory syncytial virus during community outbreaks. *J Infect Dis* 1986; 153:291–297.

69. Mufson MA, Belshe RB, Orwell C, et al: Respiratory syncytial virus epidemics: Variable dominance of subgroups A and B strains among children 1981–1986. *J Infect Dis* 1988; 157:143–148.

70. Mufson MA, Akerlind-Stopner B, Orvell C, et al: A single-season epidemic with respiratory syncytial virus subgroup B_2 during 10 epidemic years, 1978 to 1988. *J Clin Microbiol* 1991; 29:162–165.

71. Hall CB, Douglas RG: Modes of transmission of respiratory syncytial virus. *J Pediatr* 1981; 99:100–103.

72. Aherne W, Bird T, Court SDM, et al: Pathological changes in virus infections of the lower respiratory tract in children. *J Clin Pathol* 1970; 23:7–18.

73. Henderson FW, Collier AM, Clyde WA, et al: Respiratory syncytial virus infections, reinfections and immunity. *N Engl J Med* 1979; 300:530–534.

74. Glezen WP, Taber LH, Frank AL, et al: Risk of primary infection and reinfection with respiratory syncytial infection. *Am J Dis Child* 1986; 140:543–546.

75. Hall CB, Powell KR, MacDonald NE, et al: Respiratory syncytial viral infection in children with compromised immune function. *N Engl J Med* 1986; 315:77–81.

76. Henderson FW: Pulmonary infections with respiratory syncytial virus and parainfluenza viruses. *Semin Respir Infect* 1987; 2:112–121.

77. Hall CB, Hall WJ, Speers DM: Clinical and physiological manifestations of bronchiolitis and pneumonia. *Am J Dis Child* 1979; 133:798–802.

78. MacDonald NE, Hall CB, Suffin SC, et al: Respiratory syncytial viral infection in infants with congenital heart disease. *N Engl J Med* 1982; 307:397–400.

79. Kurlandsky LE, French G, Webb PM, et al: Fatal respiratory syncytial virus pneumonia in a previously healthy child. *Am Rev Respir Dis* 1988; 138:468–472.

80. Hall CB, Douglas RG, Geiman JM, et al: Nosocomial respiratory syncytial virus infections. *N Engl J Med* 1975; 293:1343–1346.

81. Hall CB, Douglas RG, Geiman JM: Possible transmission by fomites of respiratory syncytial virus. *J Infect Dis* 1980; 141:98–102.

82. Leclair JM, Freeman J, Sullivan BF, et al: Prevention of nosocomial respiratory syncytial virus infections through compliance with glove and gown isolation precautions. *N Engl J Med* 1987; 317:329–334.

83. Krasinski K, LaCouture R, Holzman RS, et al: Screening for respiratory syncytial virus and assignment to a cohort at admission to reduce nosocomial transmission. *J Pediatr* 1990; 116:894–898.

84. Fransen H, Sterner G, Forsgren M, et al: Acute lower respiratory illness in elderly patients with respiratory syncytial virus infection. *Acta Medica Scand* 1967; 182:323–330.

85. Garvie DG, Gray J: Outbreak of respiratory syncytial virus infection in the elderly. *BMJ* 1980; 281:1253–1254.

86. Hall WJ, Hall CB, Speers DM: Respiratory syncytial virus infection in adults. Clinical, viral, and serial pulmonary function studies. *Ann Intern Med* 1978; 88:203–205.

87. Vikerfors T, Grandien M, Olcen P: Respiratory syncytial virus infections in adults. *Am Rev Respir Dis* 1987; 136:561–564.

88. Zaroukian MH, Kashyap GH, Wentworth BB: Case report: Respiratory syncytial virus infection: A cause of respiratory distress syndrome and pneumonia in adults. *Am J Med Sci* 1988; 295:218–222.

89. Kasupski GJ, Leers WD: Case report: Presumed respiratory syncytial pneumonia in three immunocompromised adults. *Am J Med Sci* 1983; 285:28–33.

90. England JA, Sullivan CJ, Jordan C, et al: Respiratory syncytial virus infection in immunocompromised adults. *Ann Intern Med* 1988; 109:203–208.

91. Englund JA, Anderson LJ, Rhame FS: Nosocomial transmission of respiratory syncytial virus in immunocompromised adults. *J Clin Microbiol* 1991; 29:115–119.

92. Treuhaft MW, Soukup JM, Sullivan BJ: Practical recommendations for the detection of pediatric respiratory syncytial virus infections. *J Clin Microbiol* 1985; 22:270–273.

93. Ahluwalia G, Embree J, McNicol P, et al: Comparison of nasopharyngeal aspirate and nasopharyngeal swab specimens for respiratory syncytial virus diagnosis by cell culture, indirect immunofluorescence assay, and enzyme-linked immunosorbent assay. *J Clin Microbiol* 1987; 25:763–767.

94. Arens MQ, Swierkosz EM, Schmidt RR, et al: Enhanced isolation of respiratory syncytial virus in cell culture. *J Clin Microbiol* 1986; 23:800–802.

95. Stout C, Murphy MD, Lawrence S, et al: Evaluation of a monoclonal antibody pool for rapid diagnosis of respiratory syncytial viral infections. *J Clin Microbiol* 1989; 27:448–452.

96. Johnston SLG, Siegel CS: Evaluation of direct immunofluorescence, enzyme immunoassay, centrifugation culture, and conventional culture for the detection of respiratory syncytial virus. *J Clin Microbiol* 1990; 28:2394–2397.

97. Swenson PD, Kaplan MH: Rapid detection of respiratory syncytial virus in nasopharyngeal aspirates by a commercial enzyme immunoassay. *J Clin Microbiol* 1986; 23:485–488.

98. Waner JL, Whitekurst NJ, Todd SJ, et al: Comparison of Directigen RSV with viral isolation and direct immunofluorescence for the identification of respiratory syncytial virus. *J Clin Microbiol* 1990; 28:480–483.

99. Kumar ML, Super DM, Lembo RM, et al: Diagnostic efficacy of two rapid tests for detection of respiratory syncytial virus antigen. *J Clin Microbiol* 1987; 25:873–875.

100. Halstead DC, Todd S, Fritch G: Evaluation of five methods for respiratory syncytial virus detection. *J Clin Microbiol* 1990; 28:1021–1025.

101. Vaur L, Agut H, Garbarg-Chenon A, et al: Simplified enzyme-linked immunoadsorbent assay for specific antibodies to respiratory syncytial virus. *J Clin Microbiol* 1986; 24:596–599.

102. Hruska JF, Morrow PE, Suffin SC, et al: In vivo inhibition of respiratory syncytial virus by ribavirin. *Antimicrob Agents Chemother* 1982; 21:125–130.

103. Hall CB, McBride JT, Walsh EE, et al: Aerosolized ribavirin treatment of infants with respiratory syncytial viral infection. *N Engl J Med* 1983; 308:1443–1447.

104. Taber LH, Knight V, Gilbert BE, et al: Ribavirin aerosol treatment of bronchiolitis associated with respiratory syncytial virus infection in infants. *Pediatrics* 1983; 72:613–618.

105. Hall CB, Walsh EE, Hruska JF, et al: Ribavirin treatment of experimental respiratory syncytial viral infection. *JAMA* 1983; 249:2666–2670.

106. Hall CB, McBride JT, Galla CL, et al: Ribavirin treatment of respiratory syncytial viral infection in infants with underlying cardiopulmonary disease. *JAMA* 1985; 254:3047–3051.

107. Committee on Infectious Diseases: Ribavirin therapy of respiratory syncytial virus. *Pediatrics* 1987; 79:475–478.

108. Wald ER, Dashefsky B, Green M: In re ribavirin: A case of premature adjudication? *J Pediatr* 1988; 112:154–158.

109. Harrison R, Bellows J, Rempel D, et al: Assessing exposures of health-care personnel to aerosols of ribavirin—California. *MMWR* 1988; 37:560–563.

110. Sinnott JT, Cullison P, Sweeney MS, et al: Respiratory syncytial virus pneumonia in a cardiac transplant recipient. *J Infect Dis* 1988; 158:650–651.

111. Frankel LR, Wilson CW, Demers RR, et al: A technique for administration of ribavirin to mechanically ventilated infants with severe respiratory syncytial virus infection. *Crit Care Med* 1987; 15:1051.

112. Parrott RH, Kim HW, Arrobio JO, et al: Respiratory syncytial and parainfluenza virus vaccines: Experiences with inactivated respiratory syncytial and parainfluenza virus vaccines in man. *Pan Am Health Org Sci Pub* 1967; 147:35–41.

113. Wright PF, Shinozaki T, Fleet W, et al: Evaluation of a live, attenuated respiratory syncytial virus vaccine in infants. *J Pediatr* 1976; 88:931–936.

114. Belshe RB, VanVoris LP, Mufson MA: Parenterally administered live respiratory syncytial virus vaccine: Results of a field trial. *J Infect Dis* 1982; 145:311–319.

115. Chanock RM: Association of a new type of cytopathogenic myxovirus with infantile croup. *J Exp Med* 1956; 104:555–576.

116. Wenzel RP, McCormick DP, Beam WE: Parainfluenza pneumonia in adults. *JAMA* 1972; 221:294–295.

117. Hope-Simpson RE: Parainfluenza virus infections in the Cirencester survey: Seasonal and other characteristics. *J Hyg Cambridge* 1981; 87:393–406.

118. Glezen WP, Frank AL, Taber LH, et al: Parainfluenza virus type 3: Seasonality and risk of infection and reinfection in young children. *J Infect Dis* 1984; 150:851–857.

119. Tremonti LP, Lin J, Jackson GG: Neutralizing activity in nasal secretions and serum in resistance of volunteers to parainfluenza virus type 2. *J Immunol* 1968; 101:572–577.

120. Gross PA, Green RH, McCrea-Curnen MG: Persistent infection with parainfluenza type 3 virus in man. *Am Rev Respir Dis* 1973; 108:894–898.

121. Parkinson AJ, Muchmore HG, Kalmakoff J, et al: Parainfluenza virus upper respiratory tract illnesses in partially immune adult human subjects: A study at an Antarctic station. *Am J Epidemiol* 1979; 110:753–763.

122. Muchmore HG, Parkinson AJ, Humphries JE, et al: Persistent parainfluenza virus shedding during isolation at the South Pole. *Nature* 1981; 289:187–189.

123. DeFabritus AM, Riggio RR, David DS, et al: Parainfluenza type 3 in a transplant unit. *JAMA* 1979; 241:384–386.

124. Weintrub PS, Sullender WM, Lombard C, et al: Giant cell pneumonia caused by parainfluenza type 3 in a patient with acute myelomonocytic leukemia. *Arch Pathol Lab Med* 1987; 111:569–570.

125. VanWyke-Coelingh KL, Winter CC, Tierney EL, et al: Attenuation of bovine parainfluenza virus type 3 in nonhuman primates and its ability to confer immunity to human parainfluenza virus type 3 challenge. *J Infect Dis* 1988; 157:655–662.

126. Belshe RB, Hissom RK: Cold adaptation of parainfluenza virus type 3: Induction of three phenotypic markers. *J Med Virol* 1982; 10:235–242.

127. Rowe WP, Huebner RJ, Gilman LK, et al: Isolation of a cytopathogenic agent from human adenoids undergoing spontaneous degeneration in tissue culture. *Proc Soc Exp Biol Med* 1953; 84:570–573.

128. Hilleman MR, Werner JH: Recovery of a new agent from patients with acute respiratory illness. *Proc Soc Exp Biol Med* 1954; 85:183–188.

129. Bell JA, Rowe WP, Rosen L: Adenoviruses. *Am J Public Health* 1962; 52:902–907.

130. Assad F, Cockburn WC: A seven-year study of WHO virus laboratory report on respiratory viruses. *Bull World Health Organ* 1974; 51:437–445.

131. Zahradnik JM: Adenovirus pneumonia. *Semin Respir Infect* 1987; 2:104–111.

132. Becroft DMO: Histopathology of fatal adenovirus infection of the respiratory tract in young children. *J Clin Pathol* 1967; 20:561–569.

133. Simila S, Linna O, Lanning P, et al: Chronic lung damage caused by adenovirus type 7: A ten-year follow-up study. *Chest* 1981; 80:127–131.

134. Bryant RE, Rhoades ER: Clinical features of adenoviral pneumonia in Air Force recruits. *Am Rev Respir Dis* 1967; 96:717–723.

135. Dudding BA, Wagner SC, Zeller JA, et al: Fatal pneumonia associated with adenovirus type 7 in three military trainees. *N Engl J Med* 1972; 286:1289–1292.

136. Ladisch S, Lovejoy FH, Hierholzer JC, et al: Extrapulmonary manifestations of adenovirus type 7 pneumonia simulating Reye syndrome and the possible role of an adenovirus toxin. *J Pediatr* 1979; 95:348–355.

137. Case records of Massachusetts General Hospital: Case 6-1979. *N Engl J Med* 1979; 300:301–309.

138. Zahradnik JM, Spencer MJ, Porter DD: Adenovirus infection in the immunocompromised patient. *Am J Med* 1980; 68:725–732.

139. Shields AF, Hackman RC, Fife KH, et al: Adenovirus infections in patients undergoing bone marrow transplantation. *N Engl J Med* 1985; 312:529–533.

140. Liu C: Adenoviruses, in Belshe RB (ed): *Textbook of Human Virology.* St Louis, Mosby-Year Book, Inc, 1991, p 798.

141. Neumann R, Benersch E, Eggers HJ: Detection of adenovirus nucleic acid sequences in human tonsils in the absence of infectious virus. *Virus Res* 1987; 7:93–97.

142. Brummitt CF, Cherington JM, Katzenstein DA, et al: Nosocomial adenovirus infections: Molecular epidemiology of an outbreak due to adenovirus 3a. *J Infect Dis* 1988; 158:423–432.

143. Anderson DJ, Jordan MC: Viral pneumonia in recipients of solid organ transplants. *Semin Respir Infect* 1990; 5:38–49.

144. Pierce WE, Rosenbaum MJ, Edwards EA, et al: Live and inactivated adenovirus vaccines for the prevention of acute respiratory illness in naval recruits. *Am J Epidemiol* 1968; 87:237–246.

145. Griffin JP, Greenberg BH: Live and inactivated adenovirus vaccines. *Arch Intern Med* 1970; 125:981–986.

146. Rosenbaum MJ, Edwards EA, Hoeffler DF, et al: Recent experiences with live adenovirus vaccines in Navy recruits. *Milit Med* 1975; 140:251–257.

147. Collis PB, Dudding BA, Winter PE, et al: Adenovirus vaccines in military recruit populations: A cost-budget analysis. *J Infect Dis* 1973; 128:745–752.

148. Roebuck MO: Rhinovirus in Britain 1963–1973. *J Hyg Cambridge* 1976; 76:137–146.

149. Fox JP, Cooney MK, Hall CE, et al: Rhinoviruses in Seattle families, 1975–1979. *Am J Epidemiol* 1985; 122:830–846.

150. Monto AS, Bryan ER, Ohmit S: Rhinovirus infections in Tecumseh, Michigan: Frequency of illness and number of serotypes. *J Infect Dis* 1987; 156:43–49.

151. Warshauer DM, Dick EC, Mandel AD, et al: Rhinovirus infections in an isolated Antarctic station. *Am J Epidemiol* 1989; 129:319–340.

152. Hendley JO, Wenzel RP, Gwaltney JM: Transmission of rhinovirus colds by self-inoculation. *N Engl J Med* 1973; 288:1361–1364.

153. Gwaltney JM, Moskalski PB, Hendley JO: Hand-to-hand transmission of rhinovirus colds. *Ann Intern Med* 1978; 88:463–467.

154. Gwaltney JM, Hendley JO: Transmission of experimental rhinovirus infection by contaminated surfaces. *Am J Epidemiol* 1982; 116:828–833.

155. Dick EC, Jennings LC, Mink KA, et al: Aerosol transmission of rhinovirus colds. *J Infect Dis* 1987; 156:442–448.

156. Friday WW, Ingram RH, Hierholzer JC, et al: Airways function during mild respiratory illness: The effect of rhinovirus infection in cigarette smokers. *Ann Intern Med* 1974; 80:150–155.

157. Blair HT, Greenberg SB, Stevens PM, et al: Effects of rhinovirus infection on pulmonary function of healthy human volunteers. *Am Rev Respir Dis* 1976; 114:95–102.

158. Bush RK, Busse W, Flaherty D, et al: Effects of experimental rhinovirus 16 infection on airways and leukocyte function in normal subjects. *J Allergy Clin Immunol* 1978; 61:80–87.

159. Monto AS, Bryan ER: Susceptibility to rhinovirus infection in chronic bronchitis. *Am Rev Respir Dis* 1978; 118:1101–1103.

160. Krilou L, Pierik L, Keller E, et al: The association of rhinoviruses with lower respiratory tract disease in hospitalized patients. *J Med Virol* 1986; 19:345–352.

161. Arola M, Ziegler T, Ruskanen O, et al: Rhinovirus in acute otitis media. *J Pediatr* 1988; 113:693–695.

162. Halperin SA, Eggleston PA, Beasley P, et al: Exacerbations of asthma in adults during experimental rhinovirus infection. *Am Rev Respir Dis* 1985; 132:976–980.

163. Lemanske RF, Dick EC, Swenson CA, et al: Rhinovirus upper respiratory infection increases airway hyperreactivity and late asthmatic reactions. *J Clin Invest* 1989; 83:1–10.

164. Proud D, Naclerio RM, Gwaltney JM, et al: Kinins are generated in nasal secretions during natural rhinovirus colds. *J Infect Dis* 1990; 161:120–123.

165. Stanley ED, Jackson GG, Panusarn C, et al: Increased virus shedding with aspirin treatment of rhinovirus infection. *JAMA* 1975; 231:1248–1251.

166. Graham NMH, Burrell CJ, Douglas RM, et al: Adverse effects of aspirin, acetaminophen, and ibuprofen on immune function, viral shedding, and clinical status in rhinovirus-infected volunteers. *J Infect Dis* 1990; 162:1277–1282.

167. Gaffey MJ, Gwaltney JM, Dressler WE, et al: Intranasally administered atropine methonitrate treatment of experimental rhinovirus colds. *Am Rev Respir Dis* 1987; 135:241–244.

168. Gaffey MJ, Gwaltney JM, Sastre A, et al: Intranasally and orally administered antihistamine treatment of experiamental rhinovirus colds. *Am Rev Respir Dis* 1987; 136:556–560.

169. Hayden FG, Gwaltney JM: Intranasal interferon-α2 treatment of experimental rhinovirus colds. *J Infect Dis* 1984; 150:174–180.

170. Douglas RM, Moore BW, Miles HB, et al: Prophylactic efficacy of intranasal alpha 2-interferon against rhinovirus infections in the family setting. *N Engl J Med* 1986; 314:65–70.

171. Hayden FG, Albrecht JK, Kaiser DL, et al: Prevention of natural colds by contact prophylaxis with intranasal alpha 2-interferon. *N Engl J Med* 1986; 314:71–75.

172. Sperber SJ, Levine PA, Sorrentino JV, et al: Ineffectiveness of recombinant interferon-β serine nasal drops for prophylaxis of natural colds. *J Infect Dis* 1989; 160:700–705.

173. Dick EC, Hossain SU, Mink KA, et al: Interruption of transmission of rhinovirus colds among human volunteers using virucidal paper handkerchiefs. *J Infect Dis* 1986; 153:352–356.

174. Farr BM, Hendley JO, Kaiser DL, et al: Two randomized controlled trials of virucidal nasal tissues in the prevention of natural upper respiratory infections. *Am J Epidemiol* 1988; 128:1162–1172.

175. Rossman MG, Arnold E, Erickson JW, et al: Structure of a human common cold virus and functional relationship to other picornaviruses. *Nature* 1985; 317:145–153.

176. Smith TJ, Kremer MJ, Luo M, et al: The site of attachment in human rhinovirus 14 for antiviral agents that inhibit uncoating. *Science* 1986; 233:1286–1293.

177. McCray J, Werner G: Different rhinovirus serotypes neutralized by antipeptide antibodies. *Nature* 1987; 329:736–738.

178. Al-Nakib W, Stanway G, Forsysth M, et al: Detection of human rhinoviruses and their molecular relationship using cDNA probes. *J Med Virol* 1986; 20:289–296.

179. Hayden FG, Gwaltney JM, Colonno RJ: Modification of experimental rhinovirus colds by receptor blockade. *Antiviral Res* 1989; 9:233–247.

180. Mufson MA: Coronaviruses, in Belshe RB (ed): *Textbook of Human Virology*. St Louis, Mosby-Year Book, Inc, 1991, p 408.

181. Monto AS, Kim SK: The Tecumseh study of respiratory viruses. VI. Frequency of and relationship between outbreaks of coronavirus infection. *J Infect Dis* 1974; 129:271–276.

182. Hendley JO, Fishburne HB, Gwaltney JM: Coronavirus infections in working adults. *Am Rev Respir Dis* 1972; 105:805–811.

183. McIntosh K, Chao RK, Krause HE, et al: Coronavirus infection in acute lower respiratory tract disease in infants. *J Infect Dis* 1974; 130:502–507.

184. Wenzel RP, Hendley JO, Davis JA, et al: Coronavirus infections in military recruits: Three year study with coronavirus strains OC43 and 229E. *Am Rev Respir Dis* 1974; 109:621–624.

185. Gump DW, Phillips CA, Forsythe BR, et al: Role of infection in chronic bronchitis. *Am Rev Respir Dis* 1976; 113:465–474.

186. Riski H, Hovi T: Coronavirus infections of man associated with diseases other than the common cold. *J Med Virol* 1980; 6:259–265.

187. MacNaughton MR: Occurrence and frequency of coronavirus infections in humans as determined by enzyme-linked immunosorbent assay. *Infect Immun* 1982; 38:419–423.

188. Turner RB, Fulton A, Kosak K, et al: Prevention of experimental coronavirus colds with intranasal α-2b interferon. *J Infect Dis* 1986; 154:443–447.

189. Waring JJ, Neubuerger KT, Geever EF: Severe forms of chickenpox in adults with autopsy observations in a case with associated pneumonia and encephalitis. *Arch Intern Med* 1942; 69:384–408.

190. Krugman S, Goodrich CH, Ward R: Primary varicella pneumonia. *N Engl J Med* 1957; 257:843–848.

191. Williams B, Capers TH: The demonstration of intranuclear inclusion bodies in sputum from a patient with varicella pneumonia. *Am J Med* 1959; 26:836–839.

192. Knyvett AF: The pulmonary lesions of chickenpox. *Q J Med* 1966; 35:313–323.

193. Sander J, Serck-Hanssen A, Ulstreep JC: Fatal varicella pneumonia. *Scand J Infect Dis* 1970; 2:231–234.

194. Glick N, Levin S, Nelson K: Recurrent pulmonary infarction in adult chickenpox pneumonia. *JAMA* 1972; 222:173–177.

195. Fleisher G, Henry W, McCorley M, et al: Life-threatening complications of varicella. *Am J Dis Child* 1981; 135:896–899.

196. Morgan ER, Smalley LA: Varicella in immunocompromised children. *Am J Dis Child* 1983; 137:883–885.

197. Guess HA, Broughton DD, Melton LJ, et al: Population-based studies of varicella complications. *Pediatrics* 1986; 78(suppl):723–727.

198. Harris RF, Rhoades ER: Varicella pneumonia complicating pregnancy: Report of a case and review of the literature. *Obstet Gynecol* 1965; 25:734–740.

199. Medelon DA, Lewis GC: Varicella pneumonia during pregnancy. *Obstet Gynecol* 1969; 33:98.

200. Schlossberg D, Littman M: Varicella pneumonia. *Arch Intern Med* 1988; 148:1630–1632.

201. Lindgren KM, Douglas RG, Couch RB: Significance of *Herpesvirus hominis* in respiratory secretions of man. *N Engl J Med* 1968; 278:517–523.

202. Nash G: Necrotizing tracheobronchitis and bronchopneumonia consistent with herpetic infection. *Hum pathol* 1972; 3:283–291.

203. Cheever AW, Valsamis MP, Rabson AS: Necrotizing toxoplasma encephalitis and herpetic pneumonia complicating treated Hodgkin's disease. *N Engl J Med* 1965; 272:26–29.

204. Douglas RG, Anderson MG, Weg JG, et al: Herpes simplex virus pneumonia-occurrence in an allotransplanted lung. *JAMA* 1969; 210:902–904.

205. Ramsey PG, Fife KH, Hackman RC, et al: Herpes simplex virus pneumonia. *Ann Intern Med* 1982; 97:813–820.

206. Tuxen DV, Cade JF, McDonald MI, et al: Herpes simplex virus from the lower respiratory tract in adult respiratory distress syndrome. *Am Rev Respir Dis* 1982; 126:416–419.

207. Tuxen DV, Wilson JW, Cade JF: Prevention of lower respiratory herpes simplex virus infection with acyclovir in patients with adult respiratory distress syndrome. *Am Rev Respir Dis* 1987; 136:402–406.

208. Hubbell C, Dominquez R, Kohl S: Neonatal herpes simplex pneumonitis. *Rev Infect Dis* 1988; 10:431–438.

209. Hull HF, Blumhagen JD, Benjamin D, et al: Herpes simplex viral pneumonitis in childhood. *J Pediatr* 1984; 104:211–215.

210. Sherry MK, Klainer AS, Wolff M, et al: Herpetic tracheobronchitis. *Ann Intern Med* 1988; 109:229–233.

211. Graham BS, Snell JD: Herpes simplex virus infection of the adult lower respiratory tract. *Medicine (Baltimore)* 1983; 62:384–393.

212. Naraqi S: Cytomegaloviruses, in Belshe RB (ed): *Textbook of Human Virology.* St Louis, Mosby-Year Book, Inc, 1991, pp 908–909.

213. Weller TH, Hanshaw JB: Virologic and clinical observations on cytomegalic inclusion disease. *N Engl J Med* 1962; 266:1233–1244.

214. Marrie TJ, Tanigan DT, Haldane EV, et al: Does cytomegalovirus play a role in community-acquired pneumonia? *Clin Invest Med* 1985; 8:286–295.

215. Murray JF, Garay SM, Hopewell PC, et al: Pulmonary complications of the acquired immunodeficiency syndrome: An update. *Am Rev Respir Dis* 1987; 135:504–509.

216. Hill RB, Rowlands DT, Rifkind D: Infectious pulmonary disease in patients receiving immunosuppressive therapy for organ transplantation. *N Engl J Med* 1964; 271:1021–1027.

217. Craighead J: Pulmonary cytomegalovirus infection in the adult. *Am J Pathol* 1971; 63:487–500.

218. Beschorner WE, Hutchins GM, Burns WH, et al: Cytomegalovirus pneumonia in bone marrow transplant recipients: Miliary and diffuse patterns. *Am Rev Respir Dis* 1980; 122:107–114.

219. Shepp DH, Dandliker PS, Miranda P, et al: Activity of 9-[2-Hydroxy-1-(hydroxy methyl) ethoxy methyl] quanine in the treatment of cytomegalovirus pneumonia. *Ann Intern Med* 1985; 103:368–373.

220. Collaborative DHPG Treatment Study Group: Treatment of serious cytomegalovirus infections with 9-(1,3-dihydroxy-2-propoxymethyl) quanine in patients with AIDS and other immunodeficiencies. *N Engl J Med* 1986; 314:801–805.

221. Erici A, Jordan C, Chace BA, et al: Ganciclovir treatment of cytomegalovirus disease in transplant recipients and other immunocompromised hosts. *JAMA* 1987; 257:3082–3087.

222. O'Reilly RJ, Reich L, Gold J, et al: A randomized trial of intravenous hyperimmune globulin for prevention of cytomegalovirus (CMV) infections following marrow transplantation: Preliminary results. *Transplant Proc* 1983; 15:1405–1411.

223. Gluckman E, Lotsberg J, Devergie A, et al: Prophylaxis of herpes infections after bone-marrow transplantation by oral acyclovir. *Lancet* 1983; 2:706–707.

224. Enders J, McCarthey K, Mitus A, et al: Isolation of measles virus at autopsy in cases of giant-cell pneumonia without rash. *N Engl J Med* 1959; 21:876–881.

225. Mitus A, Enders JF, Craig JM, et al: Persistence of measles virus and depression of antibody formation in patients with giant-cell pneumonia after measles. *N Engl J Med* 1959; 261:882–889.

226. Kohn JL, Koiransky H: Successive roentgenograms of the chest in children during measles. *Am J Dis Child* 1929; 38:258–270.

227. Weinstein L, Franklin W: The pneumonia of measles. *Am J Med Sci* 1949; 217:314–324.

228. Olson RW, Hodges GR: Measles pneumonia. Bacterial suprainfection as a complicating factor. *JAMA* 1975; 232:363–365.

229. Modlin JF: Measles virus, in Belshe RB (ed): *Textbook of Human Virology.* St Louis, Mosby-Year Book, Inc, 1991, p 374.

230. O'Donovan C, Barua KN: Measles pneumonia. *Am J Trop Med Hyg* 1973; 22:72–77.

231. Sabonya RE, Hiller FC, Pingleton W, et al: Fatal measles (rubeola) pneumonia in adults. *Arch Pathol Lab Med* 1978; 102:366–371.

232. Frey HM, Krugman S: Case report: Atypical measles syndrome: Unusual hepatic, pulmonary, and immunologic aspects. *Am J Med Sci* 1981; 281:51–55.

233. Henderson JAM, Hammond DI: Delayed diagnosis in atypical measles syndrome. *Can Med Assoc J* 1985; 133:211–213.

234. Hall WJ, Hall CB: Atypical measles in adolescents: Evaluation of clinical and pulmonary function. *Ann Intern Med* 1979; 90:882–886.

CHAPTER 6

Nonspecific Airway Hyperresponsiveness: Mechanisms and Meaning*

Jonathan D. Plitman, M.D.

Senior Fellow, The Center for Lung Research, Vanderbilt University School of Medicine, Nashville, Tennessee

James R. Snapper, M.D.

Professor of Medicine, The Center for Lung Research, Vanderbilt University School of Medicine, Nashville, Tennessee

Asthma is a common problem, affecting some 3% to 5% of the adult population. It is the cause of considerable morbidity and a rising number of deaths.[1] It is appropriately the subject of intense study, yet, despite this effort, a full understanding of the pathogenesis of asthma remains elusive. Our incomplete understanding is exemplified well by the confusion and difficulties surrounding the definition of asthma.[2] What is probably the most useful definition is a rather old one. In 1962, the American Thoracic Society[3] stated, "Asthma is a disease characterized by an increased responsiveness of the trachea and bronchi to various stimuli and manifested by a widespread narrowing of the airways that changes in severity either spontaneously or as a result of therapy." This somewhat vague formulation is generally acceptable to both the physiologist and the clinician but fully satisfactory to neither. Significantly, however, it implies that nonspecific airway "twitchiness,"

*This work was supported by T32-HL07123; HL27274, and HL46971.

i.e., the tendency to narrow excessively in response to heterogeneous stimuli, may be inherent to asthma. In this chapter, we will review the physiology of nonspecific airway hyperresponsiveness and address its significance in asthma. It is impossible to be fully comprehensive in a chapter such as this and our focus inevitably is influenced by our own biases and areas of interest. Complementary reviews of this subject by various authors are available.[4-8]

WHAT IS NONSPECIFIC AIRWAY RESPONSIVENESS?

Some degree of airway responsiveness is presumably both normal and desirable. For example, a narrowed airway could protect the alveolar space from noxious airborne substances. Reduced airway radius and resulting increased airstream velocity can increase the deposition of inhaled particles in more proximal airways,[9] whence they can be removed by mucociliary transport and the cough reflex. Airway caliber also may help regulate the regional distribution of inspired air within the lung[10] and participate in ventilation-perfusion matching.

Muscle-containing airways will narrow in response to a variety of inhaled nonspecific chemical and physical stimuli. These include many pharmacologic agents (histamine, cholinergic agonists, cyclooxygenase products, leukotrienes, bradykinin, and others), irritants (e.g., cigarette smoke, ozone, sulfur dioxide), and hyperventilation of cold and/or dry air (many references; see reviews cited earlier). These stimuli are "nonspecific" in the sense that they are heterogeneous and are not allergens. Nonspecific responsiveness is distinct from "specific responsiveness," i.e., the antibody-mediated narrowing of the airways of sensitized individual after exposure to a specific antigenic stimulus. Such specific responsiveness is important in many asthmatics. We will address it in this paper, however, only to the extent to which it intersects with nonspecific airway responsiveness. As will be discussed, one interpretation is that it is within the intersection of specific and nonspecific airway responsiveness that the nature of asthma lies.

Nonspecific responsiveness varies among individuals, but the degree of responsiveness in the laboratory to one of these stimuli tends to predict the degree of responsiveness to the others.[11-14] Some of these stimuli closely resemble ones that can affect asthmatics in daily life (e.g., cold air) and others are more contrived (e.g., methacholine inhalation). The fact that responsiveness to both kinds of stimuli is comparable suggests that the responsiveness that one measures by pharmacologic bronchoprovocation is relevant to airway responsiveness "in the wild." As is true in other physiologic stimulus-response relationships,[15] the degrees of nonspecific airway responsiveness observed in a randomly selected population fall into a unimodal log-normal distribution in animals[16, 17] and in humans.[18] Where in this distribution does one draw the line between normal and excessive responsiveness? Certainly, a patient whose responsiveness is sufficient to cause symptomatic bronchospasm on exposure to nonspecific stimuli in daily life is hyperresponsive, but it is equally true that lesser degrees of responsiveness may be of clinical significance, especially in the presence of superimposed conditions such as atopy,[19] smoking,[20] and heart failure.[21] Furthermore, even a minor degree of exercise-induced airway narrowing could be of great significance to an athletic patient. From the point of view of both research and clinical utility, the choice of an arbitrary threshold of "hyperresponsiveness," as well as the selection of a method by which to measure responsiveness, is affected by many issues. These include safety, reproducibility, and predictive (diagnostic) value. Despite persistent controversy on some points, there is some technical consensus;[22, 23, 24] issues related to diagnostic value will be discussed in the following section. It is important to note that many research studies do not employ the prevalent "consensus" procedures, and this is a potentially confounding factor in the comparison of data.

Sources and Consequences of Nonspecific Airway Hyperresponsiveness

Despite the fact that nonspecific hyperresponsiveness can be found in healthy relatives of asthmatics,[25] it is unlikely that it occurs solely as a genetically determined diathesis, for significant discordance between levels of hyperresponsiveness in monozygotic twins has been observed.[26, 27] There is circumstantial evidence that nonspecific hyperresponsiveness can be the result of environmental influences. Some of it, in fact, may be allergen-related, for it seems to occur with increased frequency in nonasthmatic atopic patients.[28] Viral respiratory infection and exposure to nonantigenic irritants can result in transient increases in nonspecific responsiveness in normal individuals and asthmatics, and worsening of symptoms in asthmatics.[29-32] The effect in normal individuals does not seem to depend on underlying atopy.[30, 31]

What happens to the minority of individuals who fall in the very responsive part of the population distribution of nonspecific airway responsiveness? It is true that asthmatics often have nonspecifically hyperresponsive airways.[18, 33] It was, in fact, on asthmatics that the original observations of nonspecific hyperresponsiveness were made. In 1921, Alexander and Paddock, working at Bellevue Hospital in New York City, showed that a subcutaneous dose of pilocarpine that had no apparent effect on the respirations of normal subjects induced "asthmatic breathing" in patients with known asthma.[34] Curry, in 1949, found that asthmatics were hyperresponsive to inhaled histamine and methacholine.[35] Given that asthma and nonspecific hyperresponsiveness often coexist, one could make a (too) simple inference of causality: asthma is the result of airway narrowing in response to nonspecific stimuli innocuous to less responsive individuals (e.g., atmospheric irritants or hyperventilation). Nonspecific hyperresponsiveness also could be partially pathogenetic with respect to allergic asthma. Data in animals and humans show that specific airway responsiveness to an allergen is related not merely to the severity of allergy, but also to the underlying degree of *non*specific responsiveness.[19, 36, 37] Does nonspecific hyperresponsiveness cause asthma?

In fact, it may be valid in some situations to claim that asthma causes nonspecific hyperresponsiveness. Asthma cannot always be the cause of nonspecific hyperresponsiveness, as population surveys show that the prevalence of nonspecific hyperresponsiveness significantly exceeds that of symptomatic asthma.[38, 39] However, after experimental aeroallergen exposure resulting in a specific airway response, animals often will have residual increases in nonspecific airway responsiveness.[40, 41] This phenomenon also seems to occur in humans; nonspecific hyperresponsiveness waxes and wanes with ambient allergen exposure in sensitized individuals.[42, 43] In these examples, nonspecific hyperresponsiveness seems to be a consequence of persistent changes in the airways wrought by the specific asthmatic reaction. Further allergen exposure occurring in the presence of this increased nonspecific responsiveness could have a heightened effect. The subject now might be prone also to symptomatic bronchoconstriction on exposure to nonspecific stimuli, with resultant worsening of asthma symptoms.

The aforementioned model implies the possibility of positive feedback, which is unusual in biology. Most feedback, even in pathologic situations, is negative, thus limiting response and contributing to homeostasis. We feel, however, that the model is useful. There is probably a complex, mutually reinforcing relationship between nonspecific airway hyperresponsiveness and symptomatic asthma, both allergic and nonallergic; in a way, each seems to lack a complete identity independent of the other. The acceptance of some ambiguity may be essential to the successful study of asthma.[44] This definitional blurring of nonspecific airway hyperresponsiveness and asthma, rather than causing confusion, should enhance one's perception of nonspecific responsiveness as a key to investigating the causes of asthma.

In light of these theoretical considerations, what is the utility of laboratory bronchoprovocation in the clinical evaluation of asthma? Despite intense study, this remains a controversial issue, and opinions vary from those deeming the test essential[45] to those deeming it relatively useless.[46] Setting aside complex issues of predicting future airway disease,[20, 47] there is little, if any, utility in detecting asymptomatic hyperresponsiveness. It is thus fairly clear that bronchoprovocation is not useful as a tool for mass screening of random populations, for, in such populations, the prevalence of asymptomatic nonspecific hyperresponsiveness may roughly equal the prevalence of symptomatic hyperresponsiveness.[38, 39, 48, 49] At the other end of the spectrum, a patient with typically asthmatic historic and physical findings who responds to therapy does not need bronchoprovocation.[50]

In symptomatic patients whose diagnosis is more ambiguous, what is the role of the test? Its negative predictive value is a matter of debate. A number of studies have observed that symptomatic asthma in the absence of hyperresponsiveness is very unusual,[22, 51, 52] implying that a negative test effectively rules out asthma. Many of these data, however, were collected on clearly asthmatic patients. More applicable to a situation of clinical ambiguity might be the findings of Pattemore and colleagues,[49] who surveyed 2,053 schoolchildren. Of the group that had experienced probable asthma symptoms of variable frequency in the prior month and whose parents recalled a clinical diagnosis of asthma, 27.7% were not hyperresponsive. This study has been criticized for comparing a single bronchoprovocation to cumulative past symptoms,[50] because hyperresponsiveness in some patients varies over time, probably due to fluctuating degrees of exposure to environmental influences that can alter responsiveness.[50] In another recent study, however, 20 asthmatics of varying age and severity of symptoms were followed for 12 to 18 months with methacholine challenges every 2 to 3 weeks.[46] Methacholine responsiveness did not correlate in general with concurrent symptom severity or peak expiratory flow, although the most severely symptomatic patients did tend to be the most responsive. Some exacerbations were observed in the absence of apparent hyperresponsiveness. As a whole, these data imply that asthma can occur without demonstrable hyperresponsiveness and that bronchoprovocation may be most reliably diagnostic in the severely affected patients in whom it is diagnostically unnecessary. The relationship between nonspecific hyperresponsiveness and asthma is probably complex and modulated by many factors. Thus, laboratory bronchoprovocation, which is a fairly gross tool, may not demonstrate the relationship well in less severe cases. It should be noted particularly that a negative nonspecific bronchoprovocation may not rule out atopic or occupational asthma. Nonspecific hyperresponsiveness may develop only after prolonged exposure to the inciting agent, and may wane after cessation of exposure.[42, 43, 53–55] Although it has been studied less extensively, the predictive value of a negative bronchoprovocation may be better when the test is applied to atypical presentations of asthma, such as chronic cough.[56]

The positive predictive value of the test is compromised by the prevalence of asymptomatic hyperresponsiveness in the general population (see earlier). Also, not all patients with concurrent respiratory symptoms and hyperresponsiveness are asthmatics, in that other diseases, such as sarcoidosis, hypersensitivity pneumonitis, and heart disease, can be associated with hyperresponsiveness.[21, 57, 58] In most or all such cases, however, the underlying disease will be recognizable by means other than bronchoprovocation. Some data imply that higher levels of nonspecific hyperresponsiveness in asthmatics predict that larger amounts of medication will be required to control symptoms,[59] but there is overlap among groups, and the use of bronchoprovocation to assess disease severity or titrate therapy does not seem to be indicated.[50] Disease severity probably is assessed best using symptom reports and routine pulmonary function tests.

MECHANISMS OF HYPERRESPONSIVENESS

It is appropriate at this point to explore at some length the mechanisms that may underlie nonspecific airway hyperresponsiveness. In other words, as Rackemann wrote in 1931,[60] "The situation is somewhat analogous to that of a loaded gun. A good deal of knowledge is being obtained about the great variety of triggers . . . ; but why is the gun loaded?"

The number of potential mechanisms is large, and their enumeration and analysis is complicated additionally by interactions among them. A simple taxonomy would be useful. The semilogarithmic sigmoid dose-response curves that often are used to measure in vivo airway responsiveness resemble those used in classic in vitro studies of smooth muscle pharmacology. Because of this, and because airway smooth muscle almost certainly plays some role in airway responsiveness, it is possible to classify mechanisms of airway hyperresponsiveness in terms that usually are applied to in vitro smooth muscle hyperresponsiveness.[61, 62] We would like to examine this approach and the limitations of such in vitro/in vivo comparisons in some detail, followed by a proposed taxonomy.

Correspondence Between Models of Hyperresponsiveness

In vitro hyperresponsiveness of excitable tissues (usually referred to as "supersensitivity") has been reviewed frequently and exhaustively.[63–67] The physiologic and taxonomic concepts can be simplified and summarized as follows: If one creates a situation in which an increased amount of a stimulus interacts with its receptor (e.g., remove an access barrier between stimulus and receptor or inhibit stimulus removal), supersensitivity will result, although the intrinsic ability of the tissue to respond to stimuli is unchanged. This phenomenon is termed by various authors prejunctional, presynaptic, type I, or deviation supersensitivity. In classic in vitro smooth muscle studies, one is dealing with end-organ ligand-receptor interactions in relative isolation. As a result of this, true prejunctional supersensitivity is *specific* to the ligand-receptor system that has been manipulated. If one alters the properties of the smooth muscle such that its intrinsic ability to respond to stimuli is enhanced (e.g., amplify intracellular calcium release or make actin-myosin interaction more efficient), supersensitivity will result, although the amount of stimulus that is able to interact with receptors is unchanged. This phenomenon is termed postjunctional, postsynaptic, type II, or nondeviation supersensitivity. Increases in the number or binding avidity of surface receptors could cause this, but this generally is felt not to occur in autonomic effector organs (in contrast to denervated skeletal muscle). Rather, postjunctional smooth muscle supersensitivity is the result of changes that are, in the train of events leading to muscle contraction, past the level of the specific surface receptor. Thus, it tends to be *nonspecific*, and one can observe increased sensitivity of the tissue to heterogeneous stimuli, including those that are not truly receptor-mediated, such as electrical fields or changes in extracellular potassium concentration.

There is controversy as to the nature of characteristic dose-response curve changes in the two types of supersensitivity. Kalsner[64] emphasizes the importance of shifts of the curve along the dose axis toward lower doses in type I situations and distortion of the curve along the response axis toward increased maximal response in type II situations. Fleming,[63] however, states that dose axis shifts are "the one consistent sign of [postjunctional] supersensitivity"; there are studies that show postjunctional supersensitivity both with and without changes along the response axis.[65] Westfall[66] prefers to keep the issue of increased maximal response definitionally separate from the two types of supersensitivity. On balance, whereas both types of supersensitivity seem to cause curve shifts toward lower doses, increases in maximal response, when they occur, seem to be the province of postjunctional supersensitivity.[64, 65] If, however, one were not able to test under conditions of maximal stimulation, e.g., for reasons of stimulus toxicity to other tissues in vivo, a prejunctional change in the system could cause an increase in maximal response as well.

Potential mechanisms of in vivo airway hyperresponsiveness, in theory, can be classified as "prejunctional" and "postjunctional."[61, 62] Mechanisms that amplify the intensity of stimuli, such as increased access of inhaled substances to active sites, would be "prejunctional." Mechanisms that amplify response to a given level of stimulation, such as increased intrinsic smooth muscle contractility or reduced counterregulation by endogenous bronchodilating substances, would be "postjunctional." Extending this line of thought, one could claim that airway hyperresponsiveness is a predominantly "postjunctional" phenomenon, as it is often nonspecific. Also, Sterk and colleagues[68] have shown that laboratory bronchoprovocation can supply a maximal or nearly maximal stimulus. Thus, the observation that in vivo airway dose-response curves in hyperresponsive subjects often indicate increases in maximal response[33] could imply "postjunctionality." However, strict application of these in vitro categories in their standard senses to the analysis of in vivo nonspecific airway hyperresponsiveness is fraught with hazard. In a complex system that inherently responds to heterogeneous stimuli, factors may have both "prejunctional" and "postjunctional" effects. Furthermore, a "prejunctional" change could appear nonspecific and be mistaken for "postjunctional" when it is, in fact, "multiply specific." Also, in vivo, one is dealing with series of interacting "junctions," and "pre-" vs. "post-" can be a matter of point of view. For example, the eosinophils of asthmatics may have an increased intrinsic tendency to release smooth muscle–stimulating substances in response to nonantigenic stimuli.[69] Strictly speaking, airway hyperresponsiveness due to this would be a "prejunctional" smooth muscle phenomenon, but would behave "postjunctionally" from the standpoint of the eosinophil. One could, in fact, make the holistic claim that complete understanding might reveal that mechanisms of hyperresponsiveness in vivo interact with such complexity that this distinction is meaningless when applied to any single mechanism. Finally, the very inference of in vitro/in vivo analogy can be hazardous. As will be discussed later, in vitro responsiveness of human airway smooth muscle often does not correlate well with in vivo airway responsiveness.[70–73]

Nonetheless, at our current level of understanding, a "prejunctional vs. postjunctional" type of distinction can be a useful means of classifying and conceptualizing mechanisms of airway hyperresponsiveness. We agree with others' emphasis on "postjunctional"-type mechanisms,[61] but would prefer categories that

TABLE 1.
Taxonomy of Potential Mechanisms of Airway
Hyperresponsiveness

I. Stimulus-enhancing mechanisms.
   A. Increased aerosol deposition.
   B. Increased epithelial permeability.
II. Response-enhancing mechanisms.
   A. Altered smooth muscle.
   B. Altered airway geometry.
   C. Decreased epithelium-dependent dilation.
   D. Decreased β-adrenergic dilation.
   E. Decreased nonadrenergic noncholinergic
      dilation.
   F. Increased action of sensory neuropeptides.
   G. Altered parasympathetic function.
   H. Altered mediator receptor function.
III. Stimulus- and response-enhancing
   mechanisms.
   A. Mediators.
   B. Altered secretion and mucociliary
      clearance.
   C. Increased α-adrenergic function.

---

avoid the suggestion of complete in vitro/in vivo analogy and that account for "postjunctionality" that may not be proprietary to the smooth muscle. We will substitute the terms "stimulus-enhancing" and "response-enhancing." "Stimulus-enhancing" will refer to mechanisms whose chief putative effect is to increase the ability of an exogenous stimulus to initiate changes that result in airway narrowing. "Response-enhancing" will refer to mechanisms whose chief putative effect is to augment the ability of an endogenous structure or substance to promote airway narrowing or to diminish the ability of an endogenous structure or substance to reduce airway narrowing.

The succeeding discussion of the mechanisms will follow the order outlined in Table 1. Please note that "inflammation" is not listed as a mechanism. The role of inflammation in asthma has been the subject of intense scrutiny, and has been reviewed recently.[74] We wholly agree with its importance, but will analyze it indirectly via its manifestations, such as edema, cellular infiltration, mediator release, and epithelial damage.

Stimulus-Enhancing Mechanisms

Increased Aerosol Deposition

Deposition of airborne particles in a given airway is inversely proportional to the radius of the airway lumen and directly proportional to the velocity of the airstream within the lumen.[9] An individual with baseline airway obstruction could have reduced luminal radii and also increased airstream velocity (in order to preserve flow through a narrowed conduit). Even if the baseline narrowing were mild, and potentially clinically silent, inhaled substances could be preferentially deposited in these airways.[75] Increased airway deposition of particles could explain the relative hyperresponsiveness seen in individuals with normal but comparatively small airway luminal radii, such as infants.[76, 77] It also could explain the observation that differences in responsiveness between asthmatics and normal individuals are sometimes inapparent when bronchial stimuli are administered intravenously rather than by inhalation.[78, 79] If it were true, however, one would predict that hyperresponsiveness to inhaled agents would be proportional to baseline airway caliber. Evidence is not strong for such a relationship in normal individuals or those with asthma;[80–83] these studies have further implications in terms of the impact of airway geometry on responsiveness, and will be examined in detail below.

Increased Epithelial Permeability
   The interstices between the epithelial cells of the airways are sealed by tight junctions, which are impermeable to large molecules.[84] These cells stand between inhaled substances and subepithelial structures that could initiate an airway response, such as mediator-releasing cells,[74] afferent nerve fibers,[85] parasympathetic ganglia,[86] and airway smooth muscle itself. Damage to this barrier, with resulting increased permeability, could enhance the effects of inhaled stimuli and increase airway responsiveness. Such a mechanism may be at least a partial explanation for the nonspecific airway hyperresponsiveness that is present in human subjects after viral respiratory tract infection[32] and ozone exposure.[87]
   Epithelial damage is a pathologic hallmark of asthma. Sloughing of airway epithelial cells is noted almost universally in autopsies of fatal asthma victims.[88] In fact, Dunnill has stated,[89] "It is often extremely difficult to find normal areas of bronchial mucosa in patients dying in status asthmaticus." Epithelial damage presumably is one factor contributing to the association between airway inflammation and asthma, and, like nonspecific airway hyperresponsiveness, is often demonstrable in airway material from living asthmatics, even between attacks.[90–93]
   Guinea pigs exposed to cigarette smoke have increased airway epithelial permeability,[94, 95] and this change resolves to normal over 12 hours.[96] These animals also have airway hyperresponsiveness after cigarette smoke exposure, and the time course of the hyperresponsiveness seems grossly to parallel that of the increased permeability.[97] Sensitized monkeys also have parallel increases in permeability and airway responsiveness after exposure to allergen.[40] Bronchoscopic studies of mild asthmatics in remission have found nonspecific airway responsiveness to be proportional to the degree of epithelial damage,[92, 93] although this has not been observed unanimously.[91] The majority of data, however, do imply a possible relationship between a damaged, leaky epithelium and hyperresponsiveness. Unfortunately, more direct observations in humans do not suggest such a relationship.

Increased permeability in human smokers (measured as clearance of inhaled technetium-labelled diethylene triamine pentaacetic acid [^{99}Tc-DTPA]) does not correlate with nonspecific airway hyperresponsiveness;[98] Hogg[99] has suggested that the site of increased permeability after smoke inhalation may differ between acutely exposed animals and chronically exposed humans. Hyperresponsive asthmatics do not differ from normals in ^{99}Tc-DTPA clearance.[100, 101] Increased airway permeability, furthermore, does not explain observations of hyperresponsiveness to parenterally administered stimuli.[34] Though possibly contributing to airway hyperresponsiveness in some asthmatics, current evidence does not suggest a global relationship between airway mucosal permeability and hyperresponsiveness in humans.

Response-Enhancing Mechanisms

Altered Smooth Muscle

Airway hyperresponsiveness could result from an intrinsic abnormality of airway smooth muscle causing increased contraction in response to a given degree of stimulation. Such abnormalities include increased amounts of muscle, abnormal calcium ion handling, and increased electrical excitability across cell membranes.

In most pathologic studies, the airways of asthmatics contain increased amounts of smooth muscle,[90, 102-104] although this finding has not been universal.[105] In some older pathologic studies, this change was felt to be hypertrophic, but more recent studies show that it may be primarily hyperplastic.[103] Muscle of increased volume may contract more strongly against a given load, but it is debated whether this increase in muscle volume is a cause or a result of hyperresponsiveness.[106] It also has been suggested that airway muscle in hyperresponsive subjects may be, volume for volume, intrinsically more contractile than normal; given the central role of the calcium ion in smooth muscle contractility,[107] abnormalities in excitatory intracellular calcium handling have been suggested.[108] Many studies show that calcium channel–blocking drugs can blunt nonspecific hyperresponsiveness to stimuli such as histamine, exercise, and cold air.[109] These data, however, do not clearly suggest a defect in calcium handling, since the calcium channel–blocking agents have myriad potential inhibitory effects on normal smooth muscle, nerves, and secretory cells.[110] The possibility of increased electrical excitability relates to the existence of smooth muscle in so-called multiunit or single-unit forms.[106] In multiunit smooth muscle, cells have few gap junctions, which are channels through which depolarizations can travel directly from cell to cell. These cells are primarily dependent on neural input for activation. Multiunit behavior is typical of normal airway smooth muscle. Single-unit smooth muscle cells, on the other hand, are more self-regulated. They are prone to spontaneous changes in membrane potential and have many gap junctions. Single-unit smooth muscle cells have myogenic responses, i.e., on being stretched, they tend to contract autonomously. As Stephens[106] points out, if single-unit behavior were to predominate in the airways, the increased excitability of the muscle probably would not cause hyperresponsiveness per se, but rather would cause a reduced threshold for normal narrowing. If it were combined with increased shortening ability of the smooth muscle (? hyperplasia or hypertrophy), however, significant hyperresponsiveness could result. Increased myogenic responses in tracheal muscle have been demonstrated in a canine model of atopic asthma.[111] Although there is no direct evidence for an effect on intercellular communication, gap junctions have been observed to increase in number when normal canine tracheal muscle is treated with prostaglandin E_2 or prostacyclin.[112] Other subcellular structural alterations in hyperresponsive airway smooth muscle have been inferred,[113] but their functional significance also remains unclear. In summary, intrinsic changes in smooth muscle function can be implicated in airway hyperresponsiveness, but only circumstantially at this point.

To what extent have experimenters been able to associate clinical airway responsiveness and smooth muscle function?

There have been numerous attempts, using preoperative bronchoprovocation challenges followed by studies on surgical specimens of human airways, to establish a relationship between in vivo nonspecific airway responsiveness and in vitro muscular responsiveness. The majority of the in vitro data have been collected under isometric conditions. These studies have shown no correlation between in vivo and in vitro responsiveness to histamine in normal individuals[71, 72] and to histamine or methacholine in groups of patients with airway disease.[70, 73, 114–116] The vast majority of these patients seem to have been smokers or ex-smokers with obstructive lung disease rather than "pure" asthmatics. Given the apparent differences in dose-response relationships between airway hyperresponsiveness in chronic obstructive pulmonary disease and in asthma,[117] it may be difficult to apply these data to asthma. Similar negative results have been obtained from normal individuals in isotonic studies.[118] There are isolated reports on the in vitro isometric behavior of surgical specimens of airways from individual patients who seem to have been "pure" asthmatics, although in vivo responsiveness was not studied.[119, 120] The response of the tissue to maximal stimulation by histamine (Tmax, which is maximal tension normalized for specimen size) was greater than that of tissue from nonasthmatic control persons. A series of specimens from autopsies after fatal asthma attacks yielded similar findings.[121] The doses of histamine required to elicit half-maximal tension in these studies were no different in asthmatics and normal control individuals. In other words, the asthmatic airway tissue seemed not to be more sensitive per se, but its muscle contracted significantly more for a given level of stimulus. This could reflect the increased proportion of muscle in asthmatic airways or an inherent muscle abnormality. In either case, however, the relationship between this alteration of responsiveness and hyperresponsiveness in vivo remains unclear, in that studies on normal individuals and on patients with airway disease have shown no correlation between in vivo hyperresponsiveness and Tmax.[72, 114]

While the above studies have not revealed a consistent muscular abnormality accountable for airway hyperresponsiveness, it must be emphasized that it is tricky to infer a relationship, or the lack thereof, from these in vitro/in vivo comparisons. The function of smooth muscle is critically dependent upon mechanical conditions of which we have little understanding, let alone control, in most in vivo models. In the trachea, the long axes of the muscle fibers tend to be parallel to each other and perpendicular to the long axis of the airway, but, distal to the trachea, this relationship is much less simple.[122] As a result, the orientation of muscle fibers in bronchial tissue preparations is usually unknown, and changes in in vivo airway caliber cannot be inferred reliably from in vitro length or tension changes. Isotonic testing shows the ability of the muscle to shorten and isometric testing shows its ability to generate tension; the latter seems to correlate more closely with muscle content in in vitro specimens.[123] Almost certainly, however, an intermediate condition neither isotonic nor isometric is likely to predominate in vivo. Smooth muscle in an intact system is not held at fixed length, and it contracts against a load imposed by structures in and around the airway wall, such as cartilage, and by the outward pull of lung parenchymal recoil and transpleural pressure.[61] Like skeletal muscle, smooth muscle has a length-tension (or length-shortening) relationship, in that there is a resting length (Lmax) from which tension or shortening is maximal[124] and where, presumably, actin-myosin interaction is optimal. In vitro, resting length is a function of artificial resting tension; resting tensions vary among studies, although they often are chosen to approximate Lmax. Airway smooth muscle loading, resting length, Lmax, and shortening in vivo have not been defined clearly, and are likely to vary in different airway generations.[61, 125, 126] More precise study of smooth muscle function in hyperresponsive airways will require additional understanding of the conditions under which such muscles work.

Altered Airway Geometry

A simple way of relating airway geometry to responsiveness is the idea that airways that are more narrow at baseline may be more responsive. Poiseuille's law states that, under laminar flow conditions, the resistance to flow of a tube is related inversely to the fourth power of the luminal radius. This implies that, at lower baseline caliber, airways should have a greater increase in resistance per given increment of additional narrowing. The following typifies a common but unfairly striking example. If an airway of 6 mm luminal radius and one of 4 mm luminal radius each narrows by an additional 3 mm of radius, the resistance of the former will increase 16-fold, whereas the resistance of the latter will increase 256-fold. This example is unfair in the sense that, if one recalculates the outcome using an increment of additional narrowing that is smaller relative to the baseline radius, the dissimilarity between the two airways is much less dramatic. That is, if the 6-mm radius narrows to 5 mm and the 4-mm radius narrows to 3 mm, the resistance of the larger airway will increase roughly twofold, whereas the resistance of the smaller airway will increase roughly threefold. In any event, these examples depend on the assumption that all airways respond to similar stimuli with equal absolute increments of narrowing regardless of baseline size. Possibly more plausible is that they respond with equal percentage or fractional increments of narrowing. In this case, the factor by which resistance increases becomes the same for all airways irrespective of starting radius. If all other factors remain unchanged, airways of *any* luminal radius (R) that narrow to a fraction (F) of their baseline radius will increase their resistances by a factor equal to R^4 divided by (F $\times$ R)^4, or F^{-4}. Studies on the relationship between baseline airway caliber and responsiveness reflect this apparent complexity. Some data in asthmatics have shown a correlation between baseline airway caliber and increased responsiveness.[127] More often, however, the relationship has been subtle or inapparent, both in studies of normal individuals after prior pharmacologic bronchoconstriction with an unrelated stimulus[80] and in asthmatics without pretreatment.[81-83] Also, a study with a great number of subjects might be required to detect a consistent relationship, as the practice of expressing airway responses as "percent change from baseline," which is used commonly to normalize results, may obscure differences in responsiveness among individuals. Whether the apparent weakness of the relationship between baseline airway caliber and responsiveness reflects true physiology, limitations of experimental design, or both, remains to be determined.

The discussion above assumes a predictable linear association between smooth muscle stimulation and shortening under heterogeneous conditions in vivo, an assumption for which proof is lacking. A similar concept, but one that makes fewer assumptions about smooth muscle behavior, is one relating hyperresponsiveness to airway wall thickness, as proposed by Freedman[128] and recently analyzed[61] by Moreno and colleagues. The airway wall region bounded by smooth muscle on the outside and the luminal gas on the inside consists primarily of epithelium, glands, connective tissue, and blood vessels. These structures in turn consist mostly of water, and are essentially incompressible. Since the cross-sectional area of the wall thus does not change with smooth muscle contraction, a thicker wall will encroach more upon the lumen for a given amount of smooth muscle shortening. In the presence of an infinitely thin wall, a decrease in external diameter of somewhat over 40% will increase airway resistance tenfold. With a wall thickness of 0.4 mm, this resistance increase would require only roughly a 20% decrease in external diameter.[61] Thus, given consistent smooth muscle responses to stimuli, hyperresponsiveness could result. In asthma, wall thickening could result from various changes discussed elsewhere in this chapter, such as increases in volume of smooth muscle and secretory structure; dilation of bronchial blood vessels; infiltration with inflammatory cells; mucosal/submucosal edema; and the presence of exudate, cells, and edema fluid in the lumen. Wall thickening from changes such as these are significantly more prominent in autopsy specimens from asthma patients than from normal individuals,[129] although cigarette smoke exposure in guinea pigs, which produces airway inflammation and increased airway responsiveness,[97] was not observed to increase the cross-sectional area of the airway wall.[130]

The potential mechanical effects of edema and the bronchial vasculature merit separate mention. The internal perimeter of the incompressible airway wall is constant irrespective of smooth muscle tone and external perimeter.[131] Thus, as the smooth muscle contracts, the luminal surface of the mucosa must fold. Free liquid within the lumen could, under these conditions, accentuate increases in airway resistance in several ways. Free liquid could reduce the size of the lumen by filling the interstices between mucosal folds, and it also, by surface tension forces, could draw the folds together, further narrowing the airway.[132] Edema fluid also could increase responsiveness and narrow airways by stimulating pulmonary J-receptors and thus initiating vagally mediated reflexes.[133, 134] One can speculate that drugs that inhibit the accumulation of fluid in the airway lumen may lessen responsiveness, although direct evidence is lacking. Furosemide inhibits chloride and water secretion into the airway lumen by blocking the Na^+-Cl^- cotransporter on the basolateral aspect of the epithelial cells.[135] Inhaled furosemide has been observed to blunt specific airway responsiveness to inhaled allergen and nonspecific responsiveness to exercise,[136, 137] although it does not seem to be consistently effective on responsiveness to methacholine in asthmatics.[138, 139] It does not appear to alter airway smooth muscle contractility in vitro.[140]

Inflammatory substances can cause dilation of bronchial vessels with increased blood flow and leakage of protein-rich, exudative fluid through widened gaps in the endothelium.[141–143] This, of course, could accelerate the accumulation of edema. Dilated vessels within the perimeter of the airway smooth muscle would thicken the wall, and vasodilating drugs have been observed to have this effect on the canine trachea.[144] Such dilation also may occur with exertion and hyperpnea, and may be important in airway hyperresponsiveness to exercise.[145] Also, dilated venules in the elaborate plexuses immediately outside the perimeter of the smooth muscle might tend to uncouple the smooth muscle in intraparenchymal airways from the restraining force of parenchymal recoil and transpleural pressure.[61, 146]

These mechanisms related to edema and the vasculature, in the asthmatic, are likely to be intimately associated with a constellation of other inflammatory changes. Thus, it might be difficult to discern the pathogenetic potential of single mechanisms from among so many. However, one may be able to isolate the possible effects of fluid and vascular caliber on airway responsiveness by examining them in a much less inflammatory condition, cardiogenic pulmonary congestion. Increased left atrial pressure can result in airway, interstitial, and intra-alveolar edema. This edema could have many of the same mechanical effects as inflammatory asthmatic airway edema. The likely effect of increased left atrial pressure on the bronchial vasculature is less clear. The bronchial venous drainage from the airways beyond the trachea and most proximal bronchi empties into the pulmonary veins.[147] Thus, increased left atrial pressure can impede bronchial blood flow[148] and potentially distended bronchial vessels. Such distention could thicken airway walls. Enlarged submucosal vessels have been observed directly in the airways of patients with mitral stenosis; the degree of enlargement correlated with pulmonary capillary wedge pressure.[149] On the other hand, an acute increase in left atrial pressure was observed by Wagner and Mitzner to cause apparent bronchial vaso-constriction in sheep, in that, under conditions of constant flow, increased left atrial pressure was associated with an increase in bronchial vascular resistance that was blunted significantly by the smooth muscle paralytic agent papaverine.[150] Consistent with this finding is the morphometric observation that acute intravenous fluid overload does not cause airway wall thickening in dogs.[151] Irrespective of bronchial vascular caliber, increased "downstream" pressure in the form of in-creased left atrial pressure also may retard the clearance of chemical stimuli from the airways by bronchial blood flow. Such clearance is felt to be important in lim-iting airway responsiveness.[152, 153] Since both edema and the vascular effects of increased left atrial pressure could result in nonspecific airway hyperresponsive-ness, these factors may be important in so-called "cardiac asthma."[146]

We have observed increased airway responsiveness to inhaled histamine in awake sheep with pulmonary edema after 3.5 hours of increased left atrial pressure.[154] Rapid infusion of a large volume of intravenous normal saline can increase responsiveness to methacholine in normal humans.[155] In several recent studies, a significant percentage of patients with chronic congestive heart failure were observed to have nonspecific hyperresponsiveness.[21, 156, 157] Whereas hemo-dynamic data at cardiac catheterization in one study did not correlate with the degree of hyperresponsiveness,[157] some patients in another study did become less responsive after diuretic therapy.[156] It would be of interest to distinguish the relative importance of edema and vascular caliber. Cabanes and colleagues[21] administered the peripheral α-adrenergic agonist methoxamine to heart failure patients with airway hyperresponsiveness in an attempt to constrict bronchial blood vessels. Methacholine hyperresponsiveness was blunted, and this effect was prevented by the α-adrenergic receptor blocker phentolamine. In our studies in sheep, however, edema seemed more responsible for hyperresponsiveness. Intravenous administration of *Perilla* ketone in the sheep causes increased pulmonary microvascular permeability and resultant pulmonary edema without elevated vascular pressures.[158] A dose of *Perilla* ketone that causes edema comparable to 3.5 hours of increased left atrial pressure caused histamine hyperresponsiveness equivalent to that seen in increased left atrial pressure. A brief (0.5-hour) period of increased left atrial pressure, which should raise vascular pressures but cause little edema, caused no significant hyperresponsive-ness.[154] While inconsistencies in the data persist, it does appear that nonspecific airway hyperresponsiveness can result from noninflammatory increases in lung liquid, extravascularly and/or intravascularly. From this, one can infer a poten-tially important role for such liquid in the hyperresponsiveness observed in inflammatory airway disorders, as well.

Decreased Epithelium-Dependent Dilation

It recently has become clear that the respiratory epithelium produces a factor or factors that relax smooth muscle. This was inferred from the observation that removal of the epithelium from isolated airways causes nonspecific hyperresponsiveness to such mediators as histamine, acetylcholine, and serotonin.[159, 160] Vanhoutte[161] makes two important points. First, this effect does not appear to be due to the simple removal of a diffusion barrier, as epithelial stripping potentiates the constrictor response to electrical field stimulation, as well as impairing relaxation of the smooth muscle by such agents as isoproterenol and verapamil. Second, the effect does not appear to be due to damage of the smooth muscle by the epithelial removal process, as the contractile response to the muscle to increased extracellular potassium concentration is unchanged. Removal of epithelium also increases the responsiveness to methacholine of human airway smooth muscle and reduces its relaxation by verapamil.[162] Interestingly, there are apparent differences in the epithelium-dependent relaxation response in different airway generations.[163]

These findings suggest that asthma-related damage to the airway epithelium could result in hyperresponsiveness by reducing local concentrations of the epithelium-derived relaxing factor(s), although the role of loss of epithelium-dependent relaxation is difficult to separate from that of the many other aspects of inflammation that also could cause hyperresponsiveness. Nonetheless, this is a provocative hypothesis that merits further investigation. Such investigation would be facilitated, of course, by knowledge of the identity of the epithelium-derived relaxing factor(s). Cyclooxygenase products have been suggested by some studies,[159, 160] although removal of the epithelium enhances contractile responses even after pretreatment of the tissue with indomethacin.[164]

Nadel[165] feels that the factor may not be a direct smooth muscle relaxant per se, but rather neutral endopeptidase (NEP, enkephalinase, membrane-associated metallopeptidase), a degradative enzyme that, in the airways, may help to limit concentrations of various neuropeptides with constrictor and/or inflammatory properties. Narrowing of airways by substances that are substrates of NEP is enhanced by removal of the epithelium,[164, 166] just as such narrowing is enhanced by chemical inhibition of NEP.[167] NEP also could modulate airway responsiveness to stimuli that are not NEP substrates (e.g., histamine and acetylcholine) if these nonpeptides act via peptide intermediaries or if their action is enhanced by the concurrent presence of peptides. The hyperresponsiveness of epithelium-free airways probably is not wholly dependent on NEP substrates, however. In guinea pig tracheal tissue, the NEP inhibitor phosphoramidon does not increase the responsiveness to acetylcholine, and epithelial removal can still increase the responsiveness to the neuropeptide substance P (albeit to a lesser degree) after phosphoramidon pretreatment.[164] The potential role of neuropeptides in airway hyperresponsiveness will be discussed further later.

It is interesting to note that tracheal epithelium in some preparations releases a factor that can relax animal and human vascular smooth muscle.[168, 169] Increased bronchial vascular caliber and blood flow theoretically may reduce airway responsiveness in some circumstances, as implied earlier.[152, 153] Little is known about the identity of this vascular relaxing factor, although preliminary data imply that it is not a cyclooxygenase product.[169] Little is known of its relationship, if any, to the endothelium-derived relaxing substances present in blood vessels.

Decreased β-Adrenergic Dilation

Since originally proposed by Szentivanyi in 1968,[170] the hypothesis that airway hyperresponsiveness in asthma could result from loss of endogenous β-adrenergic function has received considerable attention. There are significant numbers of β-adrenergic receptors in human airways,[171] predominantly of the bronchodilatory β_2 variety.[172] Reduced function of this system could enhance nonspecific bronchoconstriction; pharmacologic blockade of β-adrenergic receptors does cause bronchoconstriction and increase airway responsiveness in asthmatics,[173–175] although rarely if ever in normal individuals.[176–178]

As direct adrenergic innervation to airway β_2-receptors seems to be sparse in humans,[179] the receptors may depend heavily on circulating catecholamines for stimulation. It has been proposed that asthmatics are unable to stimulate their β-receptors adequately, in that their secretion of catecholamines into the circulation in response to exercise-induced bronchoconstriction seems impaired.[180, 181] On the other hand, other studies have shown asthmatics to respond to exercise-induced bronchoconstriction with normal[182] or exaggerated[183] sympathoadrenal cathecholamine release, and asthmatics respond to metabolic sympathoadrenal stimuli normally.[184] In any event, bursts of circulating catecholamines may not be a significant reactive mechanism in the control of airway responsiveness, in that methacholine-induced bronchoconstriction does not stimulate increases in plasma catecholamines in either asthmatics or normal individuals.[185]

As β-adrenergic receptor stimulation inhibits mediator release from cells in human lung,[186, 187] reduced β-adrenergic function could exaggerate secondary mediator release in response to airway stimuli. Data on the ability of the endogenous β-adrenergic system to modulate mediator release are scant. Pharmacologic β-blockade does not raise plasma histamine in asthmatics,[188] although it should be noted that disodium cromoglycate, which may inhibit mast cell mediator release, has been observed in one study to confer some protection from propranolol challenge in such patients.[189]

Given that β-adrenergic stimuli dilate airways, could hyposensitivity to such stimuli cause airway hyperresponsiveness? There is evidence that patients with airway hyperresponsiveness may have reduced number and/or function of β-adrenergic receptors, possibly due to an interfering immune substance.[190] Data in this area must be interpreted cautiously, in that β-adrenergic hyposensitivity can be caused by the β-agonist drugs taken by asthmatic patients.[191] Recovery of full in vitro sensitivity after cessation of β-agonist therapy has been reported in some studies to occur within roughly 2 weeks,[192] but has taken from 4 weeks[193] to 8 weeks or more[194] in others.

In two studies, asthmatic human airways obtained at lung surgery[115] or at autopsy[195] were hyporesponsive to β-agonists, but this could have been due to prior therapy. In neither study, interestingly, was the tissue hyperresponsive to constrictor drugs. In some studies, a limited degree of hyposensitivity to β-agonist bronchodilation was induced in humans by β-agonist therapy, and this was not observed to enhance nonspecific airway responsiveness.[196, 197]

Because of the relative inaccessibility of airway tissue, many in vitro data have been collected on the β-adrenergic receptors of circulating leukocytes in asthmatics. These cells are subject to desensitization by β-agonist therapy,[192] but, in several studies, β-agonist therapy has been withheld for various periods. Some of these data show varying degrees of reduction in leukocyte response to β-adrenergic stimuli,[197-199] but other data show no reduction.[200-202] In one study,[199] the degree of leukocyte insensitivity to β-receptor stimulation was proportional to asthma severity (and/or possibly to the intensity of prior drug therapy). These data have been the subject of considerable debate; two additional points should be made. First, antigen bronchoprovocation in mild asthmatics with normal baseline lymphocyte β-receptors can result in reduced receptor number and function.[201] Thus, receptor abnormalities may be sequelae to, rather than causes of, airway responses. Second, it is important to note that there may not be a complete analogy between β-adrenergic receptors on leukocytes and those in airways. Intentional induction of lymphocyte hyposensitivity to β-agonists by prolonged treatment with terbutaline does not enhance bronchial responsiveness to histamine in asthmatics or normal individuals.[197] Nonspecific airway hyperresponsiveness in asthma is demonstrable in the presence of normal leukocyte β-receptor function.[202]

Atopic and asthmatic patients also have been found to have reduced sensitivity to the cardiovascular effects of the β-agonist isoproterenol.[203, 204] This phenomenon has been observed to correlate with degree of airway hyperresponsiveness in asthmatics after 30 days on no drugs.[202] These data are interesting in that vascular caliber may affect airway responsiveness, but their significance to airway function remains unknown.

Decreased Nonadrenergic Noncholinergic Dilation

Nonadrenergic noncholinergic (NANC) neural input that is inhibitory to airway smooth muscle exists in animals[205] and humans.[206] NANC bronchodilation can be demonstrated in humans in vivo in response to stimulation of respiratory irritant receptors. After cholinergic blockade, β-adrenergic blockade, and moderate pre-bronchoconstriction with an aerosolized mediator, such stimulation (either by inhalation of the hot-pepper extract capsaicin or mechanically) will produce bronchodilation in normal subjects.[207, 208] There is considerable evidence suggesting that vasoactive intestinal peptide (VIP) may be the primary NANC inhibitory neurotransmitter in the airways.[209] There is analogy here to the relaxant action of VIP in the gut, where it originally was described.[210] In vitro, VIP is much more potent than isoproterenol in relaxing human bronchi.[211] The peptide exists in nerve terminals associated with airway smooth muscle in humans and other species,[212] and receptors for it seem to exist in the human lung;[213] electric field stimulation of tracheobronchial tissue causes the release of VIP, and this release is blocked by the nerve poison tetrodotoxin.[214] In one study, inhaled VIP blunted to some extent hyperresponsiveness to inhaled histamine in asthmatics,[215] but the magnitude of this effect was much less impressive than that of in vitro bronchodilation by VIP. As Said[216] has suggested, this may be due to rapid degradation of exogenous VIP in the airways in vivo.

These findings naturally give rise to the idea that nonspecific airway hyperresponsiveness could be related to a deficiency in NANC inhibition of airway muscle. Data on this question are preliminary at present. One study[217] has found VIP neural immunoreactivity to be absent in asthmatic airways. This is a provocative finding, but whether it represents a pathogenetic phenomenon is unknown. Asthmatic airways seem to have intact NANC relaxation in vitro.[121] Mild asthmatics have been shown to have intact NANC or NANC-like bronchodilation in response to irritant stimuli after pharmacologic prebronchoconstriction.[218, 219] The definitive study of the role of VIP in the airways probably awaits the development of a more specific antagonist drug.

Increased Action of Sensory Neuropeptides

Stimulation of afferent receptors in the airways initiates reflexes that can cause smooth muscle contraction. increased production of airway liquid, and airway narrowing.[85] As noted earlier, nonspecific airway hyperresponsiveness in asthma seems to correlate with damage to the airway epithelium, at least in some studies. Such damage could render stimulation of the subepithelial afferent receptors by inhaled stimuli both more intense and less selective. Mechanisms of reflex airway narrowing, thus, are potentially germane to the pathogenesis of nonspecific airway hyperresponsiveness. Afferent activation could alter airway function in at least two ways. First, there likely would be augmented smooth muscle stimulation and liquid secretion via a vagal reflex arc, possibly mediated at the end-organs by a blend of cholinergic and noncholinergic stimulation.[85] Second, airway sensory neurons may have "response-enhancing" *efferent* actions of their own by means of so-called axon reflexes. The axon reflex[220] is a mechanism by which impulses originating at sensory nerve endings are felt to propagate antidromically along collateral branches of the same neuron, resulting in local release of neurochemical substances. Sensory nerves in the lungs can release putative neurotransmitter peptides in response to various stimuli,[221] and these peptides, if dispersed locally, could have significant effects on airway responsiveness. A number of aspects of the anatomy and physiology of sensory neuropeptides in the airways have been reviewed recently.[222, 223] We will summarize the relevant background material briefly.

The peptides of primary interest here are the so-called tachykinins or neurokinins, which are chemically related compounds felt to be derived from a common precursor.[223] These include substance P, neurokinin A (NKA), and neurokinin B (NKB). These are predominantly located, and frequently coexist, within sensory neurons, including those of the respiratory tract.[224, 225] Tachykinin-containing sensory nerve fibers are stimulated intensely (with subsequent neuropeptide depletion and prolonged insensitivity) by capsaicin.[226] Both capsaicin and exogenous tachykinins can cause noncholinergic, non–histamine-mediated contraction of airway smooth muscle, including human bronchial muscle in vitro;[227, 228] NKA is the most potent.[228] They also stimulate mucus secretion from human airways in vitro.[229] Of note, tachykinins can increase microvascular permeability and promote transudation of fluid and plasma proteins;[222, 230] they also can be potent bronchial vasodilators and increase bronchial blood flow.[142] It is primarily by virtue of these vascular effects that the putative local action of the tachykinins sometimes is called neurogenic inflammation. A nontachykinin, calcitonin gene-related peptide (CGRP), can coexist with substance P in neurons and also may be released in response to capsaicin.[237] It also has been shown to be an airway vasodilator,[142] but an airway smooth muscle effect has not been observed consistently.[231, 232] Other sensory neuropeptides of less-understood action also are found in the lung.[223]

If sensory neuropeptides are agents of airway hyperresponsiveness, epithelial damage may augment their actions by mechanisms other than those related to the exposure of sensory nerve endings already mentioned. Their effect also may be enhanced by loss of the hydrolytic membrane-associated enzyme, NEP, also discussed earlier.[233] Several animal studies also show that NEP inhibitors such as phosphoramidon and thiorphan can potentiate the airway effects of exogenous tachykinins, capsaicin, and nonselective vagus nerve stimulation.[234-237] From these results, it appears that NEP may be an important degradative enzyme for tachykinins in vivo, and thus limit their action. The NEP inhibitors used in these experiments can, to some extent, also inhibit the actions of angiotensin converting enzyme (ACE) (see later). In either case, however, the loss of membrane-associated peptidase activity via airway epithelial sloughing could potentiate the actions of the neuropeptides. Loss of NEP also might have impact on other possible substrates that may have effects on the lung, such as bradykinin (also an ACE substrate), endothelin, and atrial natriuretic peptide.[238, 239]

It is clear from an examination of the reported effects of the tachykinins how their axonal release could heighten airway responsiveness through effects on smooth muscle, luminal fluid, and the airway vasculature. The true relevance of this, however, remains to be determined. Analysis of the data is complicated by a number of issues. There is significant apparent interspecies variability in tachykinin physiology. Whereas guinea pigs, under the appropriate conditions, show significant tachykinin-related bronchoconstriction,[240, 241] rat airways seem relatively insensitive in vitro and in vivo.[222] There also seems to be regional heterogeneity in the action of tachykinins in the respiratory tract. In the presence of adrenergic and cholinergic blockade, the typical response of guinea pig bronchi to electric field stimulation is narrowing, which has been shown, at least in part, to be attributable to tachykinin release.[241] Tachykinins, on the other hand, do not seem to be involved in regulation of guinea pig tracheal mechanics in vivo,[240] where the typical response to electrical stimulation under similar conditions is relaxation.[241] These differences may reflect the relative importance of excitatory peptide (? tachykinin) effects vs. inhibitory peptide (? VIP) effects in different airways under conditions of generalized neural activation. Human airways, as noted above, can contract in response to capsaicin in vitro. When electrically stimulated, they respond in one study with only weak cholinergic contraction[227] and in other studies with NANC or NANC-like relaxation.[242, 243] Inhaled capsaicin appears to cause either moderate ipratropium-antagonized bronchial narrowing or no narrowing in human subjects.[244, 245] In fact, after prior bronchial narrowing with inhaled leukotriene D_4 (LTD$_4$), inhaled capsaicin seems to cause a NANC or NANC-like bronchodilation in both normal individuals and asthmatics.[218, 246] Inhaled substance P has not been observed to have an airway effect in normal individuals or asthmatics,[247, 248] although this may represent rapid degradation of the peptide in vivo, as the more-potent NKA did cause bronchoconstriction in asthmatics.[248] Nonspecific hyperresponsiveness after tachykinin exposure was not evaluated in these studies. In two guinea pig experiments, acute NEP inhibition did not result in airway hyperresponsiveness to inhaled muscarinic agonists,[235, 249] despite enhanced responsiveness to inhaled substance P.

When NEP was detected in the brain, it initially was thought to be a close analogue of ACE.[238] The enzymes actually are distinct in many ways, but they are both zinc-containing, membrane-associated peptidases. They also often are found together in tissues and share amino acid residues in their zinc-binding, substrate-binding, and catalytic sites.[250] ACE can cleave substance P (at bonds different from those at which substance P is hydrolyzed by NEP) and, in some systems, ACE inhibition has been observed to block the inactivation of substance P.[251] In this light, it is interesting to note that a minority of patients treated with ACE inhibitors[252, 253] develop cough and nonspecific airway hyperresponsiveness. Studies in guinea pigs have shown increased airway responsiveness to intravenous substance P in the presence of the ACE inhibitor captopril; captopril also was observed to cause a mild but significant increase in methacholine responsiveness.[249] If ACE is an important degradative enzyme for airway neuropeptides, then ACE inhibitor–induced airway hyperresponsiveness in man may be the result of increased levels of tachykinins. This mechanism may be limited to substance P, as captopril has not been observed to increase airway responsiveness in guinea pigs to intravenous NKA and NKB.[254] It is possible that some of the aforementioned effects of NEP inhibition in the airways may be due in part to ACE inhibition. The commonly used NEP inhibitors are not completely specific and inhibit ACE to varying degrees; for example, thiorphan has been observed to inhibit NEP only roughly threefold to 30-fold as potently as it does ACE.[255] The common ACE inhibitors are more selective for ACE than are the NEP inhibitors for NEP; for example, captopril inhibits ACE 50,000-fold more potentially than it does NEP.[255] In the rat kidney, however, chronic ACE inhibition has been observed to lead to significant decreases in the activity of NEP.[256] If such an effect also occurs in the lung, it represents another mechanism by which ACE inhibitors could alter airway responsiveness through allowing accumulation of tachykinins.

Altered Parasympathetic Function

Stimulation of the vagi can cause cholinergic bronchial narrowing,[257] and parasympathetic effects contribute to resting smooth muscle tone in normal airways.[258, 259] Thus, it is plausible that cholinergic hyperfunction could increase one's sensitivity to nonspecific airway stimuli. This is a theoretical explanation for the fact that cholinergic antagonists can inhibit, to varying degrees, broncho-constriction in response to stimuli as diverse as histamine, cold air inhalation, and psychological suggestion.[260–264] Asthmatics tend to have exaggerated cardiovas-cular responses to vagal maneuvers, and these responses correlate roughly with airway responsiveness to exercise.[265] Many of these examples may represent simply increased afferent activation of normal cholinergic pathways, but the existence of nonspecific hyperresponsiveness to direct muscarinic receptor ago-nists such as methacholine could imply that cholinergic function is not intrinsi-cally normal.

The physiology of the three muscarinic receptor types (M_1, M_2, M_3) in the air-ways has been reviewed recently.[266] To summarize, vagal impulses are translated into airway muscle contraction by M_3-receptors present on the smooth muscle. M_2-receptors provide feedback inhibition; they are presynaptic relative to the nerve–smooth muscle complex, and reduce smooth muscle stimulation. M_1-recep-tors in human airways are felt to have a tonic potentiating influence on cholinergic transmission via ganglionic effects. Defects in each of these receptor types could lead to nonspecific airway hyperresponsiveness.

An increase in the number, binding, or response coupling of M_3-receptors on airway smooth muscle could result in heightened smooth muscle responsiveness to a stimulus pharmacologically acting via these receptors either directly (e.g., methacholine) or indirectly (e.g., by activation of vagal reflexes). If this were the case, however, one would expect isolated samples of the affected muscle to be hyperresponsive to M_3-receptor agonists in vitro. Experimental evidence does not bear this out,[70, 73] although these data are subject to the limitations of in vitro air-way data described earlier. Since the advent of heart/lung and lung transplanta-tion, it has been noted that such transplant recipients frequently have nonspecific hyperresponsiveness to inhaled methacholine.[267, 268] Since the allograft tissue is assumed to be denervated, this hyperresponsiveness has been attributed to post-denervation M_3-receptor supersensitivity. A recent study[269] examined allograft tis-sue removed from patients undergoing a second transplant. The in vitro respon-siveness of the airways to acetylcholine and the numbers and binding characteris-tics of cholinergic receptors found there were no different from surgical control individuals. The frequency responses of the graft airways to electrical stimulation was no different from control patients, suggesting the presence of intact postganglionic nerve terminals.

The actions of presynaptic inhibitory M_2-autoreceptors on parasympathetic nerves may blunt endogenous stimulation of the M_3-receptor population. Thus, M_2-hypofunction could result in nonspecific airway hyperresponsiveness. The classic muscarinic agonist pilocarpine, at certain doses, has been shown in animals to antagonize changes in lung mechanics caused by vagal stimulation,[270, 271] and from this it has been inferred that the drug is acting as a selective M_2-agonist.[272] In atopic nonasthmatics whose airways are responsive to inhaled sulfur dioxide, treatment with inhaled pilocarpine (interestingly, in a dose that independently causes some bronchoconstriction) blunts this response.[273] It failed to do this in mild asthmatics, who were more sensitive to the constricting effects of both substances. Pilocarpine can have significant efferent cholinergic effects (e.g., bronchoconstriction, sweating, miosis, piloerection) in both animals and humans,[271, 274] so both positive and negative findings must be interpreted cautiously with respect to the M_2-receptor.

Understanding of the M_1-receptor is limited as yet, and there are few data as to its effects on airway function. A putative specific antagonist (pirenzepine) exists,[275] and this should facilitate analysis. One study has shown that inhaled pirenzepine given to atopic humans can reduce nonspecific airway responsiveness to sulfur dioxide.[276] It did not reduce responsiveness to methacholine, implying that the result was not due to incidental M_3-receptor blockade. This also may mean that the importance of M_1-receptor phenomena is limited to certain forms of airway hyperresponsiveness.

Altered Mediator Receptor Function

Presumably, mediators exert many of their actions by binding to specific receptors. Increased number/function of excitatory receptors or decreased number/function of inhibitory receptors could result in airway hyperresponsiveness. Current understanding of the receptors for most mediators is limited,[277, 278] but a significant amount of information exists concerning histamine receptors. Histamine receptors (types H_1, H_2, and H_3) are the subject of a recent extensive review.[279] For this discussion, we will summarize briefly the actions of histamine receptors that are likely to be locally relevant in the airways. H_1-receptor stimulation results in smooth muscle contraction and increased endothelial permeability with leakage of plasma proteins from vascular beds. H_2-receptor stimulation may serve a feedback inhibitory function, in that it seems to relax smooth muscle, inhibit histamine release from basophils and mast cells, and inhibit a variety of proinflammatory lymphocyte functions. The H_3-receptor, which in the brain appears to reduce histamine synthesis and release, also exists in the airways. Its significance in the airways is still being explored. Preliminary results imply that H_3-receptor stimulation may be able to inhibit postganglionic vagal neurotransmission[280] and blunt neurogenic inflammation.[281]

There is little evidence that airway smooth muscle H_1-receptors are abnormal in airway hyperresponsiveness, in that smooth muscle from hyperresponsive patients tends not to be hyperresponsive to histamine in vitro (see earlier.). In vivo observations also do not clearly support a role for H_1-stimulation in nonspecific hyperresponsiveness. Inhaled histamine does not seem to increase responsiveness to muscarinic agonists,[282] and has even been observed to decrease it.[283] Histamine H_1-receptor blockers do have some ability to attenuate nonspecific airway responsiveness, but in many studies this ability was disappointing in degree.[284, 285] Pretreatment with inhalation of the H_1-blocker chlorpheniramine, while reducing histamine hyperresponsiveness in asthmatics, does not blunt their hyperresponsiveness to methacholine.[286] More potent antihistamines subsequently have been developed,[279, 285] but studies of their effects on airway hyper-responsiveness must be interpreted carefully. Pharmacologic manipulations often prove to be less specific than initially thought. Antihistamines, for example, commonly have anticholinergic actions and anti-inflammatory effects unrelated to their actions at H_1-receptors.[285] While these mixed actions possibly may enhance the therapeutic efficacy of some of the drugs, they make them less enlightening as pharmacologic probes in the laboratory. Endothelial H_1-function has been studied intensely,[279] but no current evidence links abnormalities of it to airway function.

H_2-receptor hypofunction theoretically could augment responsiveness. Many data exist on the effect of pharmacologic H_2-blockade on airway physiology. Studies using various pharmacologic probes in sundry models have achieved inconsistent results, including increased responsiveness,[287–289] decreased responsiveness,[290] and, in the majority, no change in responsiveness.[291–294] It is possible that some of this confusion is due to nonspecificity on the part of the drugs in vivo. For example, while the in vitro potency of cimetidine as an H_2-blocker is some 560-fold greater than its potency as an H_1-blocker,[279] high-dose cimetidine has been observed to blunt guinea pig bronchoconstriction in response to subcutaneously administered histamine, presumably a direct H_1-receptor phenomenon.[289] Another possible confounding factor is the effect of the H_2-receptor on the bronchial circulation. H_2-receptor stimulation has been observed to dilate bronchial vessels and increase bronchial blood flow,[141] which, as noted, could have variable results. Thus, experimental data on the relationship between the H_2-receptor and airway function remain confusing. The issue may be clarified somewhat, however, by a clinical observation. Since the introduction of cimetidine therapy for peptide ulcer disease in 1977, H_2-blockers consistently have been among the most, if not the most, widely prescribed drugs in the world.[295] Given this, if H_2-receptor hypofunction were extremely critical to airway hyperresponsiveness, many reports of drug-related worsening of obstructive airway disease might be expected. Such apparently has not been the case. The preliminary findings on H_3-receptor function in the airways do not yet permit any more than speculation as to the role of that receptor in airway responsiveness.

Stimulus- and Response-Enhancing Mechanisms

Mediators

Soluble mediators are produced by a wide variety of cell types. Many of these cells are "classic" inflammatory ones, such as neutrophils, eosinophils, and lymphocytes. Others are less commonly thought of as inflammatory, such as mast cells, macrophages, and platelets. In fact, the ability to produce possible mediators of altered airway function is common to most of the 40-plus cell types found in the lungs (including epithelial and endothelial cells), but the quantity and type of mediator produced is often specific to a cell type and/or its location in the lungs. Mediators can stimulate contraction of smooth muscle, have multiple effects on the epithelium and vasculature, and attract or activate inflammatory cells. Changes in local concentrations of these substances, thus, could have both stimulus-enhancing and response-enhancing effects on airway responsiveness. The potential consequences of specific inflammatory changes in the airways are discussed in other parts of this chapter. A comprehensive summary of the interwoven physiologies and pharmacologies of inflammatory cells and mediators is well beyond the scope of this review. Complementary review material is available.[74, 296, 297]

Increased concentrations of various mediators, both at baseline and in response to certain nonspecific stimuli, have been observed in subjects with hyperresponsive airways. These mediators include histamine,[298, 299] prostaglandins D_2 and $F_{2\alpha}$,[300] thromboxane,[301] leukotrienes $B_4/C_4/D_4/E_4$,[302] platelet activating factor (PAF),[303] neutrophil chemotactic factor,[304] and eosinophil major basic protein.[298] Increased concentrations of mediators could be simply the result of "mass action" in that asthmatics tend to have increased numbers of several types of inflammatory cells in the respiratory tract.[74] Interestingly, inflammatory cells in asthmatics also may be excessively prone to release mediators on a cell-for-cell basis after nonantigenic stimulation. For example, samples of heterogeneous leukocytes and of purified eosinophils from asthmatics appear to have exaggerated release of histamine and leukotriene C_4, respectively, after stimulation by calcium ionophore, and this release seems to correlate with nonspecific airway hyperresponsiveness.[69, 305]

Nonspecific airway hyperresponsiveness could result from increased concentrations of mediators before ("preprovocation") and/or after ("postprovocation") the nonspecific stimulus in question. The postprovocation concept is the simpler of the two. Here, the nonspecific airway stimulus is one that itself provokes mediator release. In the presence of increased numbers and/or increased activity of inflammatory cells, heightened airway narrowing could result. Several studies suggest a relationship between postprovocation release of various mediators and an exaggerated response to a nonspecific airway stimulus.[299, 300, 302, 304] These data must be interpreted with caution, however. Quantification of mediators can be problematic in terms of technical aspects of sample collection and analysis and in terms of the relevance of the samples obtained to the local concentrations of mediators at the reactive site. The magnitude of hyperresponsiveness in some of these studies has not correlated with the magnitude of apparent postprovocation mediator release.[299, 302]

Postprovocation increases in mediator concentrations are unlikely to be a necessary element of airway hyperresponsiveness. Such increases typically are observed using certain stimuli, such as exercise, hyperpnea, and hyperosmolarity, which seem to be particularly efficient at causing mediator release.[306, 307] Other nonspecific stimuli, such as inhaled methacholine, have been observed to increase mediator concentrations less consistently,[308-310] even though hyperresponsiveness to exercise and methacholine tend to correlate.[311, 312] Hyperresponsiveness, instead, may result in many situations from increased preprovocation mediator release, i.e., from a "priming" mechanism. For the purposes of this discussion, priming will refer to the ability of a mediator to enhance responsiveness of the airways to a subsequent unrelated stimulus. The priming concentration of the mediator may or may not cause an airway response itself; it it does, the response to it and to the subsequent stimulus will be supra-additive. Priming could occur via subacute, chronic, or even intermittent increases in preprovocation mediator release. Several lines of evidence imply that this may occur. First, and probably most difficult to interpret, are studies in which nonspecific hyperresponsiveness in asthmatics seems to relate to baseline concentrations of histamine, with or without accompanying cyclooxygenase products, in bronchoalveolar lavage fluid.[298, 300, 313] Although they are interesting, these data are subject to the potential problems of mediator sampling mentioned above. Second, increased nonspecific responsiveness to a subsequent unrelated stimulus can be seen in humans in some studies after a modest inhaled dose of various mediators, such as prostaglandin D_2 in asthmatics,[282] prostaglandin $F_{2\alpha}$ in normal individuals,[314] and PAF (see later). Third, in some cases, subacute inhibition of mediator synthesis decreases nonspecific hyperresponsiveness in asthmatics, whereas acute inhibition of mediator synthesis immediately before bronchoprovocation does not. This has been observed with acute[315] vs. subacute[315-317] administration of the thromboxane A_2 synthesis inhibitor OKY-046. These data imply that prior priming of the airways by thromboxane A_2, which should be unaffected by acute thromboxane A_2 synthesis inhibition, is of importance. Preprovocation mediator effects could be relevant to all nonspecific airway stimuli. In a sense, much of the evidence that airway inflammation leads to nonspecific hyperrespon-siveness (e.g., by epithelial damage and altered airway geometry) could be looked upon as a complex case of preprovocation priming of the airways by me-diators.

Thus, nonspecific hyperresponsiveness may relate to the enhanced release of multiple mediators. Which, if any, of these relationships are causative and which are simply correlative? Ideally, in identifying "the" mediator(s) of nonspecific hyperresponsiveness, one would like evidence that exogenous doses of a given mediator in vivo increase nonspecific responsiveness to other stimuli and that selective in vivo inhibition of that mediator's synthesis or action reduces nonspecific responsiveness. One must recognize a priori that interactions between mediators[318, 319] would complicate the mechanistic interpretation of the data.

The role of histamine in the genesis of nonspecific hyperresponsiveness was discussed in the immediately preceding section.

Cyclooxygenase inhibition has had variable effects in human studies, reducing histamine hyperresponsiveness in some,[320, 321] but having no effect on exercise hyperresponsiveness in others.[322, 323] Cyclooxygenase blockade also can increase specific airway responsiveness to antigen in humans[324] and, as is well known, aspirin provokes severe bronchoconstriction in some asthmatics.[325] This diversity of results may well reflect the complex potential effects of cyclooxygenase blockade. In addition to reducing synthesis of possible responsiveness-enhancers (thromboxane A_2, prostaglandin D_2, prostaglandin $F_{2\alpha}$), it will reduce the synthesis of possible responsiveness-decreasing products such as prostacyclin and E-series prostaglandins.[326-328] Additionally, cyclooxygenase blockade may promote synthesis of potentially responsiveness-increasing noncyclooxygenase products such as leukotrienes.[329] More consistent results have been obtained using specific inhibitors of enzymes "downstream" from cyclooxygenase. As noted previously, subacute administration of the thromboxane synthetase inhibitor OKY-046 has been shown to reduce nonspecific hyperresponsiveness in asthmatics.[315-317] It is interesting to note, in this light, that thromboxane A_2 may act as a secondary mediator in airway responses to other compounds, such as leukotrienes[318, 319] and PAF.[330] The role of thromboxane A_2 in altered airway function merits further study. If thromboxane A_2 were an essential mediator of airway responsiveness irrespective of other factors, however, aspirin would abolish hyperresponsiveness in all cases. The role of thromboxane A_2 probably will be understood fully only in terms of significant interactions between mediators in individual asthmatic subjects.

The 5-lipoxygenase pathway produces leukotriene B_4 and the sulfidopeptide leukotrienes C_4, D_4, and E_4. Exogenous leukotrienes can cause bronchoconstriction,[297] but their ability to cause nonspecific airway hyperresponsiveness remains controversial. Exogenous leukotriene B_4, a potent chemotactic factor, has been found to increase nonspecific responsiveness in dogs,[331] but it did not do so in normal humans,[332] albeit at a fairly low dose. Inhalation of leukotriene D_4 has been observed variably not to increase nonspecific responsiveness[333] and to increase maximal nonspecific response[334] in human subjects. Leukotriene E_4 increased responsiveness to inhaled histamine in asthmatics, but not in normal individuals.[335] A number of inconclusive studies have investigated the effect of putative 5-lipoxygenase inhibitors[316, 336] and leukotriene receptor blockers[337, 338] on nonspecific airway hyperresponsiveness. These may have suffered, however, from lack of potency of the studied drugs. More recent data are positive. The 5-lipoxygenase inhibitor A-64077 significantly blunted the responsiveness of asthmatics to cold, dry air.[339] In this study, 5-lipoxygenase inhibition was verified by in vitro ionophore stimulation of the subjects' blood. Also, the drug MK-571, which is felt to be a potent and highly selective sulfidopeptide leukotriene receptor antagonist,[340] inhibited the airway responsiveness of asthmatics to exercise.[341]

The role of PAF in altered airway function remains obscure. It is a theoretically compelling aspirant to the role of "important mediator" in nonspecific airway hyperresponsiveness because of its multiple potential effects, such as smooth muscle contraction, increased vascular permeability, and chemotactic recruitment of inflammatory cells.[342, 343] Exogenous PAF has been observed to cause prolonged increases in nonspecific hyperresponsiveness in normal humans,[344–346] but these results have not been reproduced by all investigators.[347–349] Asthmatics have not been observed to have a meaningful increase in responsiveness after inhaling PAF.[349, 350] A relationship between endogenous PAF and airway responsiveness has yet to be established, in that increased baseline concentrations of PAF in bronchoalveolar lavage fluid do not seem to be associated with nonspecific hyperresponsiveness in asthmatics.[303] Numerous drugs that are putative PAF antagonists exist, but sufficiently selective and potent agents may not have been developed yet to delineate the role of PAF in airway hyperresponsiveness. Initial trials in humans evaluating the effects of PAF antagonists on hyperresponsiveness are negative,[351–353] but, as in the cases of the new 5-lipoxygenase inhibitor and sulfidopeptide receptor antagonist, more potent agents may yield positive results.

There is an apparent relationship in some studies between release of the eosinophil major basic protein, which is cytotoxic to airway epithelium,[354, 355] and nonspecific airway hyperresponsiveness. A causal relationship can be hypothesized. The development of antagonists is complicated by the likely concurrent action of major basic protein and other cytotoxic proteins located in the granules of eosinophils, such as eosinophil cationic protein and eosinophil peroxidase.[356]

Aside from the observation of its release during exercise-induced bronchospasm, the idea that neutrophil chemotactic factor is a proinflammatory cause of nonspecific airway hyperresponsiveness remains hypothetical. Several other mediator-like substances plausibly may be involved in airway hyperresponsiveness, but in most cases this conclusion is significantly (or wholly) speculative. An interesting example of these is the intercellular adhesion molecule-1 (ICAM-1), a ligand for leukocyte adhesion receptors that seems to be required for cellular migration into inflamed tissues.[357] In sensitized monkeys, inhaled *Ascaris* antigen caused eosinophilic airway inflammation and methacholine hyperresponsiveness with increased expression of ICAM-1 on airway epithelial cells. Intravenous treatment with monoclonal anti–ICAM-1 antibody significantly blunted the airway eosinophilia and hyperresponsiveness.[357] Another candidate is tryptase, the primary proteolytic enzyme in mast cell secretory granules, which has been observed to increase the responsiveness of canine airway smooth muscle.[358] Inhaled bradykinin causes bronchoconstriction and cough in asthmatics, and their responsiveness to bradykinin is proportional to their responsiveness to inhaled histamine.[359] On the other hand, inhaled bradykinin does not seem to potentiate subsequent responsiveness to histamine or methacholine.[282] The vasoconstrictor peptide endothelin-1 is an extraordinarily potent bronchoconstrictor. The effect of intravenous endothelin-1 on lung resistance in rats seems to be maximal at a dose of 500 picomoles per kilogram.[360] Endothelin-1 also causes contraction of isolated human bronchi.[361] In two preliminary studies, intravenous[362] and aerosolized[363] endothelin have not been observed to induce nonspecific airway hyperresponsiveness in the guinea pig. Adenosine, which relaxes animal airway smooth muscle in vitro, can cause bronchoconstriction in asthmatics. The physiology and pharmacology of purines in asthma are complex issues that have been reviewed recently.[364] Briefly, a role for endogenous adenosine in airway hyperresponsiveness is not well supported by current evidence. There seems to be only an indistinct relationship between responsiveness to adenosine and to methacholine,[365] although the correlation between adenosine and histamine responsiveness is closer.[366] Exogenous adenosine does not increase responsiveness to histamine in asthmatics.[367]

We will not address further the question of the relative roles of individual inflammatory cell types in nonspecific hyperresponsiveness. Evidence of varying degrees of completeness can be found to implicate all of the mediator-producing cells mentioned at the opening of this section. The reader once again is referred to the complementary reviews cited earlier. Interpretation of many of these studies is confounded by the limitations of experimental design, including problems of sampling and the difficulty of manipulating the function of one cell type while not affecting the function of others. Also, as is true of the mediators themselves, the interactions between cells and between mediators and cells in an intact system may be more important than the action of individual cell types.

Altered Secretion and Mucociliary Clearance

The combination of increased secretion and decreased mucociliary clearance could increase airway responsiveness by a response-enhancing increase in fluid within the airway lumen and a stimulus-enhancing increase in the time that inhaled stimuli, inflammatory cells, and mediators are allowed to dwell within the lumen.

Secretory elements usually are enlarged and/or more numerous in asthmatic airways both in vivo and postmortem.[88, 90, 102] There is considerable variability in the volume, composition, and viscosity of airway secretions produced by asthmatics,[368, 369] ranging from minimal watery mucus to copious tenacious phlegm. Many of the chemical mediators that can narrow airways can stimulate mucus secretion also,[370] but most asthma patients do not produce much mucus, a fact that has impaired the study of the relationship between airway secretions and hyperresponsiveness.[371] The majority of patients, however, do report that their periods of heaviest secretion coincide with their worst symptoms or occur during the recovery period.[372] Also, diffuse bronchial obstruction by mucous plugs is a consistent postmortem finding in cases of fatal asthma.[88]

Asthmatics seem to have impaired mucociliary clearance,[373] even when they are clinically well.[374] In the allergic sheep model,[375] the decrement in mucociliary clearance after allergen exposure outlasts the gross lung mechanics changes by days, and thus could act as a promoter of nonspecific hyperresponsiveness at a time well-removed from the initial stimulus exposure. There is evidence that mediators such as leukotrienes[376] and the eosinophil major basic protein[355, 377] can retard clearance. Interestingly, histamine, which also stimulates secretion, has been observed to accelerate mucociliary clearance in asymptomatic asthmatics.[378]

Mucociliary clearance in asthma probably is slowed by several factors. The generally accepted model of the airway lining fluid[379] is that of a more viscous, glycoprotein-containing gel layer (mucus) that rides on a periciliary sol layer consisting primarily of water and small ions. The gel layer is secreted by airway submucosal glands and epithelial secretory (goblet) cells;[379] the sol layer is felt to be the product of transport of water and ions across the epithelium.[380] Ciliary action occurs primarily within the sol layer, but the tips of the cilia interact with the gel layer.[379] Thus, derangement of the rheologic properties of either layer could impair mucociliary function. The gel layer may be abnormally viscous in some hyperresponsive states, possibly due to abnormal polysaccharides and protein cross-links.[371, 381] Epithelial damage could result in disadvantageous changes in both the sol and gel layers. Damage could reduce the ability of the epithelium to transport water and ions and to act as a diffusion barrier to larger solutes. This could alter the content of the sol layer and also increase gel viscosity, as hydration of mucus is felt to be maintained, at least in part, by Donnan's equilibria across epithelia.[382] Plasma constituents, such as clotting factors, that have transuded from leaky, inflamed bronchial vessels, theoretically could impair the rheologic properties of both layers. Clearance could be reduced further by the loss of ciliated cells due to epithelial disruption. The question of whether ciliary motion per se is diminished in asthma in vivo is unresolved. Asthmatic sputum can contain a factor that reduces ciliary motility in explants of human bronchial epithelium.[383] On the other hand, allergen challenge of ciliated cells from sensitized sheep in vitro leads to increased ciliary activity, although with reduced net mucociliary clearance.[384]

Increased α-Adrenergic Function

α-Adrenergic receptors whose stimulation results in smooth muscle contraction exist in human and animal airways, although they are not common and can be difficult to demonstrate. For example, in general, their action has been observed only in diseased airways or after treatment of the tissue with inflammatory mediators.[385, 386] If so, however, it is reasonable to speculate that an inflammatory disease of the airways might enhance their effect in vivo. There also is evidence that asthmatics may have generalized α-adrenergic hyperreactivity, as their responsiveness to α-adrenergic stimuli at other autonomic end-organs, such as the pupils and blood vessels, seems to be increased.[387, 388] α-Adrenergic hyperfunction, possibly at excitatory α_1-receptors, could play a stimulus-enhancing role by providing a parallel pathway for airway smooth muscle stimulation. Excess bronchial vasoconstriction via α-receptors could be stimulus-enhancing in some cases if it resulted in impaired clearance of stimuli from the airways.

Some studies do show that α-adrenoreceptor agonists can cause bronchoconstriction in asthmatics.[389, 390] Blockade of α- or α_1-receptors, however, fails to improve asthmatics' pulmonary function in most studies.[391-393] The relationship of α-receptors to airway hyperresponsiveness per se is obscure. In one study, inhaling the α_1-agonist phenylephrine did not increase nonspecific hyperresponsiveness to methacholine in asthmatics.[394] Decreases in hyperresponsiveness to histamine and to exercise have been observed after α-receptor blockade.[395-397] These findings are difficult to interpret, however, in light of the confounding effects of some of the drugs used.[391] Most prominent among these effects is a tendency to cause reflex release of endogenous catecholamines; phenoxybenzamine and indoramin are also antihistamines. Of note, prazosin, which is felt to be a rather "clean" α_1-blocking drug, has been observed to have only a weak effect on exercise-induced bronchoconstriction.[398] With respect to the vasoconstrictor effects of α_1-adrenergic stimulation, it appears, as discussed earlier, that this action at times may decrease airway responsiveness.[21] As is true for many of the mechanisms that may account for airway hyperresponsiveness, α-adrenergic phenomena may be important only in some individuals and, even in those individuals, may have entirely different effects depending upon whether stimulation of airway muscle or of blood vessels is more influential in a given situation, and what the effect of vasoconstriction is in that situation.

CONCLUDING STATEMENT

We hope that the foregoing discussion, in addition to providing information, has given the reader a feeling for the complexity of nonspecific airway hyperresponsiveness. The phenomenon seems to be the product of multiple factors that can interact, and this interaction can take the form of either reinforcement or antagonism in various situations. Some data relevant to the mechanisms are more complete and more convincing than others, but the current body of findings does not permit the definite inclusion or exclusion of a particular mechanism. Furthermore, mechanisms that are not of great importance to the population of asthmatics as a whole may still be of significance in individual patients. It is this complexity that endows the continuing study of nonspecific hyperresponsiveness with value.

REFERENCES

1. Benatar SR: Fatal asthma. *N Engl J Med* 1986; 314:423–429.
2. Gross NJ: What is this thing called love?—or, defining asthma. *Am Rev Respir Dis* 1980; 121:203–204.
3. American Thoracic Society: Chronic bronchitis, asthma, and pulmonary emphysema. A statement by the Committee on Diagnostic Standards for Nontuberculous Respiratory Disease. *Am Rev Respir Dis* 1962; 85:762–768.
4. Boushey HA, Holtzman MJ, Sheller JR, et al: State of the art: Bronchial hyperreactivity. *Am Rev Respir Dis* 1980; 121:389–413.

5. Leff AR: Endogenous regulation of bronchomotor tone. *Am Rev Respir Dis* 1988; 137:1198–1216.

6. Fraser RG, Paré JAP, Paré PD, et al: *Diagnosis of Diseases of the Chest,* 3rd ed, vol III. Philadelphia, WB Saunders, 1990, pp 2026–2039.

7. Coburn RF (ed): *Airway Smooth Muscle in Health and Disease.* New York, Plenum Press, 1989.

8. Widdicombe JG (chairman): International symposium on airway hyperreactivity. *Am Rev Respir Dis* 1991; 143:S1–S82.

9. Dunnill MS: *Pulmonary Pathology,* 2nd ed. Edinburgh, Churchill Livingstone, 1987.

10. Crawford ABH, Makowska M, Engel LA: Effect of bronchomotor tone on static mechanical properties of the lung and ventilation distribution in man. *J Appl Physiol* 1987; 63:2278–2285.

11. Juniper EF, Frith PA, Dunnett C, et al: Reproducibility and comparison of response to inhaled histamine and methacholine. *Thorax* 1978; 33:705–710.

12. Thomson NC, Roberts R, Bandouvakis J, et al: Comparison of bronchial responses to prostaglandin $F_{2\alpha}$ and methacholine. *J Allergy Clin Immunol* 1981; 68:392–398.

13. Adelroth E, Morris MM, Hargreave FE, et al: Airway responsiveness to leukotrienes C_4 and D_4 and to methacholine in patients with asthma and normal controls. *N Engl J Med* 1986; 315:480–484.

14. Chatham M, Bleecker ER, Smith PL, et al: A comparison of histamine, methacholine, and exercise airway reactivity in normal and asthmatic subjects. *Am Rev Respir Dis* 1982; 126:235–240.

15. Fleming WW, Westfall DP, De La Lande IS, et al: Log-normal distribution of equieffective doses of norepinephrine and acetylcholine in several tissues. *J Pharmacol Exp Ther* 1972; 181:339–345.

16. Snapper JR, Drazen JM, Loring SH, et al: Distribution of pulmonary responsiveness to aerosol histamine in dogs. *J Appl Physiol* 1978; 44:738–742.

17. Snapper JR, Lefferts PL, Stecenko AA, et al: Bronchial responsiveness to nonantigenic bronchoconstrictors in awake sheep. *J Appl Physiol* 1986; 61:752–759.

18. Cockroft DW, Berscheid BA, Murdock KY: Unimodal distribution of bronchial responsiveness to inhaled histamine in a random human population. *Chest* 1983; 83:751–754.

19. Cockcroft DW, Ruffin RE, Frith PA, et al: Determinants of allergen-induced asthma: Dose of allergen, circulating IgE antibody concentration, and bronchial responsiveness to inhaled histamine. *Am Rev Respir Dis* 1979; 120:1053–1058.

20. Dosman JA, Gomez SR, Zhou C: Relationship between airways responsiveness and the development of chronic obstructive pulmonary disease. *Med Clin North Am* 1990; 74:561–569.

21. Cabanes LR, Weber SN, Matran R, et al: Bronchial hyperresponsiveness to methacholine in patients with impaired left ventricular function. *N Engl J Med* 1989; 320:1317–1322.

22. Cockroft DW, Killian DN, Mellon JJ, et al: Bronchial reactivity to inhaled histamine: A method and clinical survey. *Clin Allergy* 1977; 7:235–243.

23. Fish JE: Bronchial challenge testing, in Middleton E Jr, Reed CR, Ellis EF, et al (eds): *Allergy: Principles and Practice,* 3rd ed. St Louis, CV Mosby, 1988, pp 447–460.

24. Chai H, Farr RS, Froehlich LA, et al: Standardization of bronchial inhalation challenge procedures. *J Allergy Clin Immunol* 1975; 56:323–327.

25. Sibbald B, Turner-Warwick M: Factors influencing the prevalence of asthma among first degree relatives of extrinsic and intrinsic asthmatics. *Thorax* 1979; 34:332–337.

26. Falliers CJ, de A Cardoso RR, Bane HN, et al: Discordant allergic manifestation in monozygotic twins: Genetic identity versus clinical, physiologic, and biochemical differences. *J Allergy* 1971; 47:207–219.

27. Zamel N, Leroux M, Vanderdoelen JL: Airway responses to inhaled methacholine in healthy nonsmoking twins. *J Appl Physiol* 1984; 56:936–939.

28. Ramsdale EH, Morris MM, Roberts RS, et al: Asymptomatic bronchial hyperresponsiveness in rhinitis. *J Allergy Clin Immunol* 1985; 75:573–577.

29. Empey DW, Laitinen LA, Jacobs L, et al: Mechanism of bronchial hyperreactivity in normal subjects following respiratory tract infection. *Am Rev Respir Dis* 1976; 113:131–139.

30. Orehek J, Massari JP, Gayrard P, et al: Effect of short-term, low-level nitrogen dioxide exposure on bronchial sensitivity of asthmatic patients. *J Clin Invest* 1976; 57:301–307.

31. Holtzman MJ, Cunningham JH, Sheller JR, et al: Effect of ozone on bronchial reactivity in atopic and non-atopic subjects. *Am Rev Respir Dis* 1979; 120:1059–1067.

32. Schoettlin CE, Landau E: Air pollution and asthmatic attacks in the Los Angeles area. *Public Health Rep* 1961; 76:545–548.

33. Woolcock AJ, Salome CM, Yan K: The shape of the dose-response curve to histamine in asthmatic and normal subjects. *Am Rev Respir Dis* 1984; 130:71–75.

34. Alexander HL, Paddock R: Bronchial asthma: Response to pilocarpin and epinephrine. *Arch Intern Med* 1921; 27:184–191.

35. Curry JJ: Comparative action of acetyl-beta-methyl choline and histamine on the respiratory tract in normals, patients with hay fever, and subjects with bronchial asthma. *J Clin Invest* 1947; 26:430–438.

36. Killian D, Cockroft DW, Hargreave FE, et al: Factors in allergen induced asthma: Relevance of the intensity of the airways allergic reaction and non-specific bronchial reactivity. *Clin Allergy* 1976; 6:219–225.

37. Snapper JR, Braasch PS, Loring SH, et al: Comparison of the responsiveness to histamine and to *Ascaris suum* challenge in dogs. *Am Rev Respir Dis* 1980; 122:775–780.

38. Weiss ST, Tager IB, Weiss JW, et al: Airways responsiveness in a population sample of adults and children. *Am Rev Respir Dis* 1984; 129:898–902.

39. Woolcock AJ, Peat JK, Salome CM, et al: Prevalence of bronchial hyperresponsiveness and asthma in a rural adult population. *Thorax* 1987; 42:361–368.

40. Boucher RC, Paré PD, Hogg JC: Relationship between airway hyperreactivity and hyperpermeability in *Ascaris*-sensitive monkeys. *J Allergy Clin Immunol* 1979; 64:197–201.

41. Marsh WR, Irwin CG, Murphy KR, et al: Increases in airway reactivity to histamine and inflammatory cells in bronchoalveolar lavage after the late asthmatic response in an animal model. *Am Rev Respir Dis* 1985; 131:875–879.

42. Sotomayor H, Badier M, Vervloet D, et al: Seasonal increase of carbachol airway responsiveness in patients allergic to grass pollen: Reversal by corticosteroids. *Am Rev Respir Dis* 1984; 130:56–58.

43. Lam S, Wong R, Yeung M: Nonspecific bronchial reactivity in occupational asthma. *J Allergy Clin Immunol* 1979; 63:28–34.

44. Snapper JR: Inflammation and airway function: The asthma syndrome. *Am Rev Respir Dis* 1990; 141:531–533.

45. Pratter MR, Irwin RS: Is the demonstration of bronchial hyperreactivity the sine qua non for diagnosing symptomatic bronchial asthma? *Allergy Proc* 1989; 10:323–327.

46. Josephs LK, Gregg I, Mullee MA, et al: Nonspecific bronchial reactivity and its relationship to the clinical expression of asthma: A longitudinal study. *Am Rev Respir Dis* 1989; 140:350–357.

47. Hopp RJ, Townley RG, Biven RE, et al: The presence of airway reactivity before the development of asthma. *Am Rev Respir Dis* 1990; 141:2–8.

48. Britton WJ, Woolcock AJ, Peat JK, et al: Prevalence of bronchial hyperresponsiveness in children: The relationship between asthma and skin reactivity to allergens in two communities. *Int J Epidemiol* 1986; 15:202–209.

49. Pattemore PK, Asher MI, Harrison AC, et al: The interrelationship among bronchial hyperresponsiveness, the diagnosis of asthma, and asthma symptoms. *Am Rev Respir Dis* 1990; 142:549–554.

50. Cockroft DW, Hargreave FE: Airway hyperresponsiveness: Relevance of random population data to clinical usefulness. *Am Rev Respir Dis* 1990; 142:497–500.

51. Hopp RJ, Bewtra AK, Nair NM, et al: Specificity and sensitivity of methacholine inhalation challenge in normal and asthmatic children. *J Allergy Clin Immunol* 1984; 74:154–158.

52. Cockroft DW, Berscheid BA, Murdock KY, et al: Sensitivity and specificity of histamine PC-20 measurements in a random population. *J Allergy Clin Immunol* 1985; 75:151.

53. Banks DE, Barkman HW Jr, Butcher BT, et al: Absence of hyperresponsiveness to methacholine in a worker with methylene diphenyl diisocyanate (MDI)-induced asthma. *Chest* 1986; 89:389–393.

54. Hargreave FE, Ramsdale EH, Pugsley SO: Occupational asthma without bronchial hyperresponsiveness. *Am Rev Respir Dis* 1984; 130:513–515.

55. Hensley MJ, Scicchitano R, Saunders NA, et al: Seasonal variation in non-specific bronchial reactivity: A study of wheat workers with a history of wheat associated asthma. *Thorax* 1988; 43:103–107.

56. Irwin RS, Curley FJ, French CL: Chronic cough: The spectrum and frequency of causes, key components of the diagnostic evaluation, and outcome of specific therapy. *Am Rev Respir Dis* 1990; 141:640–647.

57. Bechtel JJ, Starr T III, Dantzker DR, et al: Airway hyperreactivity in patients with sarcoidosis. *Am Rev Respir Dis* 1981; 124:759–761.

58. Freedman PM, Ault B: Bronchial hyperreactivity to methacholine in farmers' lung disease. *J Allergy Clin Immunol* 1981; 67:59–63.

59. Juniper EF, Frith PA, Hargreave FE: Airway responsiveness to histamine and methacholine: Relationship to minimum treatment to control symptoms of asthma. *Thorax* 1981; 36:575–579.

60. Rackemann FM: *Clinical Allergy Particularly Asthma and Hay Fever.* New York, Macmillan, 1931.

61. Moreno RH, Hogg JC, Paré PD: Mechanics of airway narrowing. *Am Rev Respir Dis* 1986; 133:1171–1180.

62. Sterk PJ, Bel EH: Bronchial hyperresponsiveness: The need for a distinction between hypersensitivity and excessive airway narrowing. *Eur Respir J* 1989; 2:267–274.

63. Fleming WW, McPhillips JJ, Westfall DP: Post-junctional supersensitivity and subsensitivity of excitable tissue to drugs. *Ergeb Physiol* 1973; 68:55–119.

64. Kalsner S: A new approach to the measurement and classification of forms of supersensitivity of autonomic effector responses. *Br J Pharmacol* 1974; 51:427–434.

65. Fleming WW: Variable sensitivity of excitable cells: Possible mechanisms and biological significance. *Rev Neurosci* 1976; 2:43–90.

66. Westfall DP: Supersensitivity of smooth muscle, in Bülbring E, Brading AF, Jones AW, et al (eds): *Smooth Muscle: An Assessment of Current Knowledge.* Austin, University of Texas Press, 1981, pp 285–309.

67. Fleming W, Westfall DP: Adaptive supersensitivity, in Trendelenburg U, Weiner N (eds): *Handbook of Experimental Pharmacology,* vol 90/I. Berlin, Springer-Verlag, 1988, pp 509–559.

68. Sterk PJ, Timmers MC, Bel EH, et al: The combined effects of histamine and methacholine on the maximal degree of airway narrowing in normal humans *in vivo. Eur Respir J* 1988; 1:34–40.

69. Schauer U, Daume U, Müller R: Relationship between LTC_4 generation of hypodense eosinophils and bronchial hyperreactivity in asthmatic children. *Int Arch Allergy Appl Immunol* 1990; 92:82–87.

70. Taylor SM, Paré PD, Armour CL, et al: Airway reactivity in chronic obstructive pulmonary disease: Failure of in vivo methacholine responsiveness to correlate with cholinergic, adrenergic, or nonadrenergic responses *in vitro. Am Rev Respir Dis* 1985; 132:30–35.

71. Vincenc KS, Black JL, Yan K, et al: Comparison of *in vivo* and *in vitro* responses to histamine in human airways. *Am Rev Respir Dis* 1983; 128:875–879.

72. Armour CL, Lazar NM, Schellenberg RR, et al: A comparison of *in vivo* and *in vitro* human airway reactivity to histamine. *Am Rev Respir Dis* 1984; 129:907–910.

73. Roberts J, Raeburn D, Rodger IW, et al: Comparison of in vivo airway responsiveness and in vitro smooth muscle sensitivity to methacholine in man. *Thorax* 1984; 39:837–843.

74. Djukanović R, Roche WR, Wilson JW, et al: Mucosal inflammation in asthma. *Am Rev Respir Dis* 1990; 142:434–457.

75. Ruffin RE, Dolovich MB, Wolff RK, et al: The effects of preferential deposition of histamine in the human airway. *Am Rev Respir Dis* 1978; 117:485–492.

76. Lesouëf PN, Geelhoed GC, Turner DJ, et al: Response of normal infants to inhaled histamine. *Am Rev Respir Dis* 1989; 139:62–66.

77. Geller DE, Morgan WJ, Cota KA, et al: Airway responsiveness to cold, dry air in normal infants. *Pediatr Pulmonol* 1988; 4:90–97.

78. Brown R, Ingram RH Jr, Wellman JJ, et al: Effects of intravenous histamine on pulmonary mechanics in non-asthmatic and asthmatic subjects. *J Appl Physiol* 1977; 42:221–227.

79. Brown R, Ingram RH Jr, McFadden ER Jr: Effects of intravenous prostaglandin $F_{2\alpha}$ on lung mechanics in non-asthmatic and asthmatic subjects. *J Appl Physiol* 1978; 44:150–155.

80. Chung KF, Snashall PD: Effect of prior bronchoconstriction on the airway response in normal subjects. *Thorax* 1984; 39:40–45.

81. Malo J-L, Pineau L, Cartier A, et al: Reference values of the provocative concentrations of methacholine that cause 6% and 20% changes in forced expiratory volume in one second in a normal population. *Am Rev Respir Dis* 1983; 128:8–11.

82. Ryan G, Latimer KM, Dolovich J, et al: Bronchial responsiveness to histamine: Relationship to diurnal variation of peak flow rate, improvement after bronchodilator, and airway calibre. *Thorax* 1982; 37:423–429.

83. Chung KF, Morgan B, Keyes SJ, et al: Histamine dose-response relationships in normal and asthmatic subjects: The importance of starting airway caliber. *Am Rev Respir Dis* 1982; 126:849–854.

84. Reid L, Jones R: Bronchial mucosal cells. *Fed Proc* 1979; 38:191–196.

85. Widdicombe JG: Vagal reflexes in the airways, in Kaliner MA, Barnes PJ (eds): *The Airways: Neural Control in Health and Disease.* New York, Marcel Dekker, 1988, pp 187–202.

86. Leff A, Munoz NM: Selective autonomic stimulation of canine trachealis with dimethylphenylpiperazinium. *J Appl Physiol* 1981; 51:428–437.

87. Golden JA, Nadel JA, Boushey HA: Bronchial hyperirritability in healthy subjects after exposure to ozone. *Am Rev Respir Dis* 1978; 118:287–294.

88. Dunnill MS: The pathology of asthma, with special reference to changes in the bronchial mucosa. *J Clin Pathol* 1960; 13:27–33.

89. Dunnill MS: *Pulmonary Pathology,* 2nd ed. Edinburgh, Churchill Livingstone, 1987, p 68.

90. Cutz E, Levison H, Cooper DM: Ultrastructure of airways in children with asthma. *Histopathology* 1978; 2:407–421.

91. Laitinen LA, Heino M, Laitinen A, et al: Damage of the airway epithelium and bronchial reactivity in patients with asthma. *Am Rev Respir Dis* 1985; 131:599–606.

92. Beasley R, Roche WR, Roberts JA, et al: Cellular events in the bronchi in mild asthma and after bronchial provocation. *Am Rev Respir Dis* 1989; 139:806–817.

93. Jeffery PK, Wardlaw AJ, Nelson FC, et al: Bronchial biopsies in asthma: An ultrastructural, quantitative study and correlation with hyperreactivity. *Am Rev Respir Dis* 1989; 140:1745–1753.

94. Boucher RC, Johnson J, Inoue S, et al: The effect of cigarette smoke on the permeability of guinea pig airways. *Lab Invest* 1980; 43:94–100.

95. Simani AS, Inoue S, Hogg JC: Penetration of the respiratory epithelium of guinea pigs following exposure to cigarette smoke. *Lab Invest* 1974; 31:75–81.

96. Hulbert WC, Walker DC, Jackson A, et al: Airway permeability to horseradish peroxidase in guinea pigs: The repair phase after injury by cigarette smoke. *Am Rev Respir Dis* 1981; 123:320–326.

97. Hulbert WM, McLean T, Hogg JC: The effect of acute airway inflammation on bronchial reactivity in guinea pigs. *Am Rev Respir Dis* 1985; 132:7–11.

98. Kennedy SM, Elwood RK, Wiggs BJR, et al: Increased airway mucosal permeability of smokers: Relationship to airways reactivity. *Am Rev Respir Dis* 1984; 129:143–148.

99. Hogg JC: Mucosal permeability and smooth muscle in asthma. *Med Clin North Am* 1990; 74:731–739.

100. Elwood RK, Kennedy S, Belzberg A, et al: Respiratory mucosal permeability in asthma. *Am Rev Respir Dis* 1983; 128:523–527.

101. O'Byrne PM, Dolovich M, Dirks R, et al: Lung epithelial permeability: Relation to nonspecific airway responsiveness. *J Appl Physiol* 1984; 57:77–84.

102. Dunnill MS, Massarella GR, Anderson JA: A comparison of the quantitative anatomy of the bronchi in normal subjects, in status asthmaticus, in chronic bronchitis, and in emphysema. *Thorax* 1969; 24:176–179.

103. Hossain S: Quantitative measurement of bronchial muscle in men with asthma. *Am Rev Respir Dis* 1973; 107:99–109.

104. Ebina M, Yaegashi H, Chiba R, et al: Hyperreactive site in the airway tree of asthmatic patients revealed by thickening of bronchial muscles: A morphometric study. *Am Rev Respir Dis* 1990; 141:1327–1332.

105. Sobonya RE: Quantitative structural alternation in long-standing allergic asthma. *Am Rev Respir Dis* 1984; 130:289–292.

106. Stephens NL: Airway smooth muscle. *Am Rev Respir Dis* 1987; 135:960–975.

107. Rodger IW: Calcium ions and contraction of airways smooth muscle, in Kay AB (ed): *Asthma: Clinical Pharmacology and Therapeutic Progress*. Oxford, Blackwell Scientific, 1986, pp 114–127.

108. Andersson K-E: Airway hyperreactivity, smooth muscle and calcium. *Eur J Respir Dis* 1983; 62(suppl 131):49–70.

109. Middleton E Jr: Calcium antagonists and asthma. *J Allergy Clin Immunol* 1985; 76:341–346.

110. Rasmussen H, Rasmussen JE: Calcium as intracellular messenger: From simplicity to complexity. *Curr Top Cell Regul* 1990; 31:1–109.

111. Antonissen LA, Mitchell RW, Kroeger EA, et al: Mechanical alterations of airway smooth muscle in a canine asthmatic model. *J Appl Physiol* 1979; 46:681–687.

112. Agrawal R, Daniel EE: Control of gap junction formation in canine trachea by arachidonic acid metabolites. *Am J Physiol* 1986; 250:C495–C505.

113. Stephens NL, Kong SK, Seow CY: Mechanisms of increased shortening of sensitized airway smooth muscle. *Prog Clin Biol Res* 1988; 263:231–254.

114. Roberts JA, Rodger IW, Thomson NC: Airway responsiveness to histamine in man: Effect of atropine on in vivo and in vitro comparison. *Thorax* 1985; 40:261–267.

115. Cerrina J, Le Roy Ladurie M, Labat C, et al: Comparison of human bronchial muscle responses to histamine *in vivo* with histamine and isoproterenol agonists *in vitro*. *Am Rev Respir Dis* 1986; 134:57–61.

116. Cerrina J, Labat C, Haye-Legrande I, et al: Human isolated bronchial muscle preparations from asthmatic patients: Effects of indomethacin and contractile agonists. *Prostaglandins* 1989; 37:457–469.

117. Ramsdale EH, Hargreave FE: Differences in airways responsiveness in asthma and chronic airflow obstruction. *Med Clin North Am* 1990; 74:741–751.

118. de Jongste JC, Sterk PJ, Willems RN, et al: Comparison of maximal bronchoconstriction *in vivo* and airway smooth muscle responses *in vitro* in non-asthmatic humans. *Am Rev Respir Dis* 1988; 138:321–326.

119. Schellenberg RR, Foster A: In vitro responses of human asthmatic airways and pulmonary vascular smooth muscle. *Int Arch Allergy Appl Immunol* 1984; 75:237–241.

120. de Jongste JC, Mons H, Bonta IL, et al: *In vitro* responses of airways from an asthmatic patient. *Eur J Respir Dis* 1987; 71:23–29.

121. Bai TR: Abnormalities in airway smooth muscle in fatal asthma. *Am Rev Respir Dis* 1990; 141:552–557.

122. Miller WS: *The Lung*, 2nd ed. Springfield, Illinois, Charles C Thomas, 1947, pp 14–16 and 28–34.

123. Armour CL, Diment LM, Black JL: Relationship between smooth muscle volume and contractile response in airway tissue. Isometric *versus* isotonic measurement. *J Pharmacol Exp Ther* 1988; 245:687–691.

124. Stephens NL, Van Niekerk W: Isometric and isotonic contractions in airway smooth muscle. *Can J Physiol Pharmacol* 1977; 55:833–838.

125. Shioya T, Munoz NM, Leff AR: Effect of resting smooth muscle length on contractile response in resistance airways. *J Appl Physiol* 1987; 62:711–717.

126. Shioya T, Munoz NM, Leff AR: Translation of contractile force to constriction in major diameter canine airways *in vivo*. *Am Rev Respir Dis* 1989; 140:687–694.

127. Ramsdale EH, Roberts RS, Morris MM, et al: Differences in responsiveness to hyperventilation and methacholine in asthma and chronic bronchitis. *Thorax* 1985; 40:422–426.

128. Freedman BJ: The functional geometry of the bronchi. *Bull Physiopathol Respir* 1972; 8:545–551.

129. James AL, Paré PD, Hogg JC: The mechanics of airway narrowing in asthma. *Am Rev Respir Dis* 1989; 139:242–246.

130. James AL, Paré PD, Hogg JC: Effects of lung volume, bronchoconstriction, and cigarette smoke on morphometric airway dimensions. *J Appl Physiol* 1988; 64:913–919.

131. James AL, Hogg JC, Dunn LA, et al: The use of the internal perimeter to compare airway size and to calculate smooth muscle shortening. *Am Rev Respir Dis* 1988; 138:136–139.

132. Yager D, Butler JP, Bastacky J, et al: Amplification of airway constriction due to liquid filling of airway interstices. *J Appl Physiol* 1989; 66:2873–2884.

133. Sellick H, Widdicombe JG: The activity of lung irritant receptors during pneumothorax, hyperpnoea and pulmonary vascular congestion. *J Physiol (Lond)* 1969; 203:359–381.

134. Roberts AM, Bhattacharya J, Schultz HD, et al: Stimulation of pulmonary vagal afferent C-fibers by lung edema in dogs. *Circ Res* 1986; 58:512–522.

135. Welsh MJ: Electrolyte transport by airway epithelia. *Physiol Rev* 1987; 67:1143–1184.

136. Bianco S, Pieroni MG, Refini RM, et al: Protective effect of inhaled furosemide on allergen-induced early and late asthmatic reactions. *N Engl J Med* 1989; 321:1069–1073.

137. Bianco S, Vaghi A, Robuschi M, et al: Prevention of exercise-induced bronchoconstriction by inhaled frusemide. *Lancet* 1988; 2:252–255.

138. Nichol GM, Alton EWFW, Nix A, et al: Effect of inhaled furosemide on metabisulfite- and methacholine-induced bronchoconstriction and nasal potential difference in asthmatic subjects. *Am Rev Respir Dis* 1990; 142:576–580.

139. Polosa R, Lau LCK, Holgate ST: Inhibition of adenosine 5'-monophosphate- and methacholine-induced bronchoconstriction in asthma by inhaled frusemide. *Eur Respir J* 1990; 3:665–672.

140. Knox AJ, Ajao P: Effect of frusemide on airway smooth muscle contractility in vitro. *Thorax* 1990; 45:856–859.

141. Long WM, Sprung CL, El Fawal H, et al: Effects of histamine on bronchial artery blood flow and bronchomotor tone. *J Appl Physiol* 1985; 59:254–261.

142. Widdicombe JG: The NANC system and airway vasculature. *Arch Int Pharmacodyn Ther* 1990; 303:83–99.

143. Persson CGA, Erjefält I, Andersson P: Leakage of macromolecules from guinea-pig tracheobronchial microcirculation. Effects of allergen, leukotrienes, tachykinins, and anti-asthma drugs. *Acta Physiol Scand* 1986; 127:95–105.

144. Kyle H, Robinson NP, Widdicombe JG: Changes in mucosal thickness in the dog trachea. *J Physiol (Lond)* 1985; 362:13P.

145. McFadden ER Jr: Hypothesis: Exercise-induced asthma as a vascular phenomenon. *Lancet* 1990; 335:880–883.

146. Fishman AP: Cardiac asthma—a fresh look at an old wheeze. *N Engl J Med* 1989; 320:1346–1348.

147. Wanner A: Circulation of the airway mucosa. *J Appl Physiol* 1989; 67:917–925.

148. Auld PAM, Rudolph AM, Golinko RJ: Factors affecting bronchial collateral flow in the dog. *Am J Physiol* 1960; 198:1166–1170.

149. Ohmichi M, Tagaki S, Nomura N, et al: Endobronchial changes in chronic pulmonary venous hypertension. *Chest* 1988; 94:1127–1132.

150. Wagner EM, Mitzner WA: Effect of left atrial pressure on bronchial vascular hemodynamics. *J Appl Physiol* 1990; 69:837–842.

151. Michel RP, Zocchi L, Rossi A, et al: Does interstitial lung edema compress airways and arteries? A morphometric study. *J Appl Physiol* 1987; 62:108–115.

152. Kelly L, Kolbe J, Mitzner W, et al: Bronchial blood flow affects recovery from constriction in dog lung periphery. *J Appl Physiol* 1986; 60:1954–1959.

153. Wagner EM, Mitzner WA: Bronchial circulatory reversal of methacholine-induced airway constriction. *J Appl Physiol* 1990; 69:1220–1224.

154. Plitman JD, Lefferts PL, Snapper JR: Effect of cardiogenic and non-cardiogenic pulmonary edema on airway responsiveness to aerosol histamine in awake sheep. *Am Rev Respir Dis* 1990; 141:A183.

155. Rolla G, Scappaticci E, Baldi S, et al: Methacholine inhalation challenge after rapid saline infusion in healthy subjects. *Respiration* 1986; 50:18–22.

156. Pison C, Malo J-L, Rouleau J-L, et al: Bronchial hyperresponsiveness to inhaled methacholine in subjects with chronic left heart failure at a time of exacerbation and after increasing diuretic therapy. *Chest* 1989; 96:230–235.

157. Sasaki F, Ishizaki T, Mifune J, et al: Bronchial hyperresponsiveness in patients with chronic congestive heart failure. *Chest* 1990; 97:534–538.

158. Coggeshall JW, Lefferts PW, Butterfield MJ, et al: Perilla ketone: A model of increased pulmonary microvascular permeability pulmonary edema in sheep. *Am Rev Respir Dis* 1987; 136:1453–1458.

159. Flavahan NA, Aarhus LL, Rimele TJ, et al: Respiratory epithelium inhibits bronchial smooth muscle tone. *J Appl Physiol* 1985; 58:834–838.

160. Hay DWP, Farmer SG, Raeburn D, et al: Airway epithelium modulates the reactivity of guinea-pig respiratory smooth muscle. *Eur J Pharmacol* 1986; 129:11-18.

161. Vanhoutte PM: Epithelium-derived relaxing factor(s) and bronchial reactivity. *Am Rev Respir Dis* 1988; 138:S24-S30.

162. Raeburn D, Hay DWP, Farmer SG, et al: Epithelium removal increases the reactivity of human isolated tracheal muscle to methacholine and reduces the effect of verapamil. *Eur J Pharmacol* 1986; 123:451-453.

163. Stuart-Smith K, Vanhoutte PM: Heterogeneity in the effects of epithelium removal in the canine bronchial tree. *J Appl Physiol* 1987; 63:2510-2515.

164. Fine JM, Gordon T, Sheppard D: Epithelium removal alters responsiveness of guinea pig trachea to substance P. *J Appl Physiol* 1989; 66:232-237.

165. Nadel JA: Some epithelial metabolic factors affecting smooth muscle. *Am Rev Respir Dis* 1988; 138:S22-S23.

166. Maggi CA, Patacchini R, Perretti F, et al: The effect of thiorphan and epithelium removal on contractions and tachykinin release by activation of capsaicin-sensitive afferents in the guinea-pig isolated bronchus. *Naunyn Schmiedebergs Arch Pharmacol* 1990; 341:74-79.

167. Sekizawa K, Tamaoki J, Nadel JA, et al: Enkephalinase inhibitor potentiates substance P- and electrically induced contraction in ferret trachea. *J Appl Physiol* 1987; 63:1401-1407.

168. Ilhan M, Sahin I: Tracheal epithelium releases a vascular smooth muscle relaxant factor: Demonstration by bioassay. *Eur J Pharmacol* 1986; 131:293-296.

169. Fernandes LB, Paterson JW, Goldie RG: Co-axial bioassay of a smooth muscle relaxant factor released from guinea-pig tracheal epithelium. *Br J Pharmacol* 1989; 96:117-124.

170. Szentivanyi A: The beta adrenergic theory of the atopic abnormality in bronchial asthma. *J Allergy* 1968; 42:203-232.

171. Carstairs JR, Nimmo AJ, Barnes PJ: Autoradiographic localisation of β-adrenoceptors in human lung. *Eur J Pharmacol* 1984; 105:189-190.

172. Goldie RG, Paterson JW, Spina D, et al: Classification of β-adrenoceptors in human isolated bronchus. *Br J Pharmacol* 1984; 81:611-615.

173. Langer I: The bronchoconstrictor action of propranolol aerosol in asthmatic subjects. *J Physiol (Lond)* 1967; 190:41P.

174. Richardson PS, Sterling GM: Effect of β-adrenergic receptor blockade on airway conductance and lung volume in normal and asthmatic subjects. *BMJ* 1969; 3:143-145.

175. Carpentiere G, Castello F, Marino S: Increased responsiveness to histamine after propranolol in subjects with asthma nonresponsive to the bronchoconstrictive effect of propranolol. *J Allergy Clin Immunol* 1988; 82:595-598.

176. Zaid G, Beall GN: Bronchial response to beta-adrenergic blockade. *N Engl J Med* 1966; 275:580-584.

177. Orehek J, Gayrard P, Grimaud C, et al: Effect of beta adrenergic blockade on bronchial sensitivity to inhaled acetylcholine in normal subjects. *J Allergy Clin Immunol* 1975; 55:164-169.

178. Tattersfield AE, Leaver DG, Pride NB: Effects of β-adrenergic blockade and stimulation on normal human airways. *J Appl Physiol* 1973; 35:613-619.

179. Richardson JB: Nerve supply to the lungs. *Am Rev Respir Dis* 1979; 119:785-802.

180. Warren JB, Keynes RJ, Brown MJ, et al: Blunted sympathoadrenal response to exercise in asthmatic subjects. *Br J Dis Chest* 1982; 76:147-150.

181. Barnes PJ, Brown MJ, Silverman M, et al: Circulating catecholamines in exercise and hyperventilation induced asthma. *Thorax* 1981; 36:435-440.

182. Gilbert IA, Lenner KA, McFadden ER Jr: Sympathoadrenal response to repetitive exercise in normal and asthmatic subjects. *J Appl Physiol* 1988; 64:2667-2674.

183. Griffiths J, Leung FY, Grzybowski S, et al: Sequential estimation of plasma catecholamines in exercise-induced asthma. *Chest* 1972; 62:527–533.

184. Morris HG, De Roche G, Earle MR: Urinary excretion of epinephrine and norepinephrine in asthmatic children. *J Allergy Clin Immunol* 1972; 50:138–145.

185. Sands MF, Douglas FL, Green J, et al: Homeostatic regulation of bronchomotor tone by sympathetic activation during bronchoconstriction in normal and asthmatic humans. *Am Rev Respir Dis* 1985; 132:993–998.

186. Assem ESK, Schild HO: Inhibition by sympathomimetic amines of histamine release induced by antigen in passively sensitized human lung. *Nature* 1969; 224:1028–1029.

187. Petersson BA: Sustained inhibition of antigen-induced histamine release from human lung by beta-2-adrenoceptor agonist terbutaline. *Allergy* 1984; 39:351–357.

188. Ind PW, Barnes PJ, Brown MJ, et al: Plasma histamine concentration during propranolol induced bronchoconstriction. *Thorax* 1985; 40:903–909.

189. Koëter GH, Meurs H, de Monchy JG, et al: Protective effect of disodium cromoglycate on propranolol challenge. *Allergy* 1982; 37:587–590.

190. Blecher M, Lewis S, Hicks JM, et al: Beta-blocking autoantibodies in pediatric bronchial asthma. *J Allergy Clin Immunol* 1984; 74:246–251.

191. Lefkowitz RJ: Beta-adrenergic receptors: Recognition and regulation. *N Engl J Med* 1976; 295:323–328.

192. Galant SP, Duriseti L, Underwood S, et al: Decreased beta-adrenergic receptors on polymorphonuclear leukocytes after adrenergic therapy. *N Engl J Med* 1978; 299:933–936.

193. Conolly ME, Greenacre JK: The lymphocyte β-adrenoceptor in normal subjects and patients with bronchial asthma: The effect of different forms of treatment on receptor function. *J Clin Invest* 1976; 58:1307–1316.

194. Busse WW, Bush RK, Cooper W: Granulocyte response *in vitro* to isoproterenol, histamine, and prostaglandin E₁ during treatment with beta-adrenergic aerosols in asthma. *Am Rev Respir Dis* 1979; 120:377–384.

195. Goldie RG, Spina D, Henry PJ, et al: *In vitro* responsiveness of human asthmatic bronchus to carbachol, histamine, β-adrenoceptor agonists and theophylline. *Br J Clin Pharmacol* 1986; 22:669–676.

196. Conolly ME, Tashkin DP, Hui KKP, et al: Selective subsensitization of beta-adrenergic receptors in central airways of asthmatics and normal subjects during long-term therapy with inhaled salbutamol. *J Allergy Clin Immunol* 1982; 70:423–431.

197. Tashkin DP, Conolly ME, Deutsch RI, et al: Subsensitization of beta-adrenoceptors in airways and lymphocytes of healthy and asthmatic subjects. *Am Rev Respir Dis* 1982; 125:185–193.

198. Parker CW, Smith JW: Alterations in cyclic adenosine monophosphate metabolism in human bronchial asthma: I. Leukocyte responsiveness to β-adrenergic agents. *J Clin Invest* 1973; 52:48–59.

199. Brooks SM, McGowan K, Bernstein IL, et al: Relationship between numbers of beta adrenergic receptors in lymphocytes and disease severity in asthma. *J Allergy Clin Immunol* 1979; 63:401–406.

200. Galant SP, Duriseti L, Underwood S, et al: Beta Adrenergic receptors of polymorphonuclear particulates in bronchial asthma. *J Clin Invest* 1980; 65:577–585.

201. Meurs H, Köeter GH, de Vries K, et al: The beta-adrenergic system and allergic bronchial asthma: Changes in lymphocyte beta-adrenergic receptor number and adenylate cyclase activity after an allergen-induced asthmatic attack. *J Allergy Clin Immunol* 1982; 70:272–280.

202. Davis PB, Simpson DM, Paget DL, et al: Beta-adrenergic responses in drug-free subjects with asthma. *J Allergy Clin Immunol* 1986; 77:871–879.

203. Shelhamer JH, Metcalf DD, Smith LJ, et al: Abnormal beta adrenergic responsiveness in allergic subjects: Analysis of isoproterenol-induced cardiovascular and plasma cyclic adenosine monophosphate responses. *J Allergy Clin Immunol* 1980; 66:52–60.

204. Shelhamer JH, Marom Z, Kaliner M: Abnormal beta-adrenergic responsiveness in allergic subjects: 2. The role of selective beta-2 adrenergic hyporeactivity. *J Allergy Clin Immunol* 1983; 71:57–71.

205. Coburn RF, Tomita T: Evidence for nonadrenergic inhibitory nerves in the guinea pig trachealis muscle. *Am J Physiol* 1973; 224:1072–1080.

206. Richardson J, Béland J: Nonadrenergic inhibitory nervous system in human airways. *J Appl Physiol* 1976; 41:764–771.

207. Ichinose M, Inoue H, Miura M, et al: Nonadrenergic bronchodilation in normal subjects. *Am Rev Respir Dis* 1988; 138:31–34.

208. Michoud M-C, Amyot R, Jeanneret-Grosjean A, et al: Reflex decrease of histamine-induced bronchoconstriction after laryngeal stimulation in humans. *Am Rev Respir Dis* 1987; 136:618–622.

209. Said SI: VIP in the airways, in Kaliner MA, Barnes PJ (eds): *The Airways: Neural Control in Health and Disease.* New York, Marcel Dekker, 1988, pp 395–416.

210. Crema A, del Tacca M, Frigo GM, et al: Presence of a non-adrenergic inhibitory system in the human colon. *Gut* 1968; 9:633–637.

211. Palmer JBD, Cuss FMC, Barnes PJ: VIP and PHM and their role in nonadrenergic inhibitory responses in isolated human airways. *J Appl Physiol* 1986; 61:1322–1328.

212. Dey RD, Shannon WA Jr, Said SI: Localization of VIP-immunoreactive nerves in airways and pulmonary vessels of dogs, cats, and human subjects. *Cell Tissue Res* 1981; 220:231–238.

213. Taton G, Delhaye M, Camus J-C, et al: Characterization of the VIP- and secretin-stimulated adenylate cyclase system from human lung. *Pflugers Arch* 1981; 391:178–182.

214. Matsuzaki Y, Hamasaki Y, Said SI: Vasoactive intestinal peptide: A possible transmitter of nonadrenergic relaxation of guinea pig airways. *Science* 1980; 210:1252–1253.

215. Barnes PJ, Dixon CMS: The effect of inhaled vasoactive intestinal peptide on bronchial reactivity to histamine in humans. *Am Rev Respir Dis* 1984; 130:162–166.

216. Said SI: VIP as a modulator of lung inflammation and airway constriction. *Am Rev Respir Dis* 1991; 143:S22–S24.

217. Ollerenshaw SL, Jarvis DL, Woolcock A, et al: Absence of immunoreactive vasoactive intestinal polypeptide from lungs of patients with asthma. *N Engl J Med* 1989; 320:1244–1248.

218. Lammers J-W, Minette P, McCusker MT, et al: Capsaicin-induced bronchodilation in mild asthmatic subjects: Possible role of nonadrenergic inhibitory system. *J Appl Physiol* 1989; 67:856–861.

219. Michoud M-C, Jeanneret-Grosjean A, Cohen A, et al: Reflex decrease in histamine-induced bronchoconstriction after laryngeal stimulation in asthmatic patients. *Am Rev Respir Dis* 1988; 138:1548–1552.

220. Burnstock G: Autonomic neural control mechanisms with special reference to the airways, in Kaliner MA, Barnes PJ (eds): *The Airways: Neural Control in Health and Disease.* New York, Marcel Dekker, 1988, pp 1–22.

221. Saria A, Martling C-R, Yan Z, et al: Release of multiple tachykinins from sensory nerves in the lung by bradykinin, histamine, dimethyl phenyl piperazinium, and vagal nerve stimulation. *Am Rev Respir Dis* 1988; 137:1330–1335.

222. Lundberg JM, Lundblad L, Ånggård A, et al: Bioactive peptides in capsaicin-sensitive C-fiber afferents of the airways: Functional and pathophysiological implications, in Kaliner MA, Barnes PJ (eds): *The Airways: Neural Control in Health and Disease.* New York, Marcel Dekker, 1988, pp 417–445.

223. Said S: Polypeptide-containing neurons and their function in airway smooth muscle, in Coburn RF (ed): *Airway Smooth Muscle in Health and Disease.* New York, Plenum Press, 1989, pp 55–76.

224. Hua X-Y, Theodorsson-Norheim E, Brodin E, et al: Multiple tachykinins (neurokinin A, neuropeptide A and substance P) in capsaicin-sensitive sensory neurons in the guinea pig. *Regul Pept* 1985; 13:1–19.

225. Lundberg JM, Hökfelt T, Martling C-R, et al: Substance P-immunoreactive sensory nerves in the lower respiratory tract of various mammals including man. *Cell Tissue Res* 1984; 235:251–261.

226. Buck SH, Burks TF: The neuropharmacology of capsaicin: Review of some recent observations. *Pharmacol Rev* 1986; 38:179–226.

227. Lundberg JM, Martling C-R, Saria A: Substance P and capsaicin induced bronchial smooth muscle contraction in human airways. *Acta Physiol Scand* 1983; 119:49–53.

228. Martling C-R, Theodorsson-Norheim E, Lundberg JM: Occurrence and effects of multiple tachykinins: Substance P, neurokinin A, neuropeptide K in human lower airways. *Life Sci* 1987; 40:1633–1643.

229. Rogers DF, Aursudkij B, Barnes PJ: Effects of tachykinins on mucus secretion in human bronchi in vitro. *Eur J Pharmacol* 1989; 174:283–286.

230. Persson CGA, Erjefält I A-L: Nonneural and neural regulation of plasma exudation in airways, in Kaliner MA, Barnes PJ (eds): *The Airways—Neural Control in Health and Disease.* New York, Marcel Dekker, 1988, pp 523–549.

231. Lundberg JM, Franco-Cereceda A, Hua X, et al: Co-existence of substance P and calcitonin gene-related peptide-like immunoreactivities in sensory nerves in relation to cardiovascular and bronchoconstrictor effects of capsaicin. *Eur J Pharmacol* 1985; 108:315–319.

232. Palmer JBD, Cuss FMC, Mulderry PK, et al: Calcitonin gene-related peptide is localised to human airway nerves and potently constricts human airway smooth muscle. *Br J Pharmacol* 1987; 91:95–101.

233. Nadel JA, Borson DB: Modulation of neurogenic inflammation by neutral endopeptidase. *Am Rev Respir Dis* 1991; 143:S33–S36.

234. Dusser DJ, Umeno E, Graf PD, et al: Airway neutral endopeptidase-like enzyme modulates tachykinin-induced bronchoconstriction in vivo. *J Appl Physiol* 1988; 65:2585–2591.

235. Thompson JE, Sheppard D: Phosphoramidon potentiates the increase in lung resistance mediated by tachykinins in guinea pigs. *Am Rev Respir Dis* 1988; 137:337–340.

236. Stimler-Gerard NP: Neutral endopeptidase-like enzyme controls the contractile activity of substance P in guinea pig lung. *J Clin Invest* 1987; 79:1819–1825.

237. Kohrogi H, Graf PD, Sekizawa K, et al: Neutral endopeptidase inhibitors potentiate substance P- and capsaicin-induced cough in awake guinea pigs. *J Clin Invest* 1988; 82:2063–2068.

238. Erdös EG, Skidgel RA: Neutral endopeptidase 24.11 (enkephalinase) and related regulators of peptide hormones. *FASEB J* 1989; 3:145–151.

239. Skolovsky M, Galron R, Kloog Y, et al: Endothelins are more sensitive than sarafotoxins to neutral endopeptidase: Possible physiological significance. *Proc Natl Acad Sci U S A* 1990; 87:4702–4706.

240. Martling C-R, Saria A, Andersson P, et al: Capsaicin pretreatment inhibits vagal cholinergic and non-cholinergic control of airway mechanics in the guinea pig. *Naunyn Schmiedebergs Arch Pharmacol* 1984; 325:343–348.

241. Karlsson JA: In vivo and in vitro studies of the non-adrenergic non-cholinergic nervous system of the guinea-pig airways. *Arch int Pharmacodyn Ther* 1986; 280(suppl 2):191–207.

242. Taylor SM, Paré PD, Schellenberg RR: Cholinergic and nonadrenergic mechanisms in human and guinea pig airways. *J Appl Physiol* 1984; 56:958–965.

243. de Jongste JC, Mons H, Bonta IL, et al: Nonneural components in the response of fresh human airways to electric field stimulation. *J Appl Physiol* 1987; 63:1558–1566.

244. Collier JG, Fuller RW: Capsaicin inhalation in man and the effects of sodium cromoglycate. *Br J Pharmacol* 1984; 81:113–117.

245. Fuller RW, Dixon CMS, Barnes PJ: Bronchoconstrictor response to inhaled capsaicin in humans. *J Appl Physiol* 1985; 58:1080–1084.

246. Lammers J-W, Minette P, McCusker MT, et al: Nonadrenergic bronchodilator mechanisms in normal human subjects in vivo. *J Appl Physiol* 1988; 64:1817–1822.

247. Fuller RW, Maxwell DL, Dixon CMS, et al: Effects of substance P on cardiovascular and respiratory function in subjects. *J Appl Physiol* 1987; 62:1473–1479.

248. Joos G, Pauwels R, van der Straeten M: Effect of inhaled substance P and neurokinin A on the airways of normal and asthmatic subjects. *Thorax* 1987; 42:779–783.

249. Shore SA, Stimler-Gerard NP, Coats SR, et al: Substance P-induced bronchoconstriction in the guinea pig: Enhancement by inhibitors of neutral metalloendopeptidase and angiotensin-converting enzyme. *Am Rev Respir Dis* 1988; 137:331–336.

250. Erdös EG, Skidgel RA: Renal metabolism of angiotensin I and II. *Kidney Int* 1990; 38(suppl 30):S24–S27.

251. Skidgel RA, Defendini R, Erdös EG: Angiotensin converting enzyme and its role in neuropeptide metabolism, in Turner AJ (ed): *Neuropeptides and Their Peptidases*. Chichester, Ellis Horwood, 1987, pp 165–182.

252. Lindgren BR, Rosenqvist U, Ekström T: Increased bronchial reactivity and potentiated skin responses in hypertensive subjects suffering from coughs during ACE-inhibitor therapy. *Chest* 1989; 95:1225–1230.

253. Kaufman J, Casanova JE, Riendl P, et al: Bronchial hyperreactivity and cough due to angiotensin-converting enzyme inhibitors. *Chest* 1989; 95:544–548.

254. Shore SA, Drazen JM: Degradative enzymes modulate airway responses to intravenous neurokinins A and B. *J Appl Physiol* 1989; 67:2504–2511.

255. Thorsett ED, Wyvratt MJ: Inhibition of zinc peptidases that hydrolyze neuropeptides, in Turner AJ (ed): *Neuropeptides and Their Peptidases*. Chichester, Ellis Horwood, 1987, pp 229–292.

256. Drummer OH, Kourtis S, Johnson H: Effect of chronic enalapril treatment on enzymes responsible for the catabolism of angiotensin I and formation of angiotensin II. *Biochem Pharmacol* 1990; 39:513–518.

257. Colebatch HJH, Halmagyi DFJ: Effect of vagotomy and vagal stimulation on lung mechanics and circulation. *J Appl Physiol* 1963; 18:881–887.

258. Severinghaus JW, Stupfel M: Respiratory dead space increase following atropine in man, and atropine, vagal or ganglionic blockade and hypothermia in dogs. *J Appl Physiol* 1955; 8:81–87.

259. Widdicombe JG: Action potentials in parasympathetic and sympathetic efferent fibres to the trachea and the lungs of dogs and cats. *J Physiol* 1966; 186:56–88.

260. Holtzman MJ, Sheller JR, Dimeo MA, et al: Effect of ganglionic blockade on bronchial reactivity in atopic subjects. *Am Rev Respir Dis* 1980; 122:17–25.

261. Sheppard D, Epstein J, Skoogh BE, et al: Variable inhibition of histamine-induced bronchoconstriction by atropine in subjects with asthma. *J Allergy Clin Immunol* 1984; 73:82–87.

262. O'Byrne PM, Thomson NC, Latimer KM, et al: The effect of inhaled hexamethonium bromide and atropine sulphate on airway responsiveness to histamine. *J Allergy Clin Immunol* 1985; 76:97–103.

263. Sheppard D, Epstein J, Holtzman MJ, et al: Effect of route of atropine delivery on bronchospasm from cold air and methacholine. *J Appl Physiol* 1983; 54:130–133.

264. McFadden ER Jr, Luparello T, Lyons HA, et al: The mechanism of action of suggestion in the induction of acute asthma attacks. *Psychosom Med* 1969; 31:134–143.

265. Kallenbach JM, Webster T, Dowdeswell R, et al: Reflex heart rate control in asthma: Evidence of parasympathetic overactivity. *Chest* 1985; 87:644–648.

266. Barnes PJ: Muscarinic receptors in airways: Recent developments. *J Appl Physiol* 1990; 68:1777–1785.

267. Banner NR, Heaton R, Hollingshead L, et al: Bronchial reactivity to methacholine after combined heart-lung transplantation. *Thorax* 1988; 43:955–959.

268. Maurer JR, McLean PA, Cooper JD, et al: Airway hyperreactivity in patients undergoing lung and heart/lung transplantation. *Am Rev Respir Dis* 1989; 139:1038–1041.

269. Stretton CD, Mak JCW, Belvisi MG, et al: Cholinergic control of human airways *in vitro* following extrinsic denervation of the human respiratory tract by heart-lung transplantation. *Am Rev Respir Dis* 1990; 142:1030–1033.

270. Blaber LC, Fryer AD, Maclagan J: Neuronal muscarinic receptors attenuate vagally-induced contraction of feline bronchial smooth muscle. *Br J Pharmacol* 1985; 86:723–728.

271. Fryer AD, Maclagan J: Muscarinic inhibitory receptors in pulmonary parasympathetic nerves in the guinea-pig. *Br J Pharmacol* 1984; 83:973–978.

272. Minette PA, Barnes PJ: Prejunctional inhibitory muscarinic receptors on cholinergic nerves in human and guinea pig airways. *J Appl Physiol* 1988; 64:2532–2537.

273. Minette PAH, Lammers J-W, Dixon CMS, et al: A muscarinic agonist inhibits reflex bronchoconstriction in normal but not in asthmatic subjects. *J Appl Physiol* 1989; 67:2461–2465.

274. Taylor P: Muscarinic agonists, in Gilman AG, Rall TW, Nies AS, et al (eds): *Goodman and Gilman's The Pharmacological Basis of Therapeutics,* 8th ed. New York, Pergamon, 1990, pp 122–130.

275. Brown JH: Atropine, scopolamine, and related antimuscarinic drugs, in Gilman AG, Rall TW, Nies AS, et al (eds): *Goodman and Gilman's The Pharmacological Basis of Therapeutics,* 8th ed. New York, Pergamon, 1990, pp 150–165.

276. Lammers J-W, Minette P, McCusker M, et al: The role of pirenzepine-sensitive (M_1) muscarinic receptors in vagally mediated bronchoconstriction in humans. *Am Rev Respir Dis* 1989; 139:446–449.

277. Goldie RG: Receptors in asthmatic airways. *Am Rev Respir Dis* 1990; 141:S151–S156.

278. Barnes PJ: Cell-surface receptors in airway smooth muscle, in Coburn RF (ed): *Airway Smooth Muscle in Health and Disease.* New York, Plenum Press, 1989, pp 77–97.

279. Hill SJ: Distribution, properties, and functional characteristics of three classes of histamine receptor. *Pharmacol Rev* 1990; 42:45–83.

280. Ichinose M, Stretton CD, Schwartz J-C, et al: Histamine H_3-receptors inhibit cholinergic neurotransmission in guina-pig airways. *Br J Pharmacol* 1989; 97:13–15.

281. Ichinose M, Belvisi MG, Barnes PJ: Histamine H_3-receptors inhibit neurogenic microvascular leakage in airways. *J Appl Physiol* 1990; 68:21–25.

282. Fuller RW, Dixon CMS, Dollery CT, et al: Prostaglandin D_2 potentiates airway responsiveness to histamine and methacholine. *Am Rev Respir Dis* 1986; 133:252–254.

283. Manning PJ, O'Byrne PM: Histamine bronchoconstriction reduces airway responsiveness in asthmatic subjects. *Am Rev Respir Dis* 1988; 137:1323–1325.

284. White J, Eiser NM: The role of histamine and its receptors in the pathogenesis of asthma. *Br J Dis Chest* 1983; 77:215–226.

285. Rafferty P, Holgate ST: Histamine and its antagonists in asthma. *J Allergy Clin Immunol* 1989; 84:144–151.

286. Woenne R, Kattan M, Orange RP, et al: Bronchial hyperreactivity to histamine and methacholine in asthmatic children after inhalation of SCH 1000 and chlorpheniramine. *J Allergy Clin Immunol* 1978; 62:119–124.

287. Tashkin PD, Ungerer R, Wolfe R, et al: Effect of orally administered cimetidine on histamine- and antigen-induced bronchospasm in subjects with asthma. *Am Rev Respir Dis* 1982; 125:691–695.

288. Nathan RA, Segall N, Glover GC, et al: The effects of H_1 and H_2 antihistamines on histamine inhalation challenges in asthmatic patients. *Am Rev Respir Dis* 1979; 120:1251–1258.

289. Drazen JM, Venugopalan CS, Soter NA: H_2 receptor mediated inhibition of immediate type hypersensitivity reaction *in vivo*. *Am Rev Respir Dis* 1978; 117:479–484.

290. Eiser NM, Guz A, Mills J, et al: Effect of H_1- and H_2-receptor antagonists on antigen bronchial challenge. *Thorax* 1978; 33:534.

291. Thomson NC, Kerr JW: Effect of inhaled H_1 and H_2 receptor antagonists in normal and asthmatic subjects. *Thorax* 1980; 35:428–434.

292. White J, Smith AP, Leopold D, et al: Effects of H_2 antagonists in asthma. *Br J Dis Chest* 1980; 74:315.

293. Nogrady SG, Bevan C: H2 receptor blockade and bronchial hyperreactivity to histamine in asthma. *Thorax* 1981; 36:268–271.

294. Maconochie JG, Woodings EP, Richards DA: Effects of H_1- and H_2-receptor blocking agents on histamine-induced bronchoconstriction in non-asthmatic subjects. *Br J Clin Pharmacol* 1979; 7:231–236.

295. Souney PF, Stoukides CA: Pharmacoeconomic aspects and formulary considerations related to histamine$_2$-receptor antagonists. *DICP* 1989; 23(suppl 10):S29–S35.

296. Holgate AT, Robinson C, Church MK: Mediators of immediate hypersensitivity, in Middleton E Jr, Reed CR, Ellis EF, et al (eds): *Allergy: Principles and Practice*, 3rd ed. St Louis, CV Mosby, 1988, pp 135–163.

297. Shore SA, Austen KF, Drazen JM: Eicosanoids and the lung, in Massaro D (ed): *Lung Cell Biology*. New York, Marcel Dekker, 1989, pp 1011–1089.

298. Wardlaw AJ, Dunnette S, Gleich GJ, et al: Eosinophils and mast cells in bronchoalveolar lavage in subjects with mild asthma: Relationship to bronchial hyperreactivity. *Am Rev Respir Dis* 1988; 137:62–69.

299. Anderson SD, Bye PTP, Schoeffel RE, et al: Arterial plasma histamine levels at rest and during and after exercise in patients with asthma: Effect of terbutaline aerosol. *Thorax* 1981; 36:259–267.

300. Gravelyn TR, Pan PM, Eschenbacher WL: Mediator release in an isolated airway segment in subjects with asthma. *Am Rev Respir Dis* 1988; 137:641–646.

301. Seltzer J, Bigby BG, Stulbarg M, et al: O_3-induced change in bronchial reactivity to methacholine and airway inflammation in humans. *J Appl Physiol* 1986; 60:1321–1326.

302. Pliss LB, Ingenito EP, Ingram RH Jr, et al: Assessment of bronchoalveolar cell and mediator response to isocapnic hyperpnea in asthma. *Am Rev Respir Dis* 1990; 142:73–78.

303. Stenton SC, Court EN, Kingston WP, et al: Platelet-activating factor in bronchoalveolar lavage fluid from asthmatic subjects. *Eur Respir J* 1990; 3:408–413.

304. Lee TH, Nagy L, Nagakura T, et al: Identification and partial characterization of an exercise-induced neutrophil chemotactic factor in bronchial asthma. *J Clin Invest* 1982; 69:889–899.

305. Neijens H, Raatgeep R, Degenhart H, et al: Altered leukocyte response in relation to the basic abnormality in children with asthma and bronchial hyperresponsiveness. *Am Rev Respir Dis* 1984; 130:744–747.

306. Flint KC, Hudspith BN, Leung KBP, et al: The hyperosmolar release of histamine from bronchoalveolar mast cells and its inhibition by sodium cromoglycate. *Thorax* 1985; 40:717.

307. Souhrada JF: Exercise-induced bronchoconstriction, in Coburn RF (ed): *Airway Smooth Muscle in Health and Disease*. New York, Plenum Press, 1989, pp 301–313.

308. Atkins PC, Rosenblum F, Dunsky EH, et al: Comparison of plasma histamine and cyclic nucleotides after antigen and methacholine inhalation in man. *J Allergy Clin Immunol* 1980; 66:478–485.

309. Atkins PC, Norman M, Weiner H, et al: Release of neutrophil chemotactic activity during immediate hypersensitivty reactions in humans. *Ann Intern Med* 1977; 86:415–418.

310. Chan-Yeung M, Chan H, Tse KS, et al: Histamine and leukotrienes release in bronchoalveolar fluid during plicatic acid-induced bronchoconstriction. *J Allergy Clin Immunol* 1989; 84:762–768.

311. Weiss JW, Rossing TH, McFadden ER Jr, et al: Relationship between bronchial responsiveness to hyperventilation with cold and methacholine in asthma. *J Allergy Clin Immunol* 1983; 72:140–144.

312. O'Byrne PM, Ryan G, Morris M, et al: Asthma induced by cold air and its relation to nonspecific bronchial responsiveness to methacholine. *Am Rev Respir Dis* 1982; 125:281–285.

313. Casale TB, Wood D, Richerson HB, et al: Elevated bronchoalveolar lavage fluid histamine levels in allergic asthmatics are associated with methacholine bronchial hyperresponsiveness. *J Clin Invest* 1987; 79:1197–1203.

314. Heaton RW, Henderson AF, Dunlop LS, et al: The influence of pretreatment with prostaglandin $F_{2\alpha}$ on bronchial sensitivity to inhaled histamine and methacholine in normal subjects. *Br J Dis Chest* 1984; 78:168–173.

315. Fujimura M, Sasaki F, Nakatsumi Y, et al: Effects of a thromboxane synthetase inhibitor (OKY-046) and a lipoxygenase inhibitor (AA-861) on bronchial responsiveness to acetylcholine in asthmatic subjects. *Thorax* 1986; 41:955–959.

316. Fujimura M, Nishioka S, Kumabashiri I, et al: Effects of aerosol administration of a thromboxane synthetase inhibitor (OKY-046) on bronchial responsiveness to acetylcholine in asthmatic subjects. *Chest* 1990; 98:276–279.

317. Fujimura M, Sakamoto S, Matsuda T: Attenuating effect of a thromboxane synthetase inhibitor (OKY-046) on bronchial responsiveness to methacholine is specific to bronchial asthma. *Chest* 1990; 98:656–660.

318. Fujimura M, Miyake Y, Uotani K, et al: Secondary release of thromboxane A2 in aerosol leukotriene C4-induced bronchoconstriction in guinea pigs. *Prostaglandins* 1988; 35:427–435.

319. Miller RF, Purvis AW, Lefferts PL, et al: Meclofenamate blocks the pulmonary arterial vasopressor effects of leukotriene B_4 in awake sheep. *Prostaglandins* 1988; 36:601–606.

320. Walters EH: Prostaglandins and the control of airways responses to histamine in normal and asthmatic subjects. *Thorax* 1983; 38:188–194.

321. Walters EH: Effect of inhibition of prostaglandin synthesis on induced bronchial hyperresponsiveness. *Thorax* 1983; 38:195–199.

322. Rudolf M, Grant BJB, Saunders KB, et al: Aspirin in exercise-induced asthma. *Lancet* 1975; 1:450.

323. Schacter EN, Kreisnian H, Bouhuys A: Prostaglandin-synthesis inhibition and exercise bronchospasm. *Ann Intern Med* 1978; 89:287–288.

324. Fish JE, Ankin MG, Adkinson NF Jr, et al: Indomethacin modification of immediate-type immunologic airway responses in allergic asthmatic and non-asthmatic subjects. *Am Rev Respir Dis* 1981; 123:609–614.

325. Giraldo B, Blumenthal MN, Spink WW: Aspirin intolerance and asthma: A clinical and immunological study. *Ann Intern Med* 1969; 71:479–496.

326. Mathé AA, Hedqvist P: Effect of prostaglandins F_2 alpha and E_2 on airway conductance in healthy subjects and asthmatic patients. *Am Rev Respir Dis* 1975; 111:313–320.

327. Cuthbert MF: Effect on airways resistance of prostaglandin E_1 given by aerosol to healthy and asthmatic volunteers. *BMJ* 1969; 4:723–726.

328. Hardy CC, Bradding P, Robinson C, et al: Bronchoconstrictor and antibronchoconstrictor properties of inhaled prostacyclin in asthma. *J Appl Physiol* 1988; 64:1567–1574.

329. Dworski R, Sheller JR, Wickersham NE, et al: Allergen-stimulated release of mediators into sheep bronchoalveolar lavage fluid: Effect of cyclooxygenase inhibition. *Am Rev Respir Dis* 1989; 139:46–51.

330. Chung KF, Aizawa H, Leikauf G, et al: Airway hyperresponsiveness induced by platelet-activating factor: Role of thromboxane generation. *J Pharmacol Exp Ther* 1986; 236:580–584.

331. O'Byrne PM, Leikauf GD, Aizawa H, et al: Leukotriene B_4 induces airway hyperresponsiveness in dogs. *J Appl Physiol* 1985; 59:1941–1946.

332. Black PN, Fuller RW, Taylor GW, et al: Effect of inhaled leukotriene B_4 alone and in combination with prostaglandin D_2 on bronchial responsiveness to histamine in normal subjects. *Thorax* 1989; 44:491–495.

333. Barnes NC, Piper PJ, Costello JF: Actions of inhaled leukotrienes and their interactions with other allergic mediators. *Prostaglandins* 1984; 28:629–631.

334. Bel EH, Van der Veen H, Kramps JA, et al: Maximal airway narrowing to inhaled leukotriene D_4 in normal subjects: Comparison and interaction with methacholine. *Am Rev Respir Dis* 1987; 136:979–984.

335. Arm JP, Spur BW, Lee TH: The effects of inhaled leukotriene E_4 on the airway responsiveness to histamine in subjects with asthma and normal subjects. *J Allergy Clin Immunol* 1988; 82:654–660.

336. Mann JS, Robinson C, Sheridan AQ, et al: Effect of inhaled Piriprost (U-60,257) a novel leukotriene inhibitor, on allergen and exercise induced bronchoconstriction in asthma. *Thorax* 1986; 41:746–752.

337. Bel EH, Timmers MC, Dijkman JH, et al: The effect of an inhaled leukotriene antagonist, L-648,051, on early and late asthmatic reactions and subsequent increase in airway responsiveness in man. *J Allergy Clin Immunol* 1990; 85:1067–1075.

338. Dinh Xuan AT, Regnard J, Similowski T, et al: Effects of SK&F 104353, a leukotriene receptor antagonist, on the bronchial responses to histamine in subjects with asthma: A comparative study with terfenadine. *J Allergy Clin Immunol* 1990; 85:865–871.

339. Israel E, Dermarkarian R, Rosenberg M, et al: The effects of a 5-lipoxygenase inhibitor on asthma induced by cold, dry air. *N Engl J Med* 1990; 323:1740–1744.

340. Jones TR, Zamboni R, Belley M, et al: Pharmacology of L-660,711 (MK-751): A novel potent and selective leukotriene D_4 receptor antagonist. *Can J Physiol Pharmacol* 1989; 67:17–28.

341. Manning PJ, Watson RM, Margolskee DJ, et al: Inhibition of exercise-induced bronchoconstriction by MK-571, a potent leukotriene D_4-receptor antagonist. *N Engl J Med* 1990; 323:1736–1739.

342. O'Donnell SR, Barnett CJK: Microvascular leakage to platelet activating factor in guinea-pig trachea and bronchi. *Eur J Pharmacol* 1987; 138:385–396.

343. Page CP, Coyle AJ: The interaction between PAF, platelets and eosinophils in bronchial asthma. *Eur Respir J* 1989; 2:483s–487s.

344. Cuss FM, Dixon CM, Barnes PJ: Effects of inhaled platelet activating factor on pulmonary function and bronchial responsiveness in man. *Lancet* 1986; 2:189–192.

345. Chung KF, Dent G, Barnes PJ: Effects of salbutamol on bronchoconstriction, bronchial hyperresponsiveness, and leucocyte responses induced by platelet activating factor in man. *Thorax* 1989; 44:102–107.

346. Wardlaw AJ, Chung KF, Moqbel R, et al: Effects of inhaled PAF in humans on circulating and bronchoalveolar lavage fluid neutrophils: Relationship to bronchoconstriction and changes in airway responsiveness. *Am Rev Respir Dis* 1990; 141:386–392.

347. Lai CKW, Jenkins JR, Polosa R, et al: Inhaled PAF fails to induce airway hyperresponsiveness to methacholine in normal human subjects. *J Appl Physiol* 1990; 68:919–926.

348. Hopp RJ, Bewtra AK, Agrawal DK, et al: Effect of platelet-activating factor inhalation on non-specific bronchial reactivity in man. *Chest* 1989; 96:1070–1072.

349. Hopp RJ, Bewtra AK, Nabe M, et al: Effect of PAF-acether inhalation on non-specific bronchial reactivity and adrenergic response in normal and asthmatic subjects. *Chest* 1990; 98:936–941.

350. Chung KF, Barnes PJ: Effects of platelet activating factor on airway calibre, airway responsiveness, and circulating cells in asthmatic subjects. *Thorax* 1989; 44:108–115.

351. Bel EH, De Smet M, Rossing TH, et al: The effect of a specific oral PAF-antagonist, MK-287, on antigen-induced early and late asthmatic reactions in man. *Am Rev Respir Dis* 1991; 143:A811.

352. Wilkens H, Wilkens JH, Bosse S, et al: Effects of an inhaled PAF-antagonist (WEB 2086 BS) on allergen-induced early and late asthmatic responses and increased bronchial responsiveness to methacholine. *Am Rev Respir Dis* 1991; 143:A812.

353. Dermarkarian RM, Israel E, Rosenberg MA, et al: The effect of SCH-37370, a dual platelet activating factor (PAF) and histamine antagonist, on the bronchoconstriction induced in asthmatics by cold, dry air isocapnic hyperventilation (ISH). *Am Rev Respir Dis* 1991; 143:A812.

354. Frigas E, Loegering DA, Solley GO, et al: Elevated levels of the eosinophil granule major basic protein in the sputum of patients with bronchial asthma. *Mayo Clin Proc* 1981; 56:345–353.

355. Frigas E, Loegering DA, Gleich GJ: Cytotoxic effects of the guinea pig eosinophil major basic protein on tracheal epithelium. *Lab Invest* 1980; 42:35–43.

356. Gleich GJ, Adolphson CR: The eosinophil leukocyte: Structure and function. *Adv Immunol* 1986; 39:177–253.

357. Wegner CD, Gundel RH, Reilly P, et al: Intercellular adhesion molecule-1 (ICAM-1) in the pathogenesis of asthma. *Science* 1990; 247:456–459.

358. Sekizawa K, Caughey GH, Lazarus SC, et al: Mast cell tryptase causes airway smooth muscle hyperresponsiveness in dogs. *J Clin Invest* 1989; 83:175–179.

359. Fuller RW, Dixon CMS, Cuss FMC, et al: Bradykinin-induced bronchoconstriction in humans: Mode of action. *Am Rev Respir Dis* 1987; 135:176–180.

360. Matsuse T, Fukuchi Y, Suruda T, et al: Effect of endothelin-1 on pulmonary resistance in rats. *J Appl Physiol* 1990; 68:2391–2393.

361. Advenier C, Sarria B, Naline E, et al: Contractile activity of three endothelins (ET-1, ET-2 and ET-3) on the human isolated bronchus. *Br J Pharmacol* 1990; 100:168–172.

362. Macquin-Mavier I, Levame M, Istin N, et al: Mechanisms of endothelin-mediated bronchoconstriction in the guinea pig. *J Pharmacol Exp Ther* 1989; 250:740–745.

363. Lagente V, Boichot E, Mencia-Huerta J, et al: Failure of aerosolized endothelin (ET-1) to induce bronchial hyperreactivity in the guinea pig. *Fundam Clin Pharmacol* 1990; 4:275–280.

364. Holgate ST, Finnerty JP, Polosa R: Mechanisms of purine-induced bronchoconstriction in asthma. *Arch Int Pharmacodyn Ther* 1990; 303:122–131.

365. Mann JS, Cushley MJ, Holgate ST: Adenosine-induced bronchoconstriction in asthma: Role of parasympathetic stimulation and adrenergic inhibition. *Am Rev Respir Dis* 1985; 132:1–6.

366. Mann JS, Holgate ST, Renwick AG, et al: Airway effects of purine nucleosides and nucleotides and release with bronchial provocation in asthma. *J Appl Physiol* 1986; 61:1667–1676.

367. Phillips GD, Holgate ST: Absence of a late-phase response or increase in histamine responsiveness following bronchial provocation with adenosine 5'-monophosphate in atopic and non-atopic asthma. *Clin Sci* 1988; 75:429–436.

368. Charman J, Reid L: Sputum viscosity in chronic bronchitis, bronchiectasis, asthma and cystic fibrosis. *Biorheology* 1972; 9:185–199.

369. Lopez-Vidriero MT, Reid L: Chemical markers of mucous and serum glycoproteins in mucoid and purulent sputum form various hypersecretory diseases. *Am Rev Respir Dis* 1978; 117:465–477.

370. Kaliner MA, Shelhamer JH, Borson DB, et al: Respiratory mucus, in Kaliner MA, Barnes PJ (eds): *The Airways: Neural Control in Health and Disease.* New York, Marcel Dekker, 1988, pp 575–593.

371. Lopez-Vidriero MT, Reid LM: Bronchial mucus in asthma, in Weiss EB, Segal MS, Stein M (eds): *Bronchial Asthma: Mechanisms and Therapeutics,* 2d ed. Little, Brown, Boston, 1985, pp 218–235.

372. Openshaw PJM, Turner-Warwick M: Observations on sputum production in patients with variable airflow obstruction: Implications for the diagnosis of asthma and chronic bronchitis. *Respir Med* 1989; 83:25–31.

373. Mezey RJ, Cohn MA, Fernandez RJ, et al: Mucociliary transport in allergic patients with antigen-induced bronchospasm. *Am Rev Respir Dis* 1978; 118:677–684.

374. Pavia D, Bateman JRM, Sheahan NF, et al: Tracheobronchial mucociliary clearance in asthma: Impairment during remission. *Thorax* 1985; 40:171–175.

375. Allegra L, Abraham WM, Chapman GA, et al: Duration of mucociliary dysfunction following antigen challenge. *J Appl Physiol* 1983; 55:726–730.

376. Ahmed T, Greenblatt DW, Birch S, et al: Abnormal mucociliary transport in allergic patients with antigen-induced bronchospasm: Role of slow reacting substance of anaphylaxis. *Am Rev Respir Dis* 1981; 124:110–114.

377. Hastie AT, Loegering DA, Gleich GJ, et al: The effect of purified eosinophil major basic protein on mammalian ciliary activity. *Am Rev Respir Dis* 1987; 135:848–853.

378. Garrard CS, Mussatto DJ, Lourenço RV: Lung mucociliary transport in asymptomatic asthma: Effects of inhaled histamine. *J Lab Clin Med* 1989; 113:190–195.

379. Wanner A: Clinical aspects of mucociliary transport. *Am Rev Respir Dis* 1977; 116:73–125.

380. Phipps RJ: Production of airway secretions. *Semin Respir Med* 1984; 5:314–318.

381. Wanner A: Mucociliary function in bronchial asthma, in Weiss EB, Segal MS, Stein M (eds): *Bronchial Asthma: Mechanisms and Therapeutics,* 2nd ed. Boston, Little, Brown, 1985, pp 270–279.

382. Tam PY, Verdugo P: Control of mucus hydration as a Donnan equilibrium process. *Nature* 1981; 292:340–342.

383. Dulfano MJ, Luk CK: Sputum and ciliary inhibition in asthma. *Thorax* 1982; 37:646–651.

384. Maurer DR, Sielczak M, Oliver W Jr, et al: Role of ciliary motility in acute allergic mucociliary dysfunction. *J Appl Physiol* 1982; 52:1018–1023.

385. Kneussl MP, Richardson JB: Alpha-adrenergic receptors in human and canine tracheal and bronchial smooth muscle. *J Appl Physiol* 1978; 45:307–311.

386. Barnes PJ, Skoogh B-E, Brown JK, et al: Activation of α-adrenergic response in tracheal smooth muscle: A postreceptor mechanism. *J Appl Physiol* 1983; 54:1469–1476.

387. Henderson WR, Shelhamer JH, Reingold DB, et al: Alpha-adrenergic hyper-responsiveness in asthma: Analysis of vascular and pupillary responses. *N Engl J Med* 1979; 300:642–647.

388. Davis PB: Pupillary responses and airway reactivity in asthma. *J Allergy Clin Immunol* 1986; 77:667–672.

389. Snashall PD, Boother FA, Sterling GM: The effect of α-adrenoceptor stimulation on the airways of normal and asthmatic man. *Clin Sci* 1978; 54:283–289.

390. Black JL, Salome CM, Yan K, et al: Comparison between airways response to an α adrenoceptor agonist and histamine in asthmatic and non-asthmatic subjects. *Br J Clin Pharmacol* 1982; 14:464–465.

391. Barnes PJ, Ind PW, Dollery CT: Inhaled prazosin in asthma. *Thorax* 1981; 36:378–381.

392. Campbell IA, Dyson AJ: Indoramin—an α adrenoceptor antagonist for airway obstruction. *Br J Dis Chest* 1977; 71:105–108.

393. Utting JA: Alpha-adrenergic blockade in severe asthma. *Br J Dis Chest* 1979; 73:317–318.

394. Thomson NC, Daniel EE, Hargreave FE: Role of smooth muscle alpha$_1$-receptors in nonspecific bronchial responsiveness in asthma. *Am Rev Respir Dis* 1982; 126:521–525.

395. Bianco S, Griffin JP, Jamburoff PL, et al: Prevention of exercise-induced asthma by indoramin. *BMJ* 1974; 4:18–20.

396. Gaddie J, Legge JS, Petrie G, et al: The effect of an alpha-adrenergic receptor blocking drug on histamine sensitivity in bronchial asthma. *Br J Dis Chest* 1972; 66:141–146.

397. Kerr JW, Govindoraj M, Patel KR: Effect of alpha-receptor blocking drugs and disodium cromoglycate on histamine hypersensitivity in bronchial asthma. *BMJ* 1970; 2:139–141.

398. Barnes PJ, Wilson NM, Vickers H: Prazosin, an alpha$_1$-adrenoceptor antagonist, partially inhibits exercise-induced asthma. *J Allergy Clin Immunol* 1981; 68:411–415.

CHAPTER 7

Conventional and High-Resolution Computed Tomography of Chronic Infiltrative Lung Disease

Charles V. Zwirewich, M.D.

Clinical Instructor, Department of Radiology, University of British Columbia, Vancouver General Hospital, Vancouver, British Columbia, Canada

Nestor L. Müller, M.D., Ph.D.

Associate Professor, Department of Radiology, University of British Columbia, Vancouver General Hospital, Vancouver, British Columbia, Canada

The term "chronic diffuse infiltrative lung disease" (CILD) embraces a large number of different diagnoses, the clinical and functional features of which may be similar. While the chest radiograph continues to be the principal imaging modality used in the evaluation of patients with CILD, it has significant limitations in the detection and characterization of the pathologic changes in this group of disorders.

Epler and coworkers found that 9.6% of patients with CILD confirmed by open lung biopsy had normal chest radiographs. The diseases most commonly associated with a normal radiograph were extrinsic allergic alveolitis, desquamative interstitial pneumonia (DIP), and asbestosis.[1] A number of studies also have shown that the severity of abnormalities on the radiograph correlates poorly with the degree of clinical and functional impairment.[2-5] Finally, although the chest radiograph may show patterns suggestive of a particular disease, it rarely allows a confident diagnosis. In a review of the chest radiographs of 365 patients with diffuse infiltrative lung disease, McLoud and coworkers[6] determined that the correct pathologic diagnosis could be predicted in only 50% of cases based on the plain film findings alone.

Recently, computed tomography (CT) has been shown to reflect accurately the morphologic features of focal and diffuse infiltrative lung diseases.[7-14] CT is more sensitive than the chest radiograph in the detection of lung disease. Abnormal and characteristic CT findings in patients with normal radiographs have been described in fibrosing alveolitis,[15] DIP,[16] extrinsic allergic alveolitis,[16] asbestosis,[17-19] lymphangitic carcinomatosis,[20] sarcoidosis,[12, 21] and lymphangioleiomyomatosis.[22] The CT findings also have been shown to correlate better than the radiograph with the degree of clinical and functional impairment in CILD.[19, 22-24] The CT appearances of some disorders in the appropriate clinical setting may be sufficiently characteristic to establish a specific diagnosis. Finally, if biopsy is required, CT is helpful in determining the optimal biopsy site.

The chronic infiltrative lung diseases may be classified by their radiologic, CT, or pathologic characteristics, or by a combination thereof. For the purposes of this review, the diseases will be classified into four categories: chronic interstitial pneumonias, granulomatous diseases, neoplastic infiltration, and occupational lung diseases (Table 1). Although more than 100 entities may lead to chronic infiltrative lung disease, the diseases described in this review account for approximately 80% to 90% of all cases of chronic infiltrative lung disease seen at our institution.

In this chapter, we will review basic concepts of CT technique and the characteristic patterns of several of the most common chronic infiltrative disorders. Specific clinical indications for the use of CT, the correlation between CT and indices of clinical and functional impairment, the diagnostic accuracy of CT, and the role of CT in determining the optimal type and site of lung biopsy will be discussed.

TABLE 1.
Chronic Infiltrative Lung Diseases

I. Chronic interstitial pneumonias.
   A. Idiopathic pulmonary fibrosis.
   B. Bronchiolitis obliterans organizing
      pneumonia (BOOP).
II. Granulomatous lung diseases.
   A. Sarcodoisis.
   B. Extrinsic allergic alveolitis.
III. Neoplastic disorders.
   A. Lymphangitic carcinomatosis.
IV. Occupational lung diseases.
   A. Asbestosis.
   B. Silicosis.

COMPUTED TOMOGRAPHIC TECHNIQUE

Conventional Computed Tomography

A CT image is a two-dimensional representation of a three-dimensional cross-sectional slice, the third dimension being slice thickness. The CT image represents a mathematic reconstruction of the x-ray attenuation characteristics within the patient. All structures within a unit volume of the slice (voxel) are represented as a single unit on the image (pixel). The x-ray characteristics of structures within a given voxel are averaged to produce the image. Conventional CT scanning utilizes a slice thickness (collimation) ranging from 8 to 10 mm, performed at 10-mm intervals through the chest at end inspiration with the patient supine. Volume averaging within the 1-cm thickness of the slice results in loss of spatial resolution. For many CT applications in the chest, this is not critical; however, it may limit the ability of CT to detect and accurately characterize the abnormalities in chronic infiltrative lung disease.

High-Resolution Computed Tomography

High-resolution CT (HRCT) employs thin collimation scans (1 to 2 mm in thickness) and a high-resolution reconstruction algorithm. The thin section virtually eliminates volume averaging. The high-resolution reconstruction algorithm maximizes spatial resolution and image contrast, thus giving an image with much sharper demarcation between normal and abnormal parenchyma. Spatial resolution can be improved further by targeting the image to one lung or a portion of one lung.[13, 25] HRCT provides spatial resolution at the submillimeter level[25] and comparable to that of macroscopic inspection.[10] It improves detection of fine parenchymal detail, allowing better characterization of morphologic abnormalities in lung disease.

The number of HRCT images obtained in any given patient varies between different institutions and also depends on the particular clinical indication for the CT scan.[13, 26, 27] HRCT scans performed at the level of the aortic arch, tracheal carina, and 1 cm above the diaphragm may be used to supplement the conventional CT examination. Scans at these three levels give a representative sample of each of the three lung zones.[7] Alternatively, the entire CT examination may be performed using 1.5-mm scans obtained at 10-mm intervals. In patients with known or suspected occupational exposure to asbestos, adequate examination of the lung parenchyma may be achieved by 4 to 6 1.5-mm HRCT scans obtained through the mid and lower lung zones in the supine and prone position during maximal inspiration.[17, 18] Prone scans are necessary in patients with suspected asbestosis in order to distinguish reversible density from fixed structural abnormalities in dependent portions of the lung bases where pulmonary fibrosis is most likely to occur.[17, 18]

HIGH-RESOLUTION COMPUTED TOMOGRAPHIC FEATURES OF SOME OF THE MORE COMMON CHRONIC INFILTRATIVE LUNG DISEASES

Chronic Interstitial Pneumonias

Liebow classified the chronic interstitial pneumonias into five types: usual interstitial pneumonia (UIP), DIP, lymphocytic interstitial pneumonia (LIP), giant-cell interstitial pneumonia (GIP), and bronchiolitis with interstitial pneumonia (BIP).[28] UIP, as the name implies, is the most common type of chronic interstitial pneumonia.[28, 29] Clinically, the term often is used synonymously with idiopathic pulmonary fibrosis (IPF) and cryptogenic fibrosing alveolitis. Identical pathologic and CT findings may be seen in patients with collagen vascular diseases. It is a matter of controversy whether DIP is a distinct entity from UIP or the early stage of a process in which UIP is the late stage.[29-31]

LIP is uncommon, seen mainly in patients with dysproteinemia, autoimmune disease (particularly Sjögren's syndrome), and, more recently, the acquired immune deficiency syndrome (AIDS).[32-35] Many cases initially classified as LIP now are considered to be lymphomas,[29] and Spencer considers LIP a "prelymphomatous" state.[36] GIP is very rare and found almost exclusively in workers exposed to hard-metal, an alloy of tungsten carbide and cobalt.[37] Therefore, it is better considered a form of pneumoconiosis. The term BIP has been replaced by the expression bronchiolitis (with or without bronchiolitis obliterans) with patchy organizing pneumonia (BOOP), as the pneumonia is not purely interstitial.[29] BOOP often has been confused with UIP, but it has distinct radiologic and pathologic features.[38-41]

Because both LIP and GIP are uncommon, they will not be discussed. This review will summarize findings of the two most common nongranulomatous chronic inflammatory lung diseases: IPF and bronchiolitis obliterans organizing pneumonia (BOOP).

Idiopathic Pulmonary Fibrosis

IPF (cryptogenic fibrosing alveolitis, UIP) is a disease of unknown etiology characterized by progressive shortness of breath, dry cough, and late inspiratory crackles or "velcro" rales on auscultation. Pulmonary function tests characteristically show a restrictive pattern with reduction in lung volumes and impaired gas exchange.[42, 43] Generally, these patients have a progressive course, with death within 3 to 6 years after the onset of symptoms.[43] IPF is characterized pathologically by the presence of alveolar septal inflammation and progressive interstitial fibrosis that may culminate in an "end-stage" lung characterized by extensive honeycombing and volume loss.

The characteristic appearance of IPF on CT is that of a patchy distribution of irregular reticular opacities situated in the subpleural regions and lung bases. These produce irregular pleural, vascular, and bronchial interfaces with normal lung[10, 15, 27] and represent areas of irregular fibrosis pathologically.[7] Honeycomb cysts measuring 2 to 20 mm in diameter are seen in 90% of cases by CT as compared to only 30% on the radiograph.[23] The peripheral predominance pathologically and on CT is identified in the vast majority of cases regardless of the stage of disease (Fig 1).

It is well known that the severity of interstitial lung disease on the chest radio-

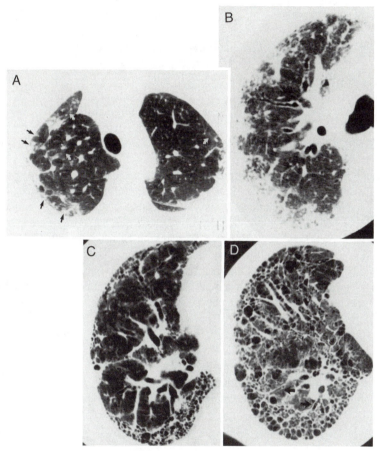

FIG 1.
HRCT scans (1.5-mm collimation) illustrating the spectrum of findings in IPF. **A,** early changes consist of hazy airspace opacification mainly in the subpleural lung regions *(curved arrows)* and mild fibrosis characterized by bilateral subpleural reticular densities and irregular thickening of the interlobular septa *(arrows)*. **B** and **C,** with progression of the disease process, HRCT shows the characteristic peripheral subpleural distribution of reticular densities and honeycombing. **D,** this peripheral predominance is maintained even in the presence of advanced fibrosis and honeycombing. Traction bronchiectasis is evident in the right lower lobe *(arrows)*. (Part B from Müller NL, Miller RR: *Am Rev Respir Dis* 1990; 142:1206–1215. Used by permission.)

graph correlates poorly with the degree of clinical and functional impairment in patients with IPF.[8, 17, 24, 44–46] The extent of disease as assessed on CT, however, correlates well with the severity of dyspnea ($r = .62$, $P < .001$) and with the severity of impairment in gas transfer as evaluated by the single-breath carbon monoxide diffusing capacity ($r = .64$, $P < .001$).[24]

The long-term survival and response to corticosteroid therapy in IPF correlate with the severity of histologic changes and the degree of active inflammation pathologically. The best response to steroid therapy is observed among patients with minimal fibrosis and marked disease activity as characterized by the presence of alveolar septal inflammation and intra-alveolar histiocytes.[8, 13, 42, 43, 45, 47] The hallmark of disease activity on CT is the presence of patchy areas of hazy increased density (ground-glass opacities).[8] In mild cases of IPF, these ground-glass densities may be limited to the posterior basal segments as crescentic areas of subpleural density that may be inapparent on the radiograph.[15] In more advanced cases of IPF, patchy areas of mild and marked inflammatory activity frequently coexist with areas of mild and severe fibrosis in the same patient and often in the same lobe.

Although open lung biopsy represents the gold standard in determining the degree of disease activity, it is an invasive procedure and may underestimate the severity of alveolar inflammation if representative areas of lung are not sampled. To determine whether CT might be helpful in the assessment of disease activity, Müller and coworkers[8] reviewed the CT scans of 12 patients with IPF who had correlation of the level of disease activity by open lung biopsy. A four-point scoring system was used to assess the intensity of disease activity on CT based on the presence and relative density of airspace opacification compared to normal lung. Observers correctly identified five patients with marked disease activity and five of seven with low disease activity. Airspace opacification was patchy in distribution, predominantly peripheral, and seen better on 1.5-mm collimation scans. The pathologic severity score was significantly greater among patients with high CT scores than among those with low CT scores ($P < .01$). Similar findings have been reported recently by Klein and associates.[48]

In summary, the pathologic changes in IPF not only are demonstrated more clearly by HRCT than by standard radiography, but disease extent as assessed by CT correlates well with the severity of dyspnea and functional impairment. In the appropriate clinical setting, HRCT findings of predominantly subpleural fibrosis can be characteristic enough to obviate the need for open lung biopsy. When the CT features are not diagnostic, CT can be useful in guiding the surgeon to the optimal biopsy site. Although data are preliminary at this time, HRCT may prove useful in the assessment of disease activity.

Bronchiolitis Obliterans Organizing Pneumonia

Bronchiolitis obliterans is a lung disease characterized by the presence of granulation tissue polyps within the lumen of bronchioles and alveolar ducts. It may lead to extensive obliteration of the small airways by scarring. The inflammatory process may involve the surrounding alveoli, resulting in a component of organizing pneumonia.

Bronchiolitis obliterans is a nonspecific reaction that may be caused by a variety of insults, including (1) inhalation of toxic fumes[49-53]; (2) bacterial, mycoplasma, or viral infection[54, 55]; (3) connective tissue diseases, particularly rheumatoid arthritis and polymyositis[56-59]; or (4) bone marrow and heart-lung transplantation.[60-63] Davidson et al.[64] and Epler et al.[38] described the most important form of bronchiolitis obliterans in the setting of CILD, which is idiopathic BOOP or cryptogenic organizing pneumonia.

Clinically, patients with BOOP typically present with a several-month history of dry cough and malaise.[38-40] They may have low-grade fever and shortness of breath. The most common findings on physical examination are rales and crackles. Pulmonary function tests characteristically show a restrictive pattern. Clinically and functionally, the findings may be similar to UIP, although the duration of symptoms is usually shorter, systemic symptoms are more common, and finger

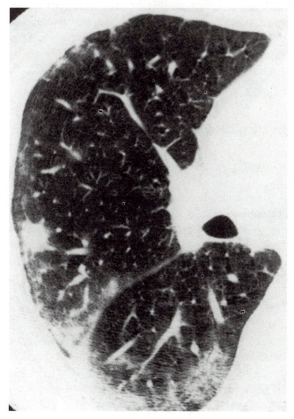

FIG 2.
HRCT image (1.5-mm collimation) in a 55-year-old man with BOOP. Airspace consolidation is present in a predominantly peripheral distribution.

clubbing is seen rarely. The patients usually respond well to corticosteroid therapy and have a good prognosis.

The characteristic radiologic features of BOOP consist of patchy, nonsegmental unilateral or, more commonly, bilateral areas of airspace consolidation.[38-41] Irregular linear opacities (reticular pattern) may be present, but they are uncommonly a major feature. Small nodular opacities may be seen as the only finding or, more commonly, in association with areas of airspace consolidation.

More recently, Müller et al.[65] reviewed the radiographic and CT features in 14 patients with BOOP. Six patients were immunocompromised due to leukemia or bone marrow transplantation and 8 patients were not immunocompromised. Ten patients had patchy unilateral or bilateral airspace consolidation, 7 had small nodular opacities, and 2 had irregular linear opacities. A predominantly subpleural distribution of the airspace consolidation was apparent on CT in 6 patients as compared to 2 on radiograph. In some patients, the airspace consolidation was more marked around the bronchi. Bronchial wall thickening and dilatation were seen in 6 patients, and 4 had small pleural effusions. All patients had areas of airspace consolidation, small nodules, or both (Fig 2). Although most of the findings could be seen on the radiographs, the CT scans demonstrated the anatomic distribution and extent of BOOP more accurately than did the plain chest radiographs. Furthermore, the presence of subpleural consolidation seen on CT in approximately 50% of patients with BOOP may be a helpful clue to the diagnosis.

Granulomatous Lung Diseases

Sarcoidosis

Sarcoidosis is a systemic disorder of unknown etiology characterized by the presence of noncaseating granulomas. Pulmonary manifestations are seen in 90% of patients, and up to 25% have permanent function impairment.[43] Although 60% to 70% demonstrate characteristic radiologic findings consisting of bilateral hilar and paratracheal lymphadenopathy with or without parenchymal changes,[66-68] the radiograph is atypical or nonspecific in 25% to 30% and may be entirely normal in 5% to 10%.[43, 66-68]

The variable and often nonspecific radiographic findings are surprising given the characteristic pathologic appearance and distribution of sarcoidosis. Sarcoid granulomas, the hallmark of the disease, are distributed mainly along the lymphatics in the bronchovascular sheath and, to a lesser extent, in the interlobular septa and pleurae.[12, 29, 69-71] This distribution is one of the most helpful features in recognizing sarcoidosis pathologically and is responsible for the high rate of success in diagnosis by bronchial and transbronchial biopsies.[3, 29, 72] The sarcoid granulomas are microscopic in size, but often coalesce to form macroscopic nodules. The characteristic distribution of sarcoid granulomas along the lymphatics can be seen clearly in illustrations of the macroscopic pathologic appearance.[29, 70] This distribution is difficult to appreciate on the radiograph because of the superimposition of the parenchymal shadows, but it is seen clearly on CT.[12]

The characteristic pattern of sarcoidosis on CT consists of nodular opacities, usually measuring under 5 mm in diameter, distributed along the bronchovascular bundles, interlobular septa, major fissures, and subpleural regions of the lung (Fig 3).[12, 21, 73, 74] The nodules tend to have irregular margins[12, 21, 74] and involve mainly the perihilar portions of the mid and upper lung zones. The nodules represent coalescent granulomas.

As fibrosis develops, irregular linear opacities are seen that, like the granulomas, are mainly peribronchovascular.[12] The fibrosis characteristically radiates from the hila to the mid and upper lung zones. Distortion of the lung parenchyma due to fibrosis may be seen on CT before the fibrosis is apparent on the radiograph.[21]

The distribution of sarcoid granulomas along the interlobular septa results in nodular septal thickening similar to that observed in pulmonary lymphangitic carcinomatosis.[9, 20, 73] However, the distribution in sarcoidosis is mainly perihilar, the interlobular septal thickening is less extensive, and usually there is distortion of the architecture of the secondary lobule due to parenchymal fibrosis.[12, 21, 74] These features allow easy distinction of sarcoidosis from lymphangitic carcinomatosis in the majority of cases.

It is controversial whether CT correlates better than the chest radiograph with the degree of clinical and functional impairment in sarcoidosis. Müller and colleagues[75] reviewed the plain radiographs and CT scans in 27 patients with sarcoidosis and found similar correlations for CT and the radiograph with severity of dyspnea ($r = .61$ and $.58$, respectively, $P < .001$), and reduction in total lung capacity ($r = -.54$ and $-.62$, respectively, $P < .01$) and diffusing capacity ($r = -.62$ and $-.52$, respectively, $P < .01$). Bergin and coworkers[74] found that CT scores correlated better with the degree of functional impairment than did the radiograph, whereas Brauner et al.[21] conversely demonstrated in a prospective study that the CT visual score had a lower correlation than the radiographic score with total lung capacity, FEV_1, and diffusing capacity.

Preliminary data suggest that CT may play a role in the assessment of disease activity and response to corticosteroid therapy in sarcoidosis (Fig 4).[73] Up to 60% of HRCT scans in sarcoidosis may demonstrate hazy areas of increased density (ground-glass opacity). These areas appear to represent active alveolitis as assessed by gallium-67 scintigraphy.[76-78] Increased uptake of gallium in the lungs correlates with the presence and intensity of alveolitis on open lung biopsy, and with the percentage of T lymphocytes on bronchoalveolar lavage.[78]

Extrinsic Allergic Alveolitis

Extrinsic allergic alveolitis (hypersensitivity pneumonitis) is an allergic disease of the lungs caused by the inhalation of antigenic material in a variety of organic dusts.[79] Following acute heavy exposure, the most common radiologic appearance

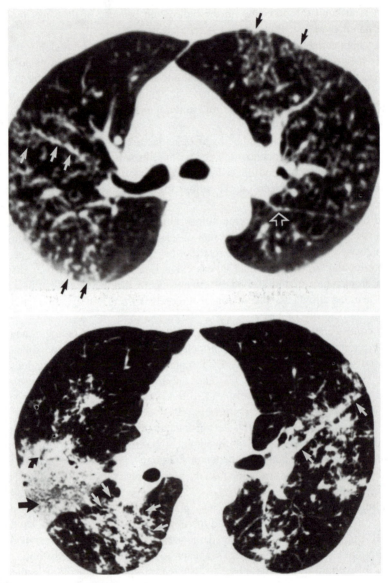

FIG 3.
CT scans illustrating the spectrum of parenchymal changes observed in sarcoidosis. Sarcoid granulomas are seen as irregular nodular opacities distributed along the bronchovascular bundles and in subpleural regions of the lung *(arrows)*. **A,** nodular pleural thickening is also evident in the left major fissure *(open arrow)*. **B,** in another patient, the right upper lobe contains an area of conglomerate granulomas shown as an ill-defined mass exhibiting central air bronchograms *(curved arrow)*. Airspace opacification is present anterior to the major fissure *(bold arrow)*. This patient had positive uptake is this area on a gallium-67 scan, indicating disease activity.

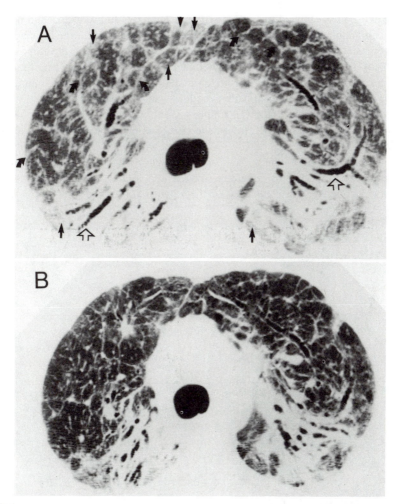

FIG 4.
HRCT scans through the upper lobes in a patient with advanced sarcoidosis. **A,** marked disease activity is evidenced by the presence of extensive hazy airspace opacification *(arrows)*. The extensive peribronchovascular distribution of fibrosis has resulted in a central conglomeration of vessels and bronchi that are displaced posteriorly, indicating volume loss. Thickened interlobular septae *(curved arrows)*, traction bronchiectasis *(open arrows)*, and lobular distortion are evident also. **B,** following the institution of corticosteroid therapy, there was marked improvement in the degree of airspace opacification. This correlated with resolution of dyspnea and improvement in arterial oxygen saturation and single-breath diffusing capacity.

is that of diffuse airspace consolidation,[80] which may reflect pulmonary edema[81] or intra-alveolar histiocytes.

The acute phase typically resolves within a few days to produce a fine nodular or reticulonodular pattern characteristic of the subacute phase, which may be totally reversible.[82, 83] The chronic phase is characterized by the development of pulmonary fibrosis, which may occur within a period of weeks or years following exposure.[83] Repeated exposure to antigen may produce a spectrum of findings, including diffuse airspace consolidation, nodules, and pulmonary fibrosis.

Silver et al.[81] reviewed the CT findings in 11 patients with extrinsic allergic alveolitis. In all of them, HRCT was superior to conventional CT in the demonstration of fine parenchymal detail. Two patients with acute extrinsic allergic alveolitis demonstrated both bilateral airspace and small rounded opacities on the chest radiograph and CT. In this subgroup, the CT scans and chest radiographs were considered equivalent in evaluation of the extent of disease. Three patients pre-

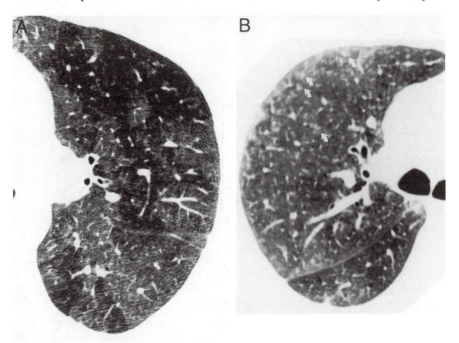

FIG 5.
Scans (1.5-mm collimation) of extrinsic allergic alveolitis in the acute and subacute phase. **A,** the patient was a 36-year-old woman who developed rapidly progressive dyspnea following the inhalation of dust containing bird droppings. The HRCT image demonstrates a patchy distribution of hazy airspace opacification (ground-glass opacity) throughout the left lung. No nodularity or fibrosis is evident. The chest radiograph was normal. The diagnosis was confirmed by serology. **B,** in a different patient, the presence of hazy airspace opacification (ground-glass pattern) coexisting with multiple small, ill-defined nodules *(arrows)* is characteristic of the subacute phase.

sented with subacute disease clinically; both the chest radiographs and CT scans showed small rounded opacities in this group, but only the CT scans identified the presence of bilateral areas of hazy increased density that did not obscure the underlying vascular margins (ground-glass opacities). In six patients with subacute symptoms superimposed on chronic extrinsic allergic alveolitis, the chest radiograph and CT scans both showed irregular linear opacities, but CT was more effective in demonstrating ground-glass opacities and scattered small nodular infiltrates.[81] The ground-glass pattern of the subacute phase of extrinsic allergic alveolitis may be missed easily on the radiograph,[1, 16] but can be seen readily on CT (Fig 5).[16]

HRCT, therefore, appears to be most helpful in the assessment of patients with subacute or chronic stages of disease in whom the characteristic hazy areas of ground-glass opacity and small ill-defined nodules are difficult to identify on the radiograph. In the appropriate clinical context, their presence should suggest the diagnosis, which may be confirmed by documenting a history of antigen exposure and examining for serum precipitins against suspected antigens.[84]

Neoplastic Disorders

Pulmonary Lymphatic Carcinomatosis

Pulmonary lymphatic carcinomatosis is defined by the presence of tumor growth within the lymphatics of the lung. The most common tumors to metastasize in this fashion include adenocarcinomas of the breast, lung, stomach, and colon, and those of unknown primary site.[66] The radiographic findings of pulmonary lymphatic carcinomatosis include thickened interlobular septae (Kerley's B lines), irregular reticular densities, subpleural edema,[10, 85] and hilar and mediastinal lymphadenopathy. Approximately 50% of proven cases have normal chest radiographs,[10] and accurate diagnosis by plain radiography is difficult because the findings frequently are nonspecific.

The distribution of proliferating tumor in lymphatics within the bronchovascular bundles, interlobular septa, and subpleural regions produces a characteristic appearance on the CT scans.[7, 75] The main findings consist of uneven, nodular thickening of bronchovascular bundles and interlobular septa producing a beaded-chain appearance (Fig 6).[10, 20, 86] Thickened interlobular septa of contiguous secondary lobules produce a pattern of polygonal arcades. These polygonal arcades frequently contain a prominent central dot on HRCT, representing tumor within lymphatics surrounding the centrilobular bronchovascular bundle (Fig 7). These polygonal arcades containing prominent central dotlike structures are one of the most characteristic features of this disorder.[9, 10, 20, 86, 87]

The clinical value of CT in the assessment of pulmonary lymphatic carcinomatosis lies in its ability to identify changes within the lung that are virtually pathognomonic in patients with a normal or nonspecific chest radiograph.[88] Among pa-

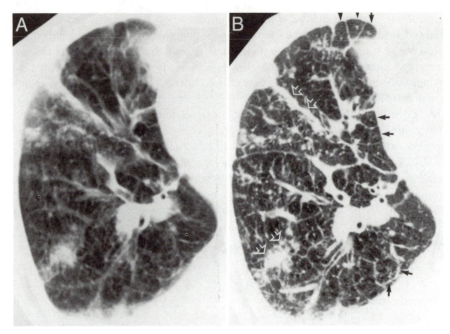

FIG 6.
A, 10-mm collimation and **B,** 1.5-mm HRCT images of pulmonary lymphangitic carcino-matosis. Uneven nodular thickening of the bronchovascular bundles *(open arrows)*, poly-gonal arcades *(arrows)*, and thickened interlobular septa are visualized more clearly on the HRCT scan. The beaded-chain appearance of tumor growth in the interlobular septa is ev-ident posteromedially *(arrows)*.

tients with a known carcinoma who develop interstitial lung disease, HRCT is valuable in differentiating pulmonary lymphatic carcinomatosis from drug effects on radiation pneumonitis, and in selecting the optimal site for transbronchial bi-opsy when a specific diagnosis is required. This is particularly important when in-volvement of the lung with pulmonary lymphatic carcinomatosis is focal, a feature reported in 50% of patients in the series by Munk and coworkers.[9]

Occupational Lung Diseases

Asbestosis
   Asbestosis refers to pulmonary fibrosis that develops in response to the deposi-tion of asbestos fibers in the lung.[18, 89] The diagnosis of asbestosis usually is made on clinical grounds without the benefit of a tissue biopsy.[46, 89] The initial reaction to asbestos fibers introduced into the lung is characterized by the immediate exu-dation of neutrophils and macrophages into the alveolar spaces at the site of fiber

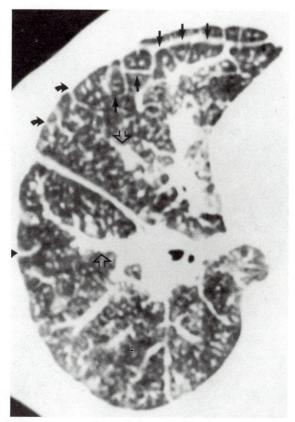

FIG 7.
Lymphangitic spread of adenocarcinoma of the lung. The classic HRCT features of this disorder include thickened interlobular septa *(curved arrows),* irregular nodular thickening along the bronchovascular bundles *(open arrows),* and polygonal arcades containing a central dot *(arrows).* (From Munk PL, Müller NL, Miller RR, et al: *Radiology* 1988; 166:705–709. Used by permission.)

deposition.[89] This is associated subsequently with varying degrees of organization and fibrosis.[90] The earliest foci of fibrosis are seen in the subpleural regions of the lung,[17] are related to the respiratory or terminal bronchioles, and may affect only occasional pulmonary subunits.[89] More advanced cases demonstrate extension of fibrosis into the alveolar walls, interlobular septa, and visceral pleurae, eventually producing diffuse interstitial fibrosis.[91] With severe disease, extensive fibrosis may be accompanied by honeycombing and traction bronchiectasis. Regardless of the stage of disease, the changes tend to be worse in the subpleural regions,[90] are bilateral, and almost always are situated posteriorly and peripherally in the lower lobes. Thus, the morphologic changes within the lung in asbestosis may be indistinguishable from those of IPF.[10, 92–94]

To establish the clinical diagnosis of asbestosis, the official statement of the

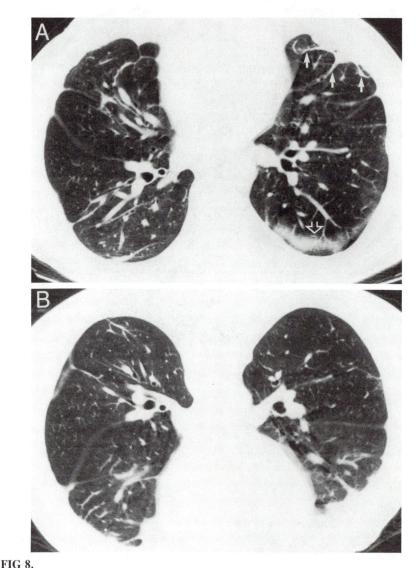

FIG 8.
Supine and prone 1.5-mm collimation HRCT scans in an asbestos-exposed patient. **A,** characteristic irregular linear opacities *(solid arrows)* representing pulmonary fibrosis are seen anteriorly in nondependent areas of the lung. These contact regions of thickened pleura. The crescentic area of subpleural dependent density *(open arrow)* in the left lower lobe is a reversible finding. **B,** it disappears when the patient is scanned in the prone position. (From Müller NL, Miller RR: *Am Rev Respir Dis* 1990; 142:1206–1215.

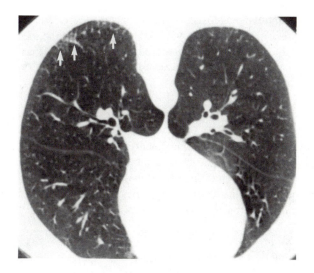

FIG 9.
Prone 1.5-mm collimation HRCT scan in a patient with mild asbestosis. Nondependent subpleural linear opacities *(interstitial short lines)* are present in the right lower lobe. Pathologically, these have been proven to represent fibrosis involving the interlobular septa and core of the secondary pulmonary lobule. Pleural plaques were evident on CT scans at other levels in this case.

American Thoracic Society, adopted in March 1986,[89] requires evidence on the radiograph of small irregular opacities meeting the International Labour Office designation type "s," "t," or "u" and of a profusion (severity) of 1/1 or greater. Although the chest radiograph, therefore, remains an essential tool in screening asbestos-exposed individuals, it has serious limitations in the detection of mild parenchymal disease. First, standard International Labour Office–classified radiographs do not include examples that define the division between normal and very mild disease,[95, 96] making it difficult to distinguish patients with minimal infiltrates from those with normal radiographs. Second, when the overall profusion of opacities on the radiograph is low, interobserver errors and variability are significant, reflecting the fact that it is difficult to identify minimal disease.[3, 92, 97] Perhaps most concerning are the findings indicating that, even when read by experienced radiologists, the radiograph may be falsely negative in 10% to 26% of cases with histologically proven asbestosis.[1, 91, 97–99]

The fact that substantial interstitial fibrosis must be present in order to be detectable on the plain radiograph, therefore, is a significant limitation in the detection of early disease using this technique.[97] This has significant ramifications in industrial litigation cases, in which the chest radiograph plays a central role in the diagnosis and an abnormal radiograph is accepted routinely as the only legal evidence of dust exposure.[100]

A number of studies have shown that HRCT can be helpful in the detection of early interstitial changes in asbestos-exposed individuals with normal chest radiographs. The presumptive diagnosis of asbestosis is made from the CT scan if pleural plaques are seen in conjunction with a variety of abnormalities in nondependent portions of the lung bases on prone and supine HRCT scans.[18] Aberle and coworkers[17, 46] have described the characteristic features of asbestosis on HRCT, which include the following:

1. Thickened intralobular lines representing fibrosis within the secondary lobule (Figs 8 and 9).
2. Parenchymal bands, nontapering linear structures measuring 2 to 5 cm in length that extend through the lung parenchyma to contact the pleural surface. These represent thickened interlobular septa (Fig 10).
3. Nondependent curvilinear subpleural lines, characterized by linear opacities within 1 cm of and paralleling the pleural surface.[101]

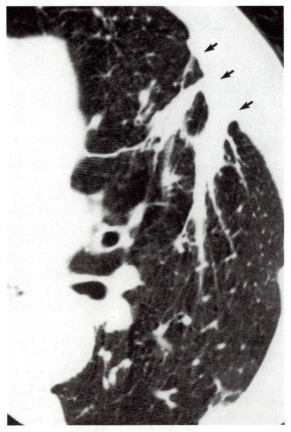

FIG 10.
HRCT scan (1.5-mm collimation) illustrates coarse parenchymal bands extending through the lung parenchyma to contact a pleural plaque *(arrows)*. Parenchymal bands represent fibrotic connective tissue septa and typically measure 2 to 5 cm in length.

4. A nondependent subpleural density, measuring 2 to 20 mm in width with sufficient opacity to obscure the morphology of underlying lung parenchyma.
5. Honeycombing.

HRCT is superior to the radiograph and conventional CT in the detection of pleural and parenchymal changes in the asbestos-exposed patient.[17, 18, 102] Aberle and coworkers compared the radiograph, HRCT, and clinical findings in 45 subjects satisfying clinical criteria for asbestosis.[46] The authors devised a CT probability score for asbestosis based upon the HRCT findings described above.[17] Among 35 patients with abnormal chest radiographs (profusion $\geq$1/0), the CT probability score was high in 86%. Among the remaining 10 patients with clinically confirmed asbestosis and normal radiographs (profusion <1/0), the CT score was high in 80%. The CT probability score showed significant inverse correlations with forced vital capacity ($P < .006$) and single-breath diffusing capacity ($P < .03$).

Staples and colleagues[19] evaluated the functional significance of an abnormal HRCT in a group of asbestos-exposed workers with normal chest radiographs (profusion <1/0). Fifty-seven patients (37%) had HRCT scans consistent with the diagnosis of asbestosis. The vital capacity and diffusing capacity were significantly lower ($P = .005$ and $P = .02$, respectively) and the clinical dyspnea score was higher ($P = .002$) among patients with HRCT findings suggestive of asbesto-

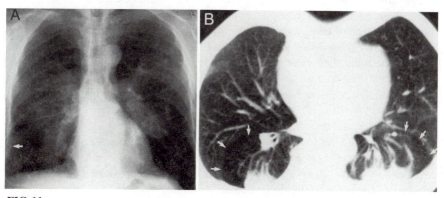

FIG 11.
Bilateral rounded atelectasis in an asymptomatic asbestos-exposed male smoker who was at high risk for lung cancer. **A,** the chest radiograph demonstrates pleural thickening *(arrow)* and bilateral ill-defined soft-tissue masses in the lower lung zones. **B,** the CT scan shows bilateral, ovoid soft-tissue masses in the lower lobes. These contact the pleural surface, which, on mediastinal windows, was diffusely thickened. Volume loss in the involved lobes is demonstrated by posterior displacement of the major fissures *(arrows)* and by reorientation of blood vessels, which appear to be gathered in a curved sheaf as they converge upon each mass. No additional pulmonary masses were evident. Thoracotomy was avoided because the CT features are characteristic of rounded atelectasis.

sis than among those with normal or nearly normal HRCT scans. The authors concluded that HRCT can identify a subset of asbestos-exposed individuals who have clinical evidence of restrictive lung disease in the presence of a normal chest radiograph.[19]

In summary, CT is superior to the chest radiograph in the imaging evaluation of asbestosis or the asbestos-exposed asymptomatic worker because it more accurately characterizes the severity and extent of pleural plaques and interstitial fibrosis, and may detect disease when other methods are equivocal or nondiagnostic and the radiograph is normal.[17, 19, 46] The severity of parenchymal changes on HRCT correlates with various clinical parameters, including the International Labour Office profusion score, reduction in forced vital capacity and single-breath diffusing capacity, and the clinical dyspnea index. Furthermore, CT is helpful in the assessment of asymptomatic focal lung masses (Fig 11) and useful in differentiating benign diffuse pleural thickening from malignant mesothelioma. HRCT also allows semiquantitative determination of the extent of parenchymal damage that is due to emphysema in asbestos-exposed patients who are smokers.[103-108]

Silicosis

Silicosis defines a fibrotic lung disease caused by the inhalation of inorganic dust containing crystalline silicon dioxide.[109] The disease process is characterized by the formation of fibrotic nodules in the lung parenchyma. Simple silicosis is characterized by the presence of nodules that are noncoalescent. In more severe cases, these nodules may become confluent, producing conglomerate masses surrounded by areas of emphysema. Under such circumstances, silicosis is said to be complicated by progressive massive fibrosis. The characteristic appearance of silicosis on both the chest radiograph and CT is that of a profusion of small nodular opacities that tend to have an upper lung zone predominance (Fig 12).[110, 111] On CT, the nodules are more numerous in the posterior portions of the lung, and vary in size from 1 to 10 mm.

Traditionally, the chest radiograph and pulmonary function tests have been employed to estimate the severity of silicosis. However, CT is superior to the radiograph in the detection of early coalescence of nodules,[110-112] which heralds the development of the complicated form of disease, the appearance of pulmonary symptoms, and deterioration in pulmonary function.[113]

Kinsella and coworkers[114] reviewed the CT scans and pulmonary function data in 30 patients with silicosis and found that it is the degree of emphysema and not the profusion of silicotic nodules that determines the level of functional impairment. Bergin et al.[110] showed that emphysema was diagnosed easily on CT scans, but frequently was difficult to assess on the plain radiograph. There was significant correlation between the CT emphysema score and both the $FEV_1\%$ predicted and the diffusing capacity ($r > .66$ and $r > .71$, respectively, $P < .001$), and impairment in lung function also correlated with superimposed emphysema rather than with the severity of nodular profusion.[110]

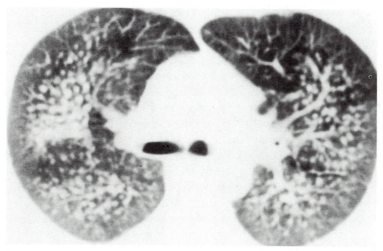

FIG 12.
CT scan (10 mm-collimation) in a patient with silicosis demonstrates multiple small, well-defined nodular opacities distributed randomly in the upper lung zones bilaterally. Early co-alescence of nodules is present in the right upper lobe. (From Mathieson JR, Mayo JR, Staples CA, et al: *Radiology* 1989; 171:111–116. Used by permission.)

Therefore, CT is superior to the radiograph in the detection of coalescence of silicotic nodules and the quantification of associated emphysema, although it clearly is not indicated in the routine assessment of these patients.

DIAGNOSTIC ACCURACY OF HIGH-RESOLUTION COMPUTED TOMOGRAPHY

Mathieson and coworkers[115] conducted a retrospective evaluation of the chest radiographs and CT scans in 118 patients with diffuse infiltrative lung disease in whom a specific diagnosis was proven pathologically. Based on the pattern and distribution of abnormalities, the CT scans and plain radiographs were compared with regard to establishing a definitive diagnosis. In a blinded fashion, three observers independently assessed the chest films and CT scans and made a confident diagnosis with 23% of the chest radiographs and 49% of the CT scans ($P < .001$). This diagnosis was correct in 77% and 93% of those readings, respectively ($P < .001$). Therefore, a confident diagnosis was made more than twice as often using the CT scans than using the chest radiographs, and the CT diagnoses were correct much more often.

CT was most accurate in the diagnosis of silicosis (93%), IPF (89%), pulmonary lymphangitic carcinomatosis (85%), and sarcoidosis (77%).[115] Whereas these findings indicate that CT is superior to the chest radiograph in accurately diagnosing specific disease processes, it is important to recognize that the CT features are rarely pathognomonic, as there is overlap in the appearance of a number of these conditions. Optimal assessment of the CT findings requires correlation with clinical, historic, functional, and laboratory data.

Among patients with clinically suspected extrinsic allergic alveolitis and a typical CT appearance, open lung biopsy may be avoided if a clear history of inhalational exposure is identified and laboratory tests indicate immunologic reactivity. In patients with IPF, particularly those with extensive honeycombing, the characteristic HRCT findings may obviate the need for biopsy. Similarly, in patients with a clinical history of asbestos exposure and HRCT scans demonstrating pleural plaques and characteristic parenchymal changes, a confident diagnosis of asbestosis can be made and biopsy avoided. With these exceptions, however, most of the causes of CILD require biopsy for definitive diagnosis.

Mathieson and coworkers[115] compared the accuracy of CT and the chest radiograph in predicting whether a transbronchial or open lung biopsy would be likely to yield a diagnostic specimen. Choice of a transbronchial biopsy was considered appropriate when the first-choice radiologic diagnosis was limited correctly to sarcoid or lymphatic spread of tumor.[3, 116] Open lung biopsy was suggested correctly when the first-choice diagnosis avoided these two entities. Among 118 patients, transbronchial biopsies were recommended correctly for diagnosis in 65% of chest radiographs and 87% of CT scans ($P < .001$). Recommendation for open lung biopsy was made correctly in 89% of chest radiographs and 99% of CT scans ($P < .001$). These data indicate that, when lung biopsy is warranted, CT is helpful in suggesting the type of biopsy as well as in guiding the surgeon to the optimal biopsy site.[85]

CONCLUSIONS

CT has revolutionized imaging of CILD by providing information about the anatomic extent, severity, and distribution of disease that is considerably superior to the chest radiograph. Specific indications for CT in patients with CILD include (1) a history suggestive of an abnormality or specific disorder in a patient with a normal or nondiagnostic chest radiograph, (2) a chest radiograph in which the appearances are out of keeping with the clinical history and the severity of symptoms or functional impairment, (3) follow-up of patients in whom the degree of clinical and functional progress is inappropriate for the type or duration of therapy, and (4) detection of specific complications related to the underlying disease process.

Although there is overlap in the CT appearances of a number of the conditions responsible for CILD, characteristic patterns have been recognized in IPF, sarcoidosis, silicosis, lymphangitic carcinomatosis, and extrinsic allergic alveolitis. The diagnostic accuracy of CT is high in several of these conditions and, when characteristic clinical, functional, and CT features are present, biopsy may be avoided in patients with IPF, asbestosis, and extrinsic allergic alveolitis. In remaining cases in which a histologic diagnosis is required, CT provides important information regarding the optimal method and site of biopsy.

CT also can show evidence of subtle pulmonary disease, inapparent on the chest radiograph, that may correlate with the severity of clinical symptoms and degree of functional impairment. Further research is necessary to determine whether CT can replace radionuclide scanning, bronchoalveolar lavage, and open lung biopsy in the assessment of disease activity in disorders characterized by the presence of active aveolitis.

REFERENCES

1. Epler GR, McLoud TC, Gaensler EA, et al: Normal chest roentgenograms in chronic diffuse infiltrative lung disease. *N Engl J Med* 1978; 298:934–939.

2. Gaensler EA, Carrington CB: Open biopsy for chronic diffuse infiltrative lung disease: Clinical, roentgenographic, and physiologic correlations in 502 patients. *Ann Thorac Surg* 1980; 30:411–426.

3. Dahlquen P, Oberholzer M: Lung biopsy: Methods, value, complications, timing, and indications. *Pathol Res Pract* 1979; 164:95–103.

4. Gaensler EA, Carrington CB, Coutu RE, et al: Radiographic-physiologic-pathologic correlations in interstitial pneumonias. *Progr Respir Res* 1975; 8:223–241.

5. Goldsmith SH, Bailey HD, Callahan EL, et al: Pulmonary metastases from breast carcinoma. *Arch Surg* 1967; 94:483–488.

6. McLoud TC, Carrington CB, Gaensler EA: Diffuse infiltrative lung disease: A new scheme for description. *Radiology* 1983; 149:353–363.

7. Müller NL, Miller RR, Webb WR, et al: Fibrosing alveolitis: CT-pathologic correlation. *Radiology* 1986; 160:585–588.

8. Müller NL, Staples CA, Miller RR, et al: Disease activity in idiopathic pulmonary fibrosis: Computed tomographic-pathologic correlation. *Radiology* 1987; 165:731–734.

9. Munk PL, Müller NL, Miller RR, et al: Pulmonary lymphangitic carcinomatosis: CT and pathologic findings. *Radiology* 1988; 166:705–709.

10. Meziane MA, Khouri NF, Hruban RH, et al: High resolution CT of the lung parenchyma with pathologic correlation. *Radiographics* 1988; 8:27–54.

11. Webb WR, Stein MG, Finkbeiner WE, et al: Normal and diseased isolated lungs: High-resolution CT. *Radiology* 1988; 166:81–87.

12. Müller NL, Kullnig P, Miller RR: The CT findings of pulmonary sarcoidosis: Analysis of 25 patients. *AJR Am J Roentgenol* 1989; 152:1179–1182.

13. Müller NL, Miller RR: Computed tomography of chronic diffuse infiltrative lung disease. Part 1. *Am Rev Respir Dis* 1990; 142:1206–1215.

14. Müller NL, Miller RR: State-of-the-art: Computed tomography of chronic diffuse infiltrative lung disease. Part 2. *Am Rev Respir Dis* 1990; 142:1440–1448.

15. Strickland B, Strickland NH: The value of high definition, narrow section computed tomography in fibrosing alveolitis. *Clin Radiol* 1988; 39:589–594.

16. Genereux GP: The Fleischner lecture: Computed tomography of diffuse pulmonary disease. *J Thorac Imaging* 1989; 4:50–87.

17. Aberle DR, Gamsu G, Ray CS, et al: Asbestos-related pleural and parenchymal fibrosis: Detection with high-resolution CT. *Radiology* 1988; 166:729–734.

18. Friedman AC, Fiel SB, Radecki PD, et al: Computed tomography of benign pleural and pulmonary parenchymal abnormalities related to asbestos exposure. *Semin Ultrasound CT MR* 1990; 11:393–408.

19. Staples CA, Gamsu G, Ray CS, et al: High resolution computed tomography and lung function in asbestos-exposed workers with normal chest radiographs. *Am Rev Respir Dis* 1989; 139:1502–1508.

20. Stein MG, Mayo J, Müller N, et al: Pulmonary lymphangitic spread of carcinoma: Appearance on CT scans. *Radiology* 1987; 162:371–375.

21. Brauner MW, Grenier P, Mompoint D, et al: Pulmonary sarcoidosis: Evaluation with high-resolution CT. *Radiology* 1989; 172:467–471.

22. Müller NL, Chiles C, Kullnig P: Pulmonary lymphangiomyomatosis: Correlation of CT with radiographic and functional findings. *Radiology* 1990; 175:335–339.

23. Murata K, Khan A, Rojas KA, et al: Optimization of computed tomography technique to demonstrate the fine structure of the lung. *Invest Radiol* 1988; 23:170–175.

24. Staples CA, Müller NL, Vedal S, et al: Usual interstitial pneumonia: Correlation of CT with clinical, functional, and radiologic findings. *Radiology* 1987; 162:377–381.

25. Mayo JR, Webb WR, Gould R, et al: High-resolution CT of the lungs: An optimal approach. *Radiology* 1987; 163:507–510.

26. Webb WR, Müller NL, Zerhouni EA: High-resolution CT of the lung: Current clinical uses. *Perspect Radiol* 1989; 2:61–69.

27. Naidich DP: Pulmonary parenchyma high-resolution CT: To be or not to be. *Radiology* 1989; 171:22–24.

28. Liebow AA: New concepts and entities in pulmonary disease, in Liebow AA (ed): *The Lung.* Baltimore, Williams & Wilkins, 1968, pp 332–365.

29. Colby TV, Carrington CB: Infiltrative lung disease, in Thurlbeck WM (ed): *Pathology of the Lung.* Stuttgart, Thieme Medical Publishers, 1988, pp 425–518.

30. Liebow AA, Steer A, Billingsley JG: Desquamative interstitial pneumonia. *Am J Med* 1965; 38:369–404.

31. Scadding JG, Hinson KFW: Diffuse fibrosing alveolitis (diffuse interstitial fibrosis of the lungs)—correlation of histology at biopsy with prognosis. *Thorax* 1967; 22:291–304.

32. Liebow AA, Carrington CB: Diffuse pulmonary lymphoreticular infiltration associated with dysproteinemia. *Med Clin North Am* 1973; 57:809–843.

33. Steimlam CV, Rosenow EC, Divertie MB, et al: Pulmonary manifestations of Sjögren's syndrome. *Chest* 1976; 70:354–361.

34. Joshi VV, Oleske JM, Minnefor AB, et al: Pathologic pulmonary findings in children with the acquired immunodeficiency syndrome. *Hum Pathol* 1985; 16:241–246.

35. Grieco MH, Chinoy-Acharya P: Lymphoid interstitial pneumonia associated with the acquired immune deficiency syndrome. *Am Rev Respir Dis* 1985; 131:952–955.

36. Spencer H (ed): *Pathology of the Lung.* Oxford, Pergamon Press, 1985, pp 1025–1032.

37. Ohori NP, Sciurba FC, Owens GR, et al: Giant-cell interstitial pneumonia and hard-metal pneumoconiosis. *Am J Surg Pathol* 1989; 13:581–587.

38. Epler GR, Colby TV, McLoud TC, et al: Idiopathic bronchiolitis obliterans with organizing pneumonia. *N Engl J Med* 1985; 312:152–159.

39. Müller NL, Guerry-Force ML, Staples CA, et al: Differential diagnosis of bronchiolitis obliterans with organizing pneumonia and usual interstitial pneumonia: Clinical, functional, and radiologic findings. *Radiology* 1987; 162:151–156.

40. Katzenstein AL, Myers JL, Prophet WD, et al: Bronchiolitis obliterans and usual interstitial pneumonia: A comparative clinicopathologic study. *Am J Surg Pathol* 1986; 10:373–381.

41. Chandler PW, Shin MS, Friedman SE, et al: Radiographic manifestations of bronchiolitis obliterans with organizing pneumonia vs usual interstitial pneumonia. *AJR Am J Roentgenol* 1986; 147:899–906.

42. Carrington CB, Gaensler EA, Coute E, et al: Natural history and treated course of usual and desquamative interstitial pneumonia. *N Engl J Med* 1978; 298:801–809.

43. Crystal RG, Bitterman PB, Rennard SI, et al: Interstitial lung diseases of unknown cause: Disorders characterized by chronic inflammation of the lower respiratory tract. *N Engl J Med* 1984; 310:154–166.

44. Crystal RG, Fulmer JD, Roberts WC, et al: Idiopathic pulmonary fibrosis: Clinical, histologic, radiographic, physiologic, scintigraphic, cytologic and biochemical aspects. *Ann Intern Med* 1976; 85:769–788.

45. Turner-Warwick M, Burrows B, Johnson A: Cryptogenic fibrosing alveolitis: Clinical features and their influence on survival. *Thorax* 1980; 35:171–180.

46. Aberle DR, Gamsu G, Ray CS: High-resolution CT of benign asbestos-related diseases: Clinical and radiographic correlation. *AJR Am J Roentgenol* 1988; 151:883–891.

47. Wright PH, Heard BE, Steel SJ, et al: Cryptogenic fibrosing alveolitis: Assessment by graded trephine lung biopsy histology compared with clinical, radiographic and physiologic features. *Br J Dis Chest* 1981; 75:61–70.

48. Klein JS, Webb WR, Gamsu G, et al: Hazy increased density in diffuse lung disease: High-resolution CT (abstract). *Radiology* 1989; 173:140.

49. Epler GR, Colby TV: The spectrum of bronchiolitis obliterans. *Chest* 1983; 83:161–162.

50. Gosink BB, Friedman PJ, Liebow AA: Bronchiolitis obliterans: Roentgenographic-pathologic correlation. *AJR Am J Roentgenol* 1973; 117:816–832.

51. Lowry T, Schuman LM: "Silo-filler's disease"—a syndrome caused by nitrogen dioxide. *JAMA* 1956; 162:153–158.

52. Cornelius EA, Betlach EH: Silo-filler's disease. *Radiology* 1960; 74:232–235.

53. Charan NB, Myers CG, Lakshminarayan S, et al: Pulmonary injuries associated with acute sulfur dioxide inhalation. *Am Rev Respir Dis* 1979; 119:555–560.

54. Laraya-Cuasay LR, DeForest A, Huff D, et al: Chronic pulmonary complications of early influenza virus infection in children. *Am Rev Respir Dis* 1977; 116:617–625.

55. Nikki P, Meretoja O, Valtonen V, et al: Severe bronchiolitis probably caused by varicella-zoster virus. *Crit Care Med* 1982; 10:344–346.

56. Geddes DM, Corrin B, Brewerton DA, et al: Progressive airway obliteration in adults and its association with rheumatoid disease. *Q J Med* 1977; 46:427–444.

57. Epler GR, Snider GL, Gaensler EA, et al: Bronchiolitis and bronchitis in connective tissue disease. *JAMA* 1979; 242:528–532.

58. Schwarz MI, Matthay RA, Sahn SA, et al: Interstitial lung disease in polymyositis and dermatomyositis: An analysis of six cases and review of the literature. *Medicine (Baltimore)* 1976; 55:89–104.

59. Herzog CA, Miller RR, Hoidal JR: Bronchiolitis and rheumatoid arthritis. *Am Rev Respir Dis* 1979; 119:555–560.

60. Ostrow D, Buskard N, Hill RS, et al: Bronchiolitis obliterans complicating bone marrow transplantation. *Chest* 1985; 87:828–830.

61. Roca J, Granena A, Rodriguez-Roisin J, et al: Fatal airway disease in an adult with chronic graft-versus-host disease. *Thorax* 1982; 37:77–78.

62. Stein-Streilen J, Lipscomb MF, Hart DA, et al: Graft-versus-host reaction in the lung. *Transplantation* 1981; 32:38–44.

63. Burke CM, Theodore J, Dawkins KD, et al: Post transplant obliterative bronchiolitis and other late lung sequelae in human heart-lung transplantation. *Chest* 1984; 86:824–829.

64. Davidson AG, Heard BE, McAllister WC, et al: Cryptogenic organizing pneumonitis. *Q J Med* 1983; 52:382–393.

65. Müller NL, Staples CA, Miller RR: Bronchiolitis obliterans organizing pneumonia: CT features in 14 patients. *Am J Roentgenol AJR* 1990; 154:983–987.

66. McLoud TC, Epler GR, Gaensler EA, et al: A radiographic classification for sarcoidosis: Physiologic correlation. *Invest Radiol* 1982; 17:129–138.

67. Scadding JG, Mitchell DN: *Sarcoidosis*. London, Chapman and Hall Medical, 1985, pp 101–180.

68. Hillerdal G, Nöu E, Osterman K, et al: Sarcoidosis: Epidemiology and prognosis, a 15-year European study. *Am Rev Respir Dis* 1984; 130:29–32.

69. Carrington CB, Gaensler EA, Mikus JP, et al: Structure and function in sarcoidosis. *Ann N Y Acad Sci* 1976; 278:265–283.

70. Heitzman ER: Sarcoidosis, in Heitzman ER (ed): *The Lung: Radiologic-Pathologic Correlations*. St Louis, CV Mosby, 1984, pp 294–310.

71. Thomas PD, Hunninghake GW: Current concepts of the pathogenesis of sarcoidosis. *Am Rev Respir Dis* 1987; 135:747–760.

72. Churg A: Lung biopsy: Handling and diagnosing limitations, in Thurlbeck WM (ed): *Pathology of the Lung*. New York, Thieme Medical Publishers, 1988, pp 67–78.

73. Lynch DA, Webb WR, Gamsu G, et al: Computed tomography in pulmonary sarcoidosis. *J Comput Assist Tomogr* 1989; 13:405–410.

74. Bergin CJ, Bell DY, Coblentz CL, et al: Sarcoidosis: Correlation of pulmonary parenchymal pattern at CT with results of pulmonary function tests. *Radiology* 1989; 171:619–624.

75. Müller NL, Mawson JB, Mathieson JR, et al: Sarcoidosis: Correlation of extent of disease at CT with clinical, functional, and radiographic findings. *Radiology* 1989; 171:613–618.

76. Newman SL, Michel RP, Wang N-S: Lingular lung biopsy: Is it representative. *Am Rev Respir Dis* 1985; 132:1084–1086.

77. Scott-Miller K, Smith EA, Kinsella M, et al: Lung disease associated with progressive systemic sclerosis. Assessment of interlobar variation by bronchoalveolar lavage and comparison with noninvasive evaluation of disease activity. *Am Rev Respir Dis* 1990; 141:301–306.

78. Line BR, Hunninghake GW, Keogh BA: Gallium-67 scanning to stage the alveolitis of sarcoidosis: Correlation with clinical studies, pulmonary function studies, and bronchoalveolar lavage. *Am Rev Respir Dis* 1981; 123:440–446.

79. Chryssanthopoulos C, Fink JN: Hypersensitivity pneumonitis. *J Asthma* 1983; 20:285–296.

80. Fraser RG, Paré JAP: *Diagnosis of Diseases of the Chest*, ed 2. Philadelphia, WB Saunders Co, 1979.

81. Silver SF, Müller NL, Miller RR, et al: Computed tomography in hypersensitivity pneumonitis. *Radiology* 1989; 173:441–445.

82. Cook PG, Wells IP, McGavin CR: The distribution of pulmonary shadowing in farmer's lung. *Clin Radiol* 1988; 39:21–27.

83. Hapke EJ, Seal RME, Thomas GO, et al: Farmer's lung. A clinical, radiographic, functional and serologic correlation of acute and chronic stages. *Thorax* 1968; 23:451–468.

84. Stechschulte DJ, Austen KF: Hypersensitivity pneumonitis, in Thorn GW, Adams RD, Braunwald E, et al (eds): *Harrison's Principles of Internal Medicine*, ed 8. New York, McGraw-Hill Book Company, 1977, pp 1345–1349.

85. Miller RR, Nelems B, Müller NL, et al: Lingular and right middle lobe biopsy in the assessment of diffuse lung disease. *Ann Thorac Surg* 1987; 44:269–273.

86. Zerhouni EA, Naidich DP, Stitik FP, et al: Computed tomography of the pulmonary parenchyma. II. Interstitial disease. *J Thorac Imaging* 1985; 1:54–64.

87. Ren H, Hruban RH, Kuhlman JE, et al: Computed tomography of inflation-fixed lungs: The beaded septum sign of pulmonary metastases. *J Comput Assist Tomogr* 1989; 12:411–416.

88. Noma S, Khan A, Herman PG, et al: High-resolution computed tomography of the pulmonary parenchyma. *Semin Ultrasound CT MR* 1990; 11:365–379.

89. Murphy RL, Becklake MR, Brooks SM, et al: *The Diagnosis of Nonmalignant Diseases Related to Asbestos.* New York, American Thoracic Society, 1986, pp 362–368.

90. Hourihane DO, McCaughey WTE: Pathological aspects of asbestosis. *Postgrad Med J* 1966; 42:613.

91. Rockoff SD, Schwartz A: Roentgenographic underestimation of early asbestosis by International Labor Organization Classification: Analysis of data and probabilities. *Chest* 1988; 93:1088–1091.

92. Gefter WB, Conant EF: Issues and controversies in the plain film diagnosis of asbestos-related disorders in the chest. *J Thorac Imaging* 1988; 3:11–28.

93. Bergin CJ, Coblentz CL, Chiles C, et al: Chronic lung diseases: Specific diagnosis by using CT. *AJR Am J Roentgenol* 1989; 152:1183–1188.

94. Fiel SB, Friedman AC, Radecki PD: Evaluation of pulmonary disease: Clinical role of conventional and high-resolution CT. *Radiol Rep* 1989; 1:188–205.

95. Kilburn KH: Does the 1980 ILO classification of pneumoconiosis need a facelift (editorial)? *Arch Environ Health* 1988; 43:261–262.

96. Rossiter CE, Browne K, Gilson JC: International classification trial of AIA set of 100 radiographs of asbestos workers. *Br J Ind Med* 1988; 45:538–543.

97. Rockoff SD, Schwartz A: Roentgenographic underestimation of early asbestosis by International Labor Office classification: Analysis of data and probabilities. *Chest* 1988; 93:1088–1091.

98. Kipen HM, Lilis R, Suzuki Y, et al: Pulmonary fibrosis in asbestos insulation workers with lung cancer: A radiological and histopathological evaluation. *Br J Ind Med* 1987; 44:96–100.

99. Gaensler EA, Carrington CB, Coutu RE, et al: Pathological, physiological, and radiological correlations in the pneumoconioses. *Ann N Y Acad Sci* 1972; 200:574–607.

100. Morgan WKC: Epidemiology and occupational lung disease, in Morgan WKC, Seaton A (eds): *Occupational Lung Diseases,* ed 2. Philadelphia, WB Saunders, 1984, pp 97–128.

101. Yoshimura H, Hatakeyama M, Otsuji H, et al: Pulmonary asbestosis: CT study of subpleural curvilinear shadow. *Radiology* 1986; 158:653–658.

102. Katz D, Kreel L: Computed tomography in pulmonary asbestosis. *Clin Radiol* 1979; 30:207–213.

103. Friedman AC, Fiel SB, Fisher MS, et al: Asbestos-related pleural disease and asbestosis: A comparison of CT and chest radiography. *AJR Am J Roentgenol* 1988; 150:269–275.

104. Kuwano K, Matsuba K, Ikeda T, et al: The diagnosis of mild emphysema. Correlation of computed tomography and pathology scores. *Am Rev Respir Dis* 1990; 141:169–178.

105. Kinsella M, Müller NL, Morrison NJ, et al: Computerized quantitation of emphysema by computed tomography (CT): Correlation with pulmonary function testing (abstract). *Am Rev Respir Dis* 1989; 4:121A.

106. Burki NK: Roentgenologic diagnosis of emphysema (editorial). Accurate or not? *Chest* 1989; 95:1178–1179.

107. Gamsu G, Aberle DR, Lynch D: Computed tomography in the diagnosis of asbestos-related thoracic disease. *J Thorac Imaging* 1989; 4:61–67.

108. Hnizdo E, Sluis-Cremer GK: Effect of tobacco smoking on the presence of asbestosis at postmortem and on the reading of irregular opacities on roentgenograms in asbestos-exposed workers. *Am Rev Respir Dis* 1988; 138:1207–1212.

109. Seaton A: Silicosis, in Morgan WKC, Seaton A (eds): *Occupational Lung Diseases,* ed 2. Philadelphia, WB Saunders, 1984, pp 250–294.

110. Bergin CJ, Müller NL, Vedal S, et al: CT in silicosis: Correlation with plain films and pulmonary function tests. *AJR Am J Roentgenol* 1986; 146:477–483.

111. Begin R, Bergeron D, Samson L, et al: CT assessment of silicosis in exposed workers. *AJR Am J Roentgenol* 1987; 148:509–514.

112. Bégin R, Ostiguy G, Groleau S, et al: Computed tomography scanning of the thorax in workers at risk of or with silicosis. *Semin Ultrasound CT MR* 1990; 11:380–392.

113. Fraser RG, Paré JAP: Silicosis, in Fraser RG, Paré JAP (eds): *Diagnosis of Diseases of the Chest*, vol 3. Philadelphia, WB Saunders, 1979, pp 1484–1502.

114. Kinsella M, Müller NL, Vedal S, et al: Emphysema in silicosis: A comparison of smokers with nonsmokers using pulmonary function testing and computed tomography. *Am Rev Respir Dis* 1990; 141:1497–1500.

115. Mathieson JR, Mayo JR, Staples CA, et al: Chronic diffuse infiltrative lung disease: Comparison of diagnostic accuracy of CT and chest radiography. *Radiology* 1989; 171:111–116.

116. Churg A: Lung biopsy: Handling and diagnosing limitations, in Thurlbeck WM (ed): *Pathology of the Lung*. New York, Thieme Medical Publishers, 1988, pp 67–78.

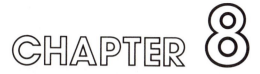

CHAPTER 8

Occupational Lung Disease

J. Bernard L. Gee, M.D.

Professor of Medicine, Pulmonary and Critical Care Section, Department of Internal Medicine, Yale University School of Medicine, New Haven, Connecticut

This review will be selective, in part reflecting the author's interests, but focusing on developments notably in the last 4 to 5 years. We begin with either a critical account or a description of some of the methods. Specific disorders follow. Finally, we hope the reader will permit some personal reflections on societal, economic, and legislative aspects of occupational lung disease (OLD).

METHODS

Radiology

The recent development of high-resolution chest computed tomographic scans (HRCTSs) by Gamsu and colleagues[1] provides a useful approach to the diagnosis of asbestosis and extends the generally recognized utility of conventional chest computed tomographic (CT) scans in recognizing and differentially diagnosing pleural abnormalities.[2] The new technique employs thin (1.0 to 1.5 mm) sections, a specific spatial frequency algorithm for increased spatial resolution, and wide window settings, permitting the assessment of the relation of pleural to parenchymal abnormalities. To avoid gravitationally determined radiologic effects, studies performed with the subject supine and prone are compared. Persistent accentuated curvilinear subpleural lines, thickened interlobular and intralobular lines, and diffuse subpleural densities are considered to represent mild asbestosis. Honeycombing also occurs. The effects are seen first in the posterior portions of the lower lobes. HRCTSs are thought to be more sensitive than both conventional chest radiographs and CT scans. Although there is a general relation to pulmonary function data, more information is needed on this relationship. Further, whereas HRCTS may establish a radiologic diagnosis of asbestosis, functional tests remain the norm for assessing the consequences of asbestosis.

The International Labor Office (ILO) radiologic classification of asbestosis into irregular opacities of various sizes and profusions of small opacities remains a most useful epidemiologic tool. Unfortunately, its use by so-called B readers who have passed the appropriate test can lead to the ascription of an unwarranted authority to certain of its users. An early study by Rossiter[3] needs emphasis, since it points out the considerable interobserver error, even among accepted "experts," particularly for x-rays with low profusions of small opacities. There are other criticisms, together with comments on pleural shadows.[4–6]

A few caveats are noteworthy. Readings of low profusions of small opacities often are unwisely proffered in low-contrast chest films in which the thoracic spine and heart shadows are indistinguishable. Soft-tissue shadows and occasionally gynecomastia lead to erroneous reading of low profusions of small opacifications.

Pulmonary Function Tests

There have been few technical developments in pulmonary function testing, but some practical issues require comment. Many laboratories fail to correct tests for race and smoking status. Black persons' dynamic and static lung volumes are generally 10% to 15% below predicted values for white individuals. Smoking diminishes diffusing capacity (D_L) values to 70% of predicted values for nonsmokers.[7, 8]

Likewise, spirometric techniques frequently are substandard, in spite of American Thoracic Society (ATS) guidelines.[9] A permanent hard copy of the record is essential if the results are to be assessed properly. Such spirometry records frequently reveal expirations of less than 6 seconds with consequent spuriously low vital capacity (VC), high forced expiratory volume in 1 second (FEV_1)/forced vital capacity (FVC) ratio and hence also low total lung capacity (TLC) values. Likewise, flow-volume records may show low or blunted peak flows indicating poor effort, which diminishes the effort-dependent portion of the FEV_1. Artifactual cut-off of the expiration, for instance by glottic closure (an asthma mimic) can be recognized readily by examining the flow-volume loops. Finally, the TLC, usually estimated from VC and a multibreath residual volume (RV) value, should agree with the observed alveolar volume (V_A) where D_L is measured by the single-breath method.

A major issue has surfaced recently. Eisen and colleagues have ascribed the lack of reproducibility of spirometric values in cohort studies to the presence of lung disease as opposed to poor test performance. This conclusion is based on several surveys[10, 11] and on Vermont granite shed workers exposed to silica.[12] Their argument is based on their reports of a greater fall in FEV_1 over the years among the inconsistent as opposed to the consistent performers of spirometry. To avoid the obvious problem of now knowing some of the FEV_1 values where reproducibility is lacking, they developed an ingenious back-extrapolation technique using the FEV_1 changes over time where the tests show acceptable reproducibility.[13] Such mathematically derived "data," together with acceptable data, were used to justify their view that poor spirometric reproducibility means disease. The use of bad data for diagnosis seems to this author to be intuitively dubious! However, Eisen's views have been endorsed by one experienced person,[14] but also criticized by others who have sought to improve spirometry performance[15] by providing visual feedback to their subjects of spirometry test results. Though this group too has 1% to 2% failures of reproducibility, they correctly state "better training, instrumentation, software and technician monitoring, etc. should be tried before one concedes that test failure is as likely to reflect ill health as it is to reflect poor cooperation, etc."

Knudson and coworkers[16] consider flow-volume curves superior to spirograms for the detection of submaximal effort and maximal effort flow-volume curves remain the evaluative norm for spirometry. In spite of the compressive effect on intrathoracic gas volume of truly maximal expiratory effort—with a small diminution of about 150 mL in FEV_1 in normal subjects—Krowka's group[17] agrees with Knudson. They state, "only FEV_1 values from maneuvers appearing to represent maximal effort should be reported." We agree with them and also strongly suggest that expiratory time or a spirogram with a time scale remain essential for FVC measures to be valid.

While not rejecting Eisen's approach out of hand since "missing" data and epidemiologic drop-outs are real problems, there are major concerns. Clinical experience shows that skilled technicians can obtain consistent results in the majority of patients. In fact, most patients with chronic obstructive pulmonary disease (COPD) show remarkably consistent spirometry. Inspection of spirometry records often shows flat peak flow records, cough artifacts, or too short expiration times to be the fault(s). Certainly, cough can result in poor performance and cough is a disease symptom. One wonders, however, to what extent such doubtless excellent computer experts have performed spirometric surveys themselves or personally examined these records. This concern is reinforced by our sad previous experience with spirometric data obtained on toluene diisocyanate (TDI) workers by some persons from this otherwise distinguished institution. For instance, our personally performed studies of a group of TDI workers[18] found higher FVC and FEV_1 values than did their earlier studies of many of the same subjects. Further questions about the validity of their Vermont workers' spirometric data were raised by Graham and Ashikaga.[19] This drew an admission from Wegman of poor spirometric techniques,[20] even though his group used these data in proposals to modify the silica standard.[21] Eisen's Table 4[12] shows that, for those Vermont workers participating in the initial 1970 study, the initial FEV_1 values (expressed as fractions of predicted values) were similar within a range of 0.90 to 0.98 in all four groups, namely those who either did or did not persistently "fail" PFTs and also those who did or did not terminate work in the sheds. Thus, on the basis of those persons actually studied at the inception of the Vermont survey, neither subsequent poor reproducibility nor work termination *directly* correlated with any initial abnormality!

Kellie et al.[22] also examined the association between spirometry reproducibility and respiratory morbidity and mortality in a large coal mine cohort. Two reproducibility criteria were used, the best two FVCs within 5% or 100 mL of one another or the best two FEV_1s within 200 mL of one another. These two criteria yielded rather different results. For instance, with the first criterion, the test failures were older (4 years), had 4 years more coal exposure, and comprised 13% of the cohort. Interestingly, they had more cough, sputum, and wheezing and reported three times more "severe shortness of breath [SOB]". Unfortunately, they do not give the FVC values for the SOB group—an important omission. For the FEV_1 criterion, 10% failed reproducibility criteria but did not differ in age, exposure time, or more significantly in symptoms from the reproducible performers except for a slight increase in the prevalence of "severe SOB" of borderline significance (again without FEV_1 values in these persons). These results are conflicting, but FVC values might well be more influenced than FEV_1s by end-expiratory airway collapse with cough, etc. It would seem that the FEV_1 is more valid. If this study is generally applicable, then a lack of reproducibility of FEV_1 is small at 10% of the population and not indicative of disease. There were no differences in the mortality odds ratios (adjusted for age, smoking, and coal dust exposure) between the consistent and inconsistent performers on either reproducibility criterion.

Other Techniques

Accounts of specific challenge techniques for occupational asthma are available.[23] Nonspecific airway challenges have been discussed from mechanistic and clinical aspects.[24] Three points may be made. First, airway reactivity reflects the law of initial values,[25] i.e., the response to a given stimulus depends on the portion of the dose:response curve at which the stimulus is proffered. Airway resistance is a fourth-power function of airway diameter, so the response curves, a fourth-power quadratic function, are hardly linear! Airway reactivity is largely a small-airway–resistive phenomenon that, during challenges, is sufficiently increased to contribute to the overall airway (large and small airways) resistance and so lower FEV_1. Alterations in small-airway caliber clearly occur in the presence of normal FEV_1s, as shown by enhanced RV and functional residual capacity (FRC) in asthmatics, and clearly demonstrate that asthmatics often start at different points of the dose: response curves compared to normal subjects. These changes in airway caliber partly reflect smooth muscle activity, but largely derive from changes in airway anatomy due to airway secretions and inflammatory and fibrotic changes in both airway mucosa and submucosa. Second, care must be taken that the volume history of the lung during this test does not influence FEV_1 changes, since airway diameter in part reflects lung compliance, which is affected by lung inflation.[26] Third, as pointed out by Krowka and coworkers,[17] the degree of expiratory effort affects the FEV_1 either by intrathoracic gas compression or by affecting the effort-dependent portion of the FEV_1. This implies that effort should be assessed in such nonspecific challenges as those requiring repeated forced expirations.

Mineralogic and metallurgical techniques are discussed under asbestos and metals, respectively. The principles underlying screening and follow-up have been reviewed by Boehlecke.[27]

METALS AND THE LUNG

A number of metals affect the lung, e.g., platinum salts and nickel cause asthma. Several comments on the contribution of some metals to lung cancer are available.[28-33] We comment briefly on some metals.

Welding

An excellent review[34] addresses the acute and chronic pulmonary effects of welding. One major effect, "fume fever," is similar whatever the welded material may be (e.g., zinc, plastic coatings), i.e., fever and leukocytosis are common, but chest x-ray findings are rare. Generally, the disorder is short-term and self-limiting. A more prolonged and serious disorder, hypersensitivity or chemical pneumonitis, also occurs and is associated with radiologic changes; when recurrent, it requires removal from the job. Cadmium used to prevent weathering is particularly dangerous. Asthma also occurs in stainless steel welders.

Among the reported chronic sequelae are chronic bronchitis, but the exact prevalence is uncertain. Smoking is so common among welders that the true incidence of COPD from welding alone is probably low. Persistent pulmonary function changes, either restrictive or obstructive, are rare. In welder's siderosis, there are small opacities on x-rays, usually without symptoms. They often resolve on leaving the job and are not associated with functional changes. The opacities are largely iron, but silica is found also. Occasional radiologic features similar to progressive massive fibrosis occur. Radiopaque tin yields dense radiologic shadows with no functional changes (stannosis). Lung cancer excesses have been described, but they are usually small (standard mortality ratio [SMR] <2.0) and generally not statistically significant. The major contributors to this subject are Kallio-maki and colleagues,[35] who used magnetopneumography to detect iron deposits; McMillan and Heath in United Kingdom naval dockyards[36]; and Doig and Duguid in England.[37] A detailed study of a European group of 11,000 welders is available.[38] The group includes stainless steel, mild steel, and shipyard workers. The SMR for lung cancer was 1.37 (confidence interval 1.11 to 1.68), but cases of the disease tended to occur early in employment and were not dose-related.

Hard Metal Diseases

"Hard metal" is formed from tungsten and carbon, which are heated to 1,400 to 1,500° C to produce tungsten carbide. Cobalt and nickel in varying proportions are incorporated then by sintering at high temperatures, producing the hard metal, which has 90% to 95% of diamond hardness. Exposure can occur during manufacture; in diamond cutters, mainly in Antwerp; and in widespread industrial use in grinding and cutting tools. Metallic dusts result from its use. When used in grinding with coolant liquids, cobalt is released into the inhalable coolants whose reuse serves to concentrate it, creating a hapten. Several disorders result.[39, 40] Occupational asthma occurs; inhalation challenge tests yield immediate, delayed, or dual responses. Sensitization occurs in a few months and symptoms persist after prolonged exposure. Chronic obstructive disease may result.[41]

Parenchymal disorders include simple interstitial disease and a form of interstitial pneumonitis diagnostically characterized by giant-cell formation.[42] Restrictive defects occur with either normal chest x-rays or a blotchy micronodular radiologic pattern. A single case with the febrile picture of hypersensitivity pneumonitis has been described.[43] The fibrosis can be detected by magnetic resonance imaging, even in the absence of conventional chest x-ray abnormalities.[43] Skin reactions, pruritus, and sensitivity rashes also occur.

The diagnosis usually is evident from a careful history. It can be confirmed by bronchoalveolar lavage (BAL), with 4% to 5% of the cell yield often being giant cells. Energy-dispersive x-ray analysis will reveal metals; tungsten is diagnostic,[43, 44] whereas cobalt is leached out and not easily detected, even in open biopsies. An open lung biopsy generally is unnecessary.

The prognosis for established parenchymal disease is poor, with little functional response to steroids. Radiologic and lung function monitoring of workers, therefore, is important. The 8-hour time-weighed average (TWA) threshold limit value (TLV) for cobalt has been lowered by the American Conference of Governmental Industrial Hygienists (ACGIH) from 0.10 to 0.05 mg/m^3. Whether this limit is adequate is uncertain, since progression of the obstructive ventilatory defect has occurred in workers exposed to average airborne cobalt concentrations of 0.06 mg/m^3.[45] The emphasis on cobalt rather than tungsten is justified by the studies of Demedts and colleagues of different metal component exposure among the Antwerp diamond cutters.[46]

Beryllium

Beryllium fumes cause acute lung injury that may pass into a chronic fibrotic stage. More common is chronic berylliosis, which simulates sarcoidosis. New developments, since a careful review,[47] address the immunologic mechanisms of berylliosis, for which multiple beryllium exposures are a prerequisite. Lymphocyte transformation tests were introduced by Williams and later by Daniele and colleagues,[48] the latter using BAL lymphocyte populations. Saltini et al.[49] elegantly extended these observations, showing that proliferation of CD4+ helper/inducer cells, obtained by BAL, is maintained by continuing presentations of beryllium antigen or beryllium hapten to beryllium-specific T cell clones. This activity required the presence of both the major histocompatibility complex (MHC) and functional interleukin-2 receptors, which were more active in BAL than in peripheral blood lymphocytes. The necessity for MHC was shown by using class-restricted antibodies. This observation is important, since it presumably underlies the clinical observation that berylliosis occurs in only a few beryllium-exposed persons. Beryllium is present continually in the lungs of patients with berylliosis and beryllium assays formerly provided a diagnostic test. Now, immunologic studies of BAL cells may avoid the necessity for an open lung biopsy and establish the presence of the appropriate immunologic mechanisms for this disorder.[50, 51] Histologic and BAL immunologic features of beryllium predictably occur prior to functional or radiologic changes.[52]

Cadmium

In addition to cadmium's acute role in welding, chronic exposure in the manufacture of certain cadmium-copper alloys produces an emphysema-like picture.[53] FEV_1 values were decreased, RV was increased, and there was a striking loss of D_L in one study. Radiologic emphysema occurred. Classification of cadmium workers by exposure categories was performed from a knowledge of airborne cadmium exposure or neutron activation analysis of liver cadmium. High cadmium exposures related to the severity of the lung functional changes. Of interest is the fact that a cigarette contains 2 μg of cadmium! Cadmium can be found in smokers' lungs, but its involvement in smoker's emphysema is improbable.[54]

Aluminum

Aluminum affects the lung as either the source ore, bauxite, or the metal and its oxide, usually in relation to abrasives. The development of pulmonary fibrosis is a potential hazard. A recent account of bauxite miners and refiners indicated the development of low-profusion, rounded opacities due to some combination of smoking and bauxite.[55] Two accounts of lung fibrosis in aluminum-containing abrasives have appeared,[56, 57] together with a case report describing aluminum oxide in a fibrous form.[58]

A sarcoidlike granuloma has been reported in a worker exposed to mixed metals including aluminum metal and oxides. The latter was the predominant metal in lung tissue.[59]

ASBESTOS-RELATED DISORDERS

Controversy over asbestos continues unabated! Our own view[60, 61] is that, whereas there will be a legacy, particularly of mesothelioma, asbestos-related disorders are on the wane in Western society. For developing countries, caution remains essential. Asbestos-related malignancies are the subject of an excellent recent text.[62]

Mineralogic Types

Among commercial types of asbestos, one distinguishes between the serpentine chrysotile asbestos (white) and the rodlike/needlelike amphiboles (crocidolite—blue; amosite—brown; tremolite and anthophyllite). The definition of a "fiber" is debated, the Environmental Protection Agency (EPA) definition being a length:diameter ratio of 3:1. However, Wylie,[63] an expert mineralogist, discusses the proper use of the term asbestiform in relation to fiber dimensions, indicating that a length:diameter ratio of 3:1 is too simplistic. She points out that these fiber features can be recognized and are related to biologic activity, which varies with fiber morphology. Most important, for tremolite, the distinction between asbestiform and cleavage fragments is recognizable and of pathologic importance.

Many occupational exposures are to several different asbestos types; mineralogic types show important differences in biologic responses. First, chrysotile is relatively biodegradable in both human and animal lungs, whereas amphiboles, notably crocidolite, persist for decades. Although the biologic effects of chrysotile during its shorter half-life are still important, the biologic longevity of amphiboles is more important. By persisting in the lung, these amphiboles act as a "cumulative dose" over decades, rendering the time since exposure an important factor and permitting a higher total deposited lung burden. The magnitude of the biologic effects broadly depends on the product of exposure time and total cumulative dose, except that this method may "smooth out" dose-response curves.

Fiber dimensions are important also. Two studies emphasize the importance of fiber length in causing experimental asbestosis, one in a sheep instillation model and the other in rat asbestos inhalation experiments. The classic studies of Stanton at the National Cancer Institute, Pott in Germany, and others from Canada and the United Kingdom show that dimensions of >8.0 μ by <0.5 μ are critical for the induction of mesotheliomas by pleural asbestos implantation. This is confirmed by autopsy asbestos lung burdens in which mesotheliomas occur largely in patients whose lungs contain these types of fibers. Finnish work with refined techniques also now shows that mesotheliomas arise from crocidolite as opposed to the locally mined anthophyllite. One recent Australian paper interprets its data differently.[64] These workers report lung fiber burdens of both crocidolite and chrysotile but not amosite to be statistically related to mesothelioma risk. However, the observations partly reflect the minimal importation of amosite into Australia. Also, only one of the lungs with mesothelioma contained chrysotile only, leaving the relative contribution of these two asbestos fibers moot.

Finally, that tremolite can cause mesothelioma is clear from the results of its presence in the whitewash used in some Greek homes and of its contamination of ore in a Montana vermiculite mine. Vermiculite is used in cat litter and, after processing, in slow-release fertilizers. However, in spite of a recent ATS report,[65] many mineralogists distinguish between tremolite fibers and their fragmentation products. Pleural inoculation experiments indicate that mesotheliomas result from the long, thin tremolite fibers.[66, 67]

Cellular and Molecular Features

Cellular and molecular features of asbestos-related disorders are summarized in three recent reviews.[60, 61, 68] The fibrosing alveolitis of asbestosis is manifest in several cell systems. Alveolar macrophages (AMs) phagocytosing fibers liberate oxidants (O_2, H_2O_2, etc.) and release plasminogen activator, which generates plasmin, a degrader of such structural proteins as fibronectin, laminin, fibrinogen, and proteoglycans. Thus, matrices can be damaged oxidatively and proteolytically. Most asbestotic human lungs contain excess neutrophils that release materials similar to those of AM and along with other tissue injury materials, e.g., collagenase and elastase. Macrophages also regulate fibroblast activity, releasing the fibroblast chemoattractant fibronectin, fibroblast growth factors such as "platelet-derived" growth factor, and an AM-derived growth factor. These factors act at different points in the cell growth cycle. Both expressions of their messenger RNA (mRNA) and the transcription rates for components of their proteins are increased in AM exposed in vitro to asbestos. Type I alveolar cells are injured and type II cells proliferate. The role of oxidants in the injury is suggested by many analogies with other lung disorders and confirmed by the modulation of developing asbestosis by such antioxidants as polyethylene glycol–linked catalase and retinols.[60] Interestingly, the latter also diminish asbestos:3.methylcholanthrene-induced cancers in tracheal implants.[60]

Benign Pleural Disorders

Benign pleural disorders are the most common pleural manifestation of asbestos exposure, are largely without functional consequences, and are characterized by discrete hyaline acellular fibrous tissue. They occur some 15 years after exposure, most commonly in the lower third of the parietal pleural and on the diagram. They frequently calcify later, becoming visible as dense rounded or linear shadows on chest x-rays. When single, plaques can simulate lung cancers or be a manifestation of "rounded atelectasis" in which pleural fibrous reactions invade the subjacent lung, entrapping some lung parenchyma and simulating a lung tumor. When multiple, small plaques can convey a nodular appearance on the chest film that must be distinguished from parenchymal asbestosis. Some authorities consider plaques to result largely from amphibole exposure,[69] even though chrysotile fibers are found readily in the visceral pleura. Calcific pleural plaques in the general population vary greatly geographically, e.g., from sepiolite in Bulgaria, from unknown causes in northwest Greece,[70] and in different locations in Corsica and Finland.[71, 72]

Pleural effusions, usually asymptomatic but sometimes with febrile pleurisy, also occur, again usually after 10 to 15 years of exposure.[73] They usually are unilateral. There are no specific diagnostic features to the pleural fluid. When they are unilateral and occur more than 20 to 25 years after the first asbestos exposure, effusions first must be considered due to either lung cancer or mesothelioma. Benign effusions usually resolve spontaneously, but they may recur. They probably cause many of the cases of asbestos-related diffuse pleural fibrosis, often associated with restrictive lung function.

The physiologic consequences of plaques and pleural fibrosis have been restudied since the classic paper of Epler and coworkers.[73] Gaensler and colleagues recently extended their study with similar findings.[74] There is no doubt that diffuse pleural fibrosis can cause significant restrictive deficits, whereas they stated that discrete plaques usually produce little defect. Bourbeau et al.[75] reported losses in FVC and FEV_1 (100 and 200 mL, respectively), but strangely with no effects on TLC or D_L, when they compared subjects without and with *any* form of pleural "thickening." They state that 5.5% of their subjects had diffuse pleural involvement for which they required involvement of a costophrenic angle. Unfortunately, they do not present functional data for isolated plaques, but indicate the plaque effects to be small and state that there was no demonstrable difference "in the exercise data in the presence or absence of simple plaques." Cardiophrenic angle obliteration is a feature of diffuse pleural disease, probably from previous effusions, indicating that these functional defects result from diffuse pleural fibrosis rather than from plaques. The splinting action of such fibrosis produces a reduction in the O_2 uptake in the subjacent lung. The diminution of diaphragm motion suggested by cardiophrenic angle obliteration is an effective respiratory splint.

More recent studies report some minor changes even with plaques. The cross-sectional study by Oliver and colleagues[76] reported plaques to be associated with a 5% loss of VC and FEV_1 amounting to 0.50 and 0.36 L, respectively. D_L as percent predicted was unaffected, but no data on V_A were quoted. Her subjects with plaques were older by 8 years and had worked 9 more years with an undetermined amount of asbestos. Hjortsberg et al. report a 5% drop in the predicted FVC in nonsmoking plaque-bearing railroad workers.[77] Schwartz and coworkers[78] also studied this issue and, along with Oliver, correctly raised the difficulty of recognizing an occult associated asbestosis (lung fibrosis). Schwartz did not always use ATS repeatability criteria in his study of sheet metal workers. Rather, he used the average of the two largest values of the FEV_1 and FVC when ATS repeatability criteria were not met. This point (see earlier) is important, since it necessarily results in some low spirometric values. The justification for basically using a lower second FVC or FEV_1 value, when errors in estimates of dynamic volumes are always in the direction of lowering the value, is obscure. Further, aside from studying only about half the members of the Sheet Metal Workers' International Association, they state that 18% of those tested did not meet the ATS criteria of "within 5%." These criterion failures tended to occur in more experienced or retired sheet metal workers in whom their own data indicate pleural changes to be more common, introducing a methodical bias into their results. The foregoing notwithstanding, the effects of plaques and/or pleural fibrosis are assessed on an individual basis with the additional consideration that a low D_L most likely reflects asbestosis. Thus, plaques at the most produce a small percent loss of VC, which is of no great functional significance.

Pleural changes are not, per se, associated with an increased risk of malignancy.[79] Using pleural changes as markers of asbestos exposure in various populations (e.g., school custodians) is reasonable, since plaques are the earliest manifestation of asbestos exposure and are associated with lower autopsy lung fiber burdens. However, some studies employing this approach are poorly controlled. For instance, internal "blindly read" control chest films must be included along with the study group lest intrareader and interreader variability nullify the study. Careful distinction of plaques from other causes of "pleural" shadows (e.g., rib fractures, fat pads,[80] muscle slipcs, etc.) is essential. Other causes of pleurisy also should be considered in such studies. One such cross-sectional study employed four x-ray views (posteroanterior, lateral, and two obliques) and reported a 21% prevalence of plaques in custodians solely exposed to asbestos in Boston schools.[81, 82] This study lacks such internal controls; a rereview of these same films by an experienced observer reported only one plaque—a 2% prevalence![83]

A well-controlled French study[84] of general (nonasbestos) workers in university buildings failed to detect differences in plaque prevalences between workers in buildings with friable asbestos and those in buildings without asbestos. The study should be extended beyond the 15-year observation period.

Asbestosis

There is little doubt that all of the aforementioned asbestos types, under some circumstances, can cause asbestosis, long fibers being the most pathogenic. Whereas the initial pathologic lesion is in the terminal bronchiolar region, most find evidence of isolated small-airway disease (i.e., in the absence of smoking-related COPD) to be either small or infrequent,[85] although Kilburn and Warshaw claim otherwise.[86] Hjortsberg and colleagues[87] report a small increase in the volume of trapped gas in the presence of plaques, suggesting small-airway changes.

Classic asbestosis with restrictive function loss is a serious disorder, but Swedish and American studies[88] show little progression of minor forms of asbestosis. The disorder is not seen in the general population and preliminary evidence suggests it does not occur at airborne fiber levels of 0.1 to 0.2 fibers per milliliter.

Lung Cancer

All lung cancer cell types occur in asbestos workers, with some lower lobe preference. The latency from first exposure is usually in excess of 20 years and the disease is essentially one of smokers. The relation between asbestosis and lung cancer has been much debated. The following evidence supports the view that asbestosis should be considered a prerequisite for the ascription of a lung cancer to asbestos: (1) *excess* lung cancers in smokers appear to be associated with radiologic or histologic asbestosis,[89, 90] (2) low-level asbestos exposure yields neither excess lung cancers nor asbestosis,[91, 92] and (3) idiopathic lung fibrosis is associated with excess lung cancers notably among cigarette smokers.[93]

Whether there is an increase in lung cancers in nonsmoking asbestos workers is arguable. There are few such cases; out of 17,800 insulation workers only 4 with lung cancer were listed as "never smoked regularly," but whether they had asbestosis is not stated. Several occupational cohorts do show variable excess lung cancer in "nonsmokers,"[94] but the validity of the smoking history is sometimes questionable.[95]

More important is the wide variation in the numbers of such cancers observed in various worker cohorts.[61, 94] Large excesses occur in South Carolina chrysotile textile workers, but very few occur in Connecticut friction product workers. Seidman and Selikoff have updated the studies of insulation workers.[96]

Mesothelioma

The major recent development in the field of mesothelioma is the relative importance of fiber type.[97] Cape Blue crocidolite was recognized as more dangerous than Transvaal asbestos as early as 1965. Since then, the experimental observations of Stanton have provoked studies of the different mesotheliomagenic potential of crocidolite and chrysotile. That crocidolite is the more potent is clear from the following: (1) Proportional mortality studies of various cohorts show a 15-fold difference in mesothelioma deaths between amphibole-exposed and chrysotile-exposed workers. (2) In cohorts previously thought to be largely or entirely chrysotile-exposed, the mesothelioma now have been shown to be associated with crocidolite detected in the autopsied lung (e.g., United Kingdom textile workers). (3) Dose responses with crocidolite >8.0 μm by <0.5 μm fibers appear likely. (4) Two worker groups (United Kingdom/Canadian gas mask workers, and U.S. cigarette filter manufacturers) employed either chrysotile or crocidolite exclusively. In the latter, mesotheliomas occurred in about 15%, but there were none where only chrysotile was used. (5) Among chrysotile miners and millers, only some 10 to 15 mesotheliomas occurred among over 9,000 deaths, in spite of these workers being subject to heavy and prolonged exposure. Indeed, Gibbs, with a considerable experience of lung burden studies, comes close to exonerating chrysotile as a cause of mesothelioma.[98] However, tremolite remains an important cause of mesothelioma, notably in Cyprus and Greece. Whether the 1% tremolite contamination of Canadian chrysotile is important needs some clarification. Such contamination does not result in mesotheliomas among the South Carolina, Pennsylvania, or United Kingdom chrysotile-using textile workers.

Asbestos and the General Population

Asbestos and the general population is an emotional subject that needs calm reflection if panic is to be avoided. It is clear that asbestosis does not occur in the general population and that plaques are distributed capriciously geographically. Since we believe that asbestosis is either a mechanistic or, at the least, a statistical prerequisite for an *asbestos*-related lung cancer, it follows that the general population will not develop such cancers. This point is reinforced by numerous studies[91, 92] of low-level asbestos-exposed workers in which there are no excess lung cancers, and by evidence suggesting that there is a dose threshold for asbestos lung cancer. The latter suggests that a sigmoid dose-response relation between airborne asbestos fiber exposure (fibers per cubic centimeter times years) and lung cancer incidence is more likely than a linear no-threshold relationship. This conforms to most pharmacobiologic dose-response relationships.

Much more important, however, are the current data[99, 100] indicating that electron microscopic measures of building airborne asbestos fibers (>5 μ in length) are 100 to 1,000 times less than the current Occupational Safety and Health Administration (OSHA) standard for workplaces at which neither asbestosis nor asbestos lung cancers have occurred so far. Studies by Sawyer in 1978 of the Yale University art and architecture building continue to be quoted[82] in 1990 as evidence of high building airborne exposure levels, e.g., 15[4] fibers per cubic centimeter! Sawyer in 1978 used phase microscopy to "count" asbestos fibers. This technique does not distinguish asbestos fibers from other fibrous structures. Sawyer recognizes this (personal communication, 1991) and now uses appropriate electron microscopic methods; he repudiates these understandable errors.

A major societal concern has been the mesothelioma risks to children exposed early in life to asbestos in schools. However, three points are relevant. First, most U.S. building asbestos is chrysotile. Second, commercial chrysotile, even in industry, causes few or no mesotheliomas. Third, the airborne fiber levels are so low as to fall well below likely threshold levels. The notion that mesothelioma does not result from asbestos exposure of the general population is supported strongly by historic records of national mesothelioma incidences. In men, death rates from mesothelioma continue to rise, reflecting their ocupational asbestos exposure. For women, who generally are not directly occupationally exposed, mesothelioma incidence is not rising in the United States, Canada, the United Kingdom, and many other European countries.[97, 101–103] These data are available for the last 20 years, a period in which rising mesothelioma rates reasonably might be expected, since building asbestos usage dates from the 1930s.

Several comparative assessments of societal risks from building assessment are available.[60, 61] These assessments, a worst-case scenario, neglect the threshold concepts but still show only minute risks. About 1 per million annual asbestos-related deaths is a reasonable *upper* limit of risk, in contrast to U.S. annual deaths of 12,000 from lung cancer from smoking! The communication of the "minitude" of this risk to lay or professional persons has proved difficult,[104] since deeply entrenched numinous societal fears exist and are amplified by many news media reports.

Several recent international symposia addressed the general problems of asbestos with special reference to the general population.[105–107] Broadly speaking, they support the views expressed here. Opinions and references on nonrespiratory cancers and asbestos exposure are found in these same symposia, our two reviews,[60, 61] and the lively but sometimes inaccurate correspondence resulting from these reviews.[108–110]

SILICA

Relation to Lung Cancer

The International Association pour Recherche Centre le Cancer (IARC) concluded that silica is carcinogenic in animals and that there is "limited" evidence for similar concerns in man.[111] Many recent papers[112] have addressed this topic, but the evidence is conflicting and inconsistent. Since the matter is the recent major development, we discuss it in some detail.

Miner Groups

Retrospective Cohorts.—McDonald's[113] study in the Lead South Dakota gold mines yielded a lung cancer SMR of 1.03 in a group of 1,310 workers. Similar results (SMR 1.00) were calculated by Brown et al.[114] on 3,328 similar gold miners. However, with either "high" levels of dust exposure or 15 years mining, these two studies showed enhanced SMRs of about 2.40 and 1.84, but these effects did not persist at even higher dust levels or even later at 20 years. No excess lung cancers were noted either by Lawler and colleagues[115] in 10,000 iron ore miners or by Koskela's group[116] in their study of 1,026 granite workers.

Case Control Studies.—The South African studies[117-119] did not yield significant elevations of lung cancer SMR. Forastiere and coworkers'[120] study in the Latium province of Italy yielded an SMR of 2.0 (1.1 to 3.5) or less depending on the exact population included. A prospective Viennese study[121] of 1,630 silica-exposed persons compared them with others not exposed to silica but seen in an occupational medical clinic. There were some differences in the groups' mortality experience, but the lung cancer SMR of 1.46 and the stomach cancer SMR of 1.90 both were considered statistically significant. The dust-exposed persons included 775 foundry workers and 475 grinders; Neuberger states that the increased lung cancer rates occurred in all subgroups, but gives no details. One still wonders about the contribution of foundry locations to lung cancer from nonsilica causes.

Silicosis

The foregoing studies of silica "workers," without reference to the presence of silicosis are weakly positive or negative. Separate studies of subjects with silicosis raise more concern, since the possibility of selection bias due to smoking is difficult to exclude. Smoking, as opposed to simple silicosis, produces symptoms, bringing these smokers to a diagnostic work-up and thereby enhancing the likelihood that they will be diagnosed as silicotic persons. To the extent this is true, the "silicotic person's" smoking habits would exceed those with unrecognized silicosis.

Forastiere's group reported[120] such studies of "silicotics" yielding an SMR of 1.5 (1.1 to 1.9) and, interestingly, also an SMR of cirrhosis of 1.9 (1.3 to 2.5). There were unexplained variations of the SMR from 0.9 to 2.5 depending on the exposure cause of silicosis (e.g., bricklaying, mining). No diagnostic criteria for silicosis were given. Kurppa et al.[122] reported on 1,127 cases of silicosis in Finland, indicating SMRs of 3.12, 7.35, 7.04, and 4.78 for lung cancer, tuberculosis, nonmalignant respiratory disease, and COPD, respectively. This study raises more questions than it answers—the high incidence of tuberculosis raises the issue of scar cancers and of other respiratory disorders of poorly adjusted smoking states. Further, lower grades of silicosis had higher lung cancer rates than those with more extensive disease, hardly a dose-response relationship. Somewhat similar data have been reported in Zambon and colleagues' study of silicotic persons from Veneto.[123] Ng and coworkers[124] reported from Hong Kong on 28 lung cancers among 1,419 men listed in a silicosis register with a lung cancer SMR of 2.03 (1.35 to 2.93) and indicated a relation between lung cancer risk and silicosis category. Again, tuberculosis death rates were even more increased to an SMR of 3.83 (1.80 to 7.00). Ninety percent of the cohort was smokers. Of the lung cancer patients (28 deaths), all were smokers and 19 had tuberculosis, the latter being statistically associated with an increased cancer risk in this cohort with an SMR of 2.52 (1.50 to 3.90). They followed Axelson's[125] method of adjusting for smoking (20-fold increase in lung cancer risk of smokers over nonsmokers). This suggests that half of the rise in silicosis-lung cancer rates is from smoking, but does not adjust for tuberculosis. It seems to this author that this study provides very weak evidence, and we agree with the authors that "smoking undoubtedly accounts for most of the excess lung cancer deaths."

The South African studies also reported a relation between silicosis and lung cancer[117-119] in necropsy studies of a group of 2,209 white gold miners for whom good respirable dust counts were available. They had worked for an average of 23.5 years and had 77 proven lung cancer deaths. Good smoking histories were available. Their analysis is complex, but employs non-lung cancer patients of the cohort as controls. The patients with lung cancer smoked more than did the controls (30 vs. 20 pack years), and had worse airway function tests and more respiratory symptoms. They report their data in terms of a smoking:dust interaction model and suggest a synergism. They also suggest a relation between lung cancer and "hilar gland silicosis," but the odds ratio for lung cancer does not relate completely to the degree of gland involvement by silicosis.

A study from Sardinia[126] of silicosis and lung cancer employed a nested case control method. They found 22 lung cancers (SMR 1.29, 0.80 to 2.00) among 724 miners (lead, zinc, and coal mines, and granite quarries). Although there was a greater risk after 15 years' latency, no statistically significant increase in SMR for lung cancer occurred either overall or when silicosis category was considered. Again, tuberculosis was increased (SMR 11.9) and so also was buccal cancer (SMR 4.0).

A Danish study[127] of some 6,000 foundry workers used the general Danish population adjusted for sex and calendar periods as controls. Overall, lung cancers numbered 166, with an SMR of 1.30 (1.12 to 1.51). The necessary adjustment for latency showed an increasing SMR, reaching 1.85 (1.39 to 2.45) at over 30 years. There were only 149 cases with radiologic silicosis; among them, only 11 lung cancers were noted, yielding an SMR of 1.7 (0.9 to 3.1). They stratified the lung cancer risk in foundry workers by prevalence of silicosis and found a positive association, with the highest lung cancer rates at the highest prevalence of silicosis with an SMR of 1.40 (1.16 to 1.77). However, "unfortunately no data on tobacco consumption were recorded" and the relation of lung cancer to silicosis could reflect a poor work environment.

Amandus and Costello[128] examined the relation between silicosis and lung cancer in 369 and 9,912 silicotic and nonsilicotic white male "mixed" metal miners. The overall respective SMRs were 1.73 (0.94 to 2.90) and 1.18 (0.98 to 1.42), the former based on 14 lung cancer cases and the latter clearly insignificant. They believe that the increased lung mortality does not reflect years underground or radon exposure. However, first, radon data were sparse. Second, there is a curious shortfall of lung cancer mortality among nonsilicotic exsmokers and nonsmokers (SMRs 0.47 and 0.24, $P < .05$); this group was a sizeable 2,715 persons. Third, while they believe their adjustments for smoking to be valid, there was only one lung cancer death among the nonsmokers with silicosis.

A second report of Amandus et al.[129] is based on 760 cases of silicosis diagnosed among North Carolina dusty trades workers. Silica was diagnosed radiologically by members of the North Carolina Industrial Commission. Cigarette smoking habits were generally known but not quantified. Reference groups included nonsilicotic metal miners, patients with coal workers pneumoconiosis (CWP), and the general U.S. and North Carolina male populations. They find lung cancer SMRs in silicotics without other occupational carcinogen exposures to be 2.3 (1.5 to 3.0) and 4.5 (3.4) for those with such additional exposures. For smokers, SMR overall was 3.4 (2.0 to 5.3); for nonsmokers, it was 1.7 (0.5 to 3.9). They state, "these SMRs for smoking silicotics should be interpreted cautiously because *general* population rates were used for calculating expected deaths so that the effect of smoking is *not* controlled"; they also discuss this aspect in detail.

To summarize, the papers reviewed provide no support for the association between silica exposure alone and lung cancer. Though the evidence is a little stronger for an association between silicosis and lung cancer, it is certainly conflicting. Even when present, the effects are generally small (SMR circa 1.5 to 2.0) and, in my opinion, probably lie within the error term ascribable to smoking. Tuberculosis and hence scar cancer risk is a confounding factor in many series and one wonders whether hilar silicosis has higher tuberculosis risks than do other forms of silicosis. Other confounding factors include radon exposure in mines, the combined risks for steelworkers where both sandblasting and exposure to coke-oven products occur and, in some work situations, added asbestos exposures. Parkinson[130] documented this increased lung cancer in coke-oven workers, which frequently include silica-exposed sandblasters. Benzpyrene adducts are found in the polymorphonuclear leukocytes of such workers, and these levels appear to be related to environmental contamination.[131, 132]

Silicosis

Silicosis is now a controllable disorder as judged by Graham and coworkers' radiologic study on the Vermont granite shed workers.[133] They also reported "no difference" in the annual losses of FEV_1 and FVC between office, quarry, and stone shed workers overall or in different silicosis categories.[134]

A paper on black South African gold miners is interesting.[135] It points out the effect of job self-selection; the healthiest persons with the best function do the heaviest and therefore the dustiest jobs. They report small significant losses of VC (234 mL), FEV_1 (320 mL), and D_L (3 mL/min/mm Hg) when categories 0 and 2 silicosis are compared. They use an unusual approach to spirometry, basically employing the ATS guidelines, with the exception that the best forced expiratory curve, before and after salbutamol, was accepted when successive measurements diminished FVC and/or FEV_1. They reported on about 60% of the available work force and give no information on the reasons for limited worker response. They believe the effects occur after statistical adjustments for age, smoking, work duration, and exposure. The pattern and extent of emphysema has been described in South African gold miners.[135] Silicosis now is reported among gemstone workers, as tiger's eye pneumoconiosis.[137]

The soluble but inert aluminum lactate has been shown to reduce quartz lung toxicity and silicosis in a sheep model.[138] Success with prednisone therapy in silicosis has been reported from India.[139]

AIRWAY DISEASES

Airway diseases are probably now the most important group of disorders; they include industrial bronchitis (cough and sputum with minimal or no airway obstruction), COPD, asthma, restrictive airways disorder syndrome [RADS] and, to a much smaller extent, emphysema and bronchiolitis obliterans.

Industrial Bronchitis

There is no doubt that cough and sputum with *and* without airway obstruction can occur both in a wide variety of dusty trades and in cigarette smokers.[140, 141] Similarly, air pollution produces these effects, but it can be controlled as it is in London by limiting SO_2 emissions from coal fires. It is likely that the simple chronic bronchitis symptoms result from larger dust particles or water-held small-particle conglomerates that are deposited selectively in the large airways, producing mucous gland and goblet cell hyperplasia. The issue now is the relative contributions of cigarettes and industrial-environmental settings, an issue that is both controversial and confusing.[142] Becklake, in a review summarizing the information up to 1989,[143] considers that the workplace is indeed an independent source of airflow limitation. She stresses the value of longitudinal studies that minimize interindividual variations and discusses the relative merits of community-wide vs. work group studies. We comment on some recent papers and on problems inherent in the relative risk assessment.

First, whereas death rates from COPD clearly do relate clinically and epidemiologically to FEV_1 and to FEV_1/FVC,[144] death rates in the general population also have been shown to correlate with FEV_1 loss in the Framingham, Massachusetts study.

This does not *necessarily* imply that the deaths result from COPD, for the Framingham and other studies clearly point out various fatality factors that intercorrelate with FEV_1, such disorders as ischemic heart disease, as in the Framingham study.

Second, Foxman's group report[145] contrasts the high prevalence of respiratory symptoms in the dusty trades, implying industrial bronchitis will little affect mortality in this study. Further, the conclusions on mortality are not affected by stratifying patients into "light" and "heavy smokers," but interaction between smoking and dusty trades was not defined. Again, Foxman states that cough and sputum do indeed relate statistically to increased mortality, but he also points out that, after smoking adjustments, these symptoms contribute little to mortality.

Third, Annesi and Kauffmann[146] report the dust effects on mortality as 40% and 60% of those of heavy and light smoking, respectively. They also state that relative longevity losses from dust and smoking alone (i.e., without the presence of cough and sputum) were 3, 6, and 10 years for dust, light smoking, and heavy smoking, respectively. In addition, they believe that there is a small statistical correlation between "cough and sputum" alone and mortality. Similarly, the population-based study[147] by Korn and colleagues considers chronic respiratory symptoms and functional changes to be associated independently with occupational exposure.

Fourth, since, even among smokers, only a small percentage get severe airway obstruction, often from emphysema, it can be difficult to adjust accurately for smoking effects. All factors—respiratory symptoms, FEV_1, age, smoking, and job duration dust levels—clearly are mutually intercorrelated. Thus, statistical "unraveling" by multivariate analysis is not a simple matter.

Fifth, this issue also arises in relation to coal miners.[148] There are two views, each expressed by collegial collaborators, as to whether coal worker's pneumoconiosis in its simple form as opposed to the complicated form of progressive massive fibrosis causes airflow limitation. Certainly, such mining increases the incidence of cough and sputum, but opinions differ on the prevalence and magnitude of airway obstruction, even though focal emphysema in the coal macule was shown many years ago by Gough.

Therefore, it seems that, acknowledging the evidence that dusty trades cause airway obstruction, the effects on FEV_1 are relatively small, generally produce little disability, and probably do not themselves affect mortality. Vitamin A and retinols probably are important chemoprophylactic agents. Dietary intake deficiencies and low blood levels have been observed in several occupational groups. Vitamin A analogies diminish experimental cancer production in tracheal implants.[60, 61] There are now indications[149] that diets poor in vitamin A enhance the risks of both simple and obstructive bronchitis.

Asthma

We reiterate[150] the proposal by Hendrick and Fabbri that occupational asthma be defined as a *new* state of bronchial reactivity induced by a workplace agent, a definition adopted by the United Kingdom Industrial Accidents Commission. While occupational exacerbation of preexisting asthma remains a real problem, the induction of a new asthmatic state carries a heavier responsibility, particularly where this state is prolonged either at or after ceasing work. Aside from compensation issues, this distinction remains a practical health issue, since known asthmatics should be excluded from certain jobs. These jobs clearly include those involving irritant nonspecific dusts, fumes, etc. (e.g., acid fumes or phenol-formaldehydes in the manufacture of chemical drums lined with protective coatings). They also include jobs involving agents known to cause occupational asthma. The latter follows from two features, the tendency for subjects with IgE-medicated sensitivity to one agent (e.g., ragweed) to become sensitive to other materials (e.g., animal dander) and the general principle of allergic asthma management (i.e., the reduction of real or potential allergic "loads"). This preventive aspect is reinforced by our knowledge that continued work with an unrecognized asthmagenic agent can lead to persistent asthma, in some instances for many years, e.g., from western red cedar[151] or TDI.[152] For the former, only 50% showed complete recovery on leaving the job and over one third deteriorated while at work for up to 7 years. Malo's detailed follow-up of snow crab processors showed that it required 1 and 2 years, respectively, for spirometry and airway reactivity to become normal after leaving the industry. Further persistence of the occupational risk was apparent, since specific IgE levels declined, with a half-life of 20 months up to 5 years of allergen avoidance; even then, 17% of the workers still had high IgE levels.[153] An additional practical point is that, since some agents largely produce airway obstruction some hours after exposure when the worker has gone home, the work association may not be recognized. Finally, though intellectually appealing, the notion that measures of nonspecific airway reactivity can be used to screen prospective employees has not been shown to be useful.

Specific Causes

We listed the major causes of airway diseases earlier.[150] New agents include a detergent ingredient, sodium iso-nonanoyl oxybenzene sulphonate,[154] and pancreatic extracts, as well as a reemphasis on psyllium. The latter is used in the manufacture of laxatives, can cause reactions in nurses, etc., and is an IgE-mediated asthma. Another IgE-mediated asthma occurs in coffee process workers.[155] Asthma also develops de novo among respiratory therapists,[156] with an illness odds ratio of 3.2 (1.9 to 5.5) even in the absence of a family history of asthma. The responsible agent(s) is unclear, since no challenge data are available, but they include glutaraldehyde, formaldehyde, earlier use of sulfites[157] in bronchodilators, and infectious agents, including fungi. Aldehydes are known to cause asthma in endoscopy units[158] and industry,[159] and among electron microscopy technicians.

Several other biologic products are intriguing, such as bat guano in the Sudan,[160] animal danders loosened by washing the cat, mouse urine protein, cockroaches, Japanese butterflies, and crabs! Individuals working in the bakery industry are at risk for asthma[161, 162] and atopic subjects should not be employed here.[163] The agents responsible include grain weevils, such fungi as *Aspergillus* and *Alternaria*, and a number of enzymes such as α-maltase[164, 165] used to treat flour and gluten.[166]

An important group of agents is used in the plastics industry (including polyurethanes, paints, varnishes, insulation, adhesives, electronics, Kevlar in the aeronautics industry, theatre and art materials, etc.) and the pharmaceutical industry provides major asthma risks. The former agents include acid anhydrides,[167] accelerator amines, incorporated phenolic aldehydes, and, most importantly, the di-isocyanates. The latter vary in molecular weight from the methylisocyanate of Bhopal infamy to TDI (the most common) to the diphenylmethane, naphthalene, and hexamethylene derivatives and more complex polymers such as "MDI" and "PAPI." In general, biologic reactivity is related inversely to molecular weight and hence directly to vapor pressure. Methylisocyanates cause direct chemical injury, with a RADS-like syndrome. TDI is a potent sensitizer; the higher–molecular weight compounds cause a hypersensitivity lung disease syndrome.[168] Airway responses include RADS from methylisocyanate or heavy "one-shot" exposure to TDI,[169] classic asthma, and perhaps long-term slow development of mild COPD.

The underlying mechanisms for TDI asthma are debated. Thompson's[170] group emphasizes the role of tachykinins, low–molecular weight peptides released from airway afferent nerves. These agents are in vogue as mechanisms affecting general asthma by affecting airway smooth muscle, inflammatory responses, and vascular endothelial permeability. Employing tachykinin antagonists and/or capsaicin to deplete substance P and other tachykinins, they produced evidence for the involvement of tachykinins in TDI asthma in guinea pigs, probably mediated by mechanisms other than altered vascular permeability.

TDI asthma reactions often include an immediate response presumably due to smooth muscle contraction, which is reversible by β-agonists. Late asthmatic reactions at about 8 hours after TDI exposure also occur; these are unaffected by β-agonists but are preventable by prior use of cromolyn or steroids. Fabbri et al.[171] employed BAL, spirometry, and methacholine challenge to examine the late TDI reaction in humans. During this phase, FEV_1 fell and airways responsiveness was predictably enhanced. BAL demonstrated enhanced sustained neutrophilia increased lavage albumin concentration, and a slight (50%) but significant increased eosinophilia. These inflammatory changes resemble late allergic cutaneous reactions and are consistent with much recent evidence for inflammation being an important component of asthma. Fabbri reviews many potential mechanisms and suggests that polymorphonuclear leukocytes and perhaps eosinophils cause the delayed asthma response. He points out that such mechanisms probably do not involve polymorphonuclear leukocyte release of cyclooxygenase products, since indomethacin does not inhibit the TDI late asthma response.

Additional Mechanisms and Assessment Techniques

A general practical review[172] describes these features. The role of low-molecular weight chemicals in forming haptens with human serum proteins is exemplified by phthalic anhydride binding to IgG4,[173] $NiSO_4$ binding to human serum albumin at what is probably a copper transportation site, and cobalt binding to form specific IgE antibody in hard metal workers with asthma.[174] Allergen characterization is advanced by electroblotting, for instance, the identification of 78- and 72-kD cockroach proteins,[175] components of castor beans,[176] and butterflies in Japan[177]!

Newman-Taylor and Tee provide some approaches to exposure assessment, indicating both the need and some methods for assessing airborne allergen levels.[178] Other methods include specific and nonspecific airway challenge studies, the serologic tests mentioned above, and radioallergosorbent inhibition.

Relation Between Smoking and Allergy

There is increasing evidence of a variable association between smoking and allergy. It appears that smoking increases the risks of developing both IgE antibody and asthma to previously naive antigens. This potentiation has been observed in hapten-induced asthma occurring with acid anhydrides used to cure epoxy resins.[179] Both United Kingdom and Australian reports on detergent worker asthma found twice as many persons with asthma and skin-prick reactivity among smokers as among nonsmokers.[180, 181] Enhanced IgE formation also has been observed[182] in "smoking" rats exposed to *airborne* ovalbumin. However, it is likely that smoking diminishes the risk of developing hypersensitivity lung disease.[183] The underlying mechanism(s) is obscure, but alteration of lung permeability by smoking leading to enhanced allergen access has been proposed by Newman-Taylor.

Diagnosis and Management

Careful inquiries about jobs and hobbies are necessary for the diagnosis of airways disease, as is a knowledge of domestic or industrial situations. Weekend or vacation improvement and job removal sometimes can help by suggesting that the asthma arises in a workplace setting. Inquiries concerning other workers' illnesses are relevant. The management is that of asthma in general, together with job changes, retraining, and occasionally the use of respirators for high-molecular weight causes of occupational asthma.

OCCUPATIONAL LUNG DISEASE IN THE RURAL ENVIRONMENT

Ten million people work in farming and related occupations. They serve 230 million U.S. citizens and provide major exports of grain, rice, fruit, and, if the French would agree to accept it, American meat! The transition from homesteading or ranching to high-productivity specialized agricultural processes has resulted in the intensification of workplace hazards. To this and the substantial risks of machinery accidents, modern chemical fertilizers, herbicides, and pesticides have added further risks to farmers, migrant workers, etc. The myriad lung risks have been well summarized by doPico,[184] and a 1988 conference held in Iowa provides information on occupational lung disease in this setting[185] together with the technical workshop deliberations. Probably, agricultural workers have the highest prevalence of disabling respiratory disease of any broad occupational group, and their work is usually physically demanding. Brief references to the several groups of disorders are all that space permits.

Airway Diseases

Asthma, simple bronchitis, and obstructive bronchitis are the most common airway diseases in agricultural workers. Reactions to grain dust, first described in 1713 by Ramazzini, are exceedingly common among farmers, grain elevator operators, etc., and are well described among others[186, 187] by Dosman and colleagues.[188] Enarson and Chan-Yeung have made important contributions to our knowledge of the health effects of wood dusts.[189]

Bronchiolitis is a well-recognized feature of disease of silo workers; NO_2 is the offending agent.

Hypersensitivity Pneumonitis

Originally described in detail by the Wisconsin group, hypersensitivity pneumonitis is now a widely recognized response to many biologic products. Characterized by fever, cough, SOB, and recurrent pneumonias, we now have useful guidelines for the clinical evaluation of this disorder, together with a list of 37 known causes, most of which are responses to biologic agents.[190] Among farmers, at least 4 per 1,000 are affected. Antibodies to the antigens (e.g., thermophilic actinomycetes) are present in the blood and clearly play some pathogenic role. However, their levels fluctuate[191] and reflect exposure[192] and not disease. Indeed, at least in pigeon breeders,[193] high antibody levels persist, yet many persons contrive to keep pigeons with minimal health effects. The mechanism for the immunorefractory "stand-off" between further exposure, antibodies, and health is unclear, but probably relates to suppressor T cell activity.[194]

Pesci and colleagues[195] give good evidence for the pathogenetic importance of immune complexes in this disorder. The Italian workers report loss of complement in hypersensitivity pneumonitis, but that it is the sole mechanism is questioned by German work.[196] They compared AM lavaged from persons with sarcoidosis, hypersensitivity pneumonitis, and controls, and found 60% of AM to manifest F_C receptors for IgE in all of ten patients with hypersensitivity pneumonitis. Control and sarcoid AMs were negative to the probing antibody, anti-FCR_{11} in Ab M 1-25. They make the intriguing suggestion that interleukin-4, a T cell–derived cytokine produced by allergen exposure in hypersensitivity pneumonitis, induces AM IgE receptors and IgE antibody. Subsequent AM activation leading to release of oxidants, inflammatory mediators, and cytokines then may cause lung injury.

Organic Dust Toxic Syndrome

There is an important distinction between hypersensitivity pneumonitis and another entity occurring in similar farm settings, namely, organic dust toxic syndrome.[197] This is not mediated by the immune system, and is characterized by an acute high dust exposure, fever, myalgias, cough, and SOB, but not by precipitating antibodies. The lung shows a neutrophilic reaction as opposed to the mononuclear granulomatous reaction of hypersensitivity pneumonitis.

Humidifier Fever

Humidifier fever may be difficult to separate from hypersensitivity pneumonitis, but it is generally short-lived, with little long-term damage and usually a normal chest x-ray. The responsible agents also differ. Two recent papers are available.[198, 199]

Animal Confinement–Related Diseases

Industrialization of livestock production has caused animal confinement-related diseases. These disorders include many risks, NH_3, H_2S, CH_4, CO_2, CO (from heaters), a wide range of biologic particulate dusts, and asphyxia from CO or O_2 depletion. These are frighteningly described by doPico.[184] The poultry industry includes the job of "chicken catcher!" The birds, caught by hand, are crated live and transferred by fork lift to a truck. A crew of 6 to 10 catchers can load 35,000 birds in an average 6-hour shift! These unhappy birds then meet the chicken hanger, who shackles them to an overhead conveyor that transports them to a slaughter area. A study of 59 chicken catchers suggested an increased prevalence of respiratory symptoms and an across-work-shift fall of 2% to 3% in FEV_1.[200] These effects on humans seem small considering the flurry of activity and contrast sharply with the SMR in the chickens! However, repetitive motion and traumatic injuries are common in chicken catchers.

Infectious Diseases

Infectious diseases include zoonoses, fungal infections, and parasite infestations.

Chemical and Toxic Gases

Chemical and toxic gases include pesticides (organophosphates), herbicides (paraquat), fumigants, fertilizers, and rodenticides (warfarin).

Byssinosis

Byssinosis was reviewed earlier and little new information is available.

OCCUPATIONAL LUNG DISEASE, SOCIETY, AND SCIENTISTS

Space forbids an account of the hue and cry over silicosis in New York state in the 1940s and 1950s with its fortissimo reprise over asbestos in the 1970s to 1990s. Disease there was and is! Legal perturbations and capricious judgments (and profits) were then and perhaps now are more in need of abatement than one present cause: asbestos! Until society, properly led by the legislatures and the judicial and scientific medical community, can impress order on the legal Brownian movement, equity will be ill-served. Ill-treated workers will go unrecompensed or Hamlet's comment on the law's delay will become only too apparent to workers and their families. Profitable industries and, with them, worker's jobs and society's wealth, will disintegrate.

These latter-day comments (they are warranted) are the context for a few personal remarks. Reading some of the correspondence[100, 108, 109] will show something of the personal element in criticisms of our reviews on asbestos. A small library in the lay press, and even comments in so-called scientific meetings, are calumnious. The chairman of a committee that issued an official statement on asbestos pleural changes[201] had to pay for his own legal counsel, sadly without the support of the very lung societies that adopted the committee's report! A learned journal now excludes reviews by persons who have received monies from interested parties, generally meaning industry. This practice is unscholarly and can readily exclude contributions to science merely because the authors' distinctive talents make their services appropriate and valuable to interested parties. The policy is not evenhanded, since it does not equally exclude those whose private or academic clinics are financially dependent on referrals from specific political liaisons. Persons are attacked as expert witnesses when they appear largely "on one side," as if it is these persons who decide who is chosen! In reality, it should be a combination of the expert's views published in the peer-reviewed scientific literature and counsel's choice that should influence their selection. For my part, as the author of this text, I am content for the reader to know something of my affiliations. In litigation, I have served both "sides," albeit very largely "defense." In 1970, I editorially supported the lowering of the asbestos workplace standard. I started the first occupational lung disease clinic in Connecticut and coauthored a bill passed by our state legislature for monitoring persons exposed to silica. We backed (through the Connecticut Lung Association and its Occupational Lung Disease Council) the primary sponsors of "worker's right to know" legislation and state financial support both to the Workmen's Compensation Commission's statistical service and to university occupational medical clinics.

Science must be the basis of public policy. Scientists should speak to that basis. Perhaps the involvement of the lung disease professional organizations in occupational lung disease policies should be extended to avoid social chaos.

REFERENCES

1. Aberle DR, Gamsu G, Ray CS, et al: Asbestos-related pleural and parenchymal fibrosis: Detection with high-resolution CT. *Radiology* 1988; 166:729–734.

2. Friedman AC, Biel SB, Fisher MS, et al: Asbestos-related pleural disease and asbestosis: A comparison of CT and chest radiography. *Am J Radiol* 1988; 150:269–275.

3. Rossiter CE: Initial repeatability trials of the UICC/Cincinnati classification of the radiographic appearances of pneumoconioses. *Br J Ind Med* 1972; 29:407–419.

4. Parker DL, Bender AP, Barklind A: Public health implications of the variability in the interpretation of "B" readings, in Berberich J (ed): *Proceedings VIIth International Pneumoconioses Conference.* Washington, DC, US Department of Health and Human Services, DHHS (NIOSH) Publication No 90-108, 1990, pp 196–200.

5. Maehle WM, Muir D, Chan JC, et al: The Canadian pneumoconiosis reading panel study, in Berberich J (ed): *Proceedings VIIth International Pneumoconioses Conference.* Washington, DC, US Department of Health and Human Services, DHHS (NIOSH) Publication No 90-108, 1990, pp 201–204.

6. Attfield MD, Hodous T, Althouse: A comparison of the profusion of small opacities reported with the 1980 and 1971 ILO classifications using readings from the coalworkers' x-ray surveillance program, in Berberich J (ed): *Proceedings VIIth International Pneumoconioses Conference.* Washington, DC, US Department of Health and Human Services, DHHS (NIOSH) Publication No 98-108, 1990, pp 207–212.

7. Rankin J, Gee JBL, Chosy LW: The influence of age and smoking on pulmonary diffusing capacity in healthy subjects. *Med Thorac* 1965; 22:366–374.

8. Knudson RJ, Kaltenborn WT, Burrows B: The effects of cigarette smoking and smoking cessation on the carbon monoxide diffusing capacity of the lung in asymptomatic subjects. *Am Rev Respir Dis* 1989; 140:645–651.

9. American Thoracic Society: ATS Statement—Snowbird workshop on standardization of spirometry. *Am Rev Respir Dis* 1979; 119:831–838.

10. Eisen EA, Oliver LC, Christiani DC, et al: Effects of spirometry standards in two occupational cohorts. *Am Rev Respir Dis* 1985; 132:120–124.

11. Eisen EA, Dockery DW, Speizer FE, et al: The association between health status and the performance of excessively variable spirometry tests in a population-based study in six U.S. cities. *Am Rev Respir Dis* 1987; 136:1371–1376.

12. Eisen EA, Wegman DH, Louis TA: Effects of selection in a prospective study of forced expiratory volume in Vermont granite workers. *Am Rev Respir Dis* 1983; 128:587–591.

13. Eisen EA: Standardizing spirometry: Problems and prospects. *Occup Med* 1987; 2:213–225.

14. Becklake MR: Epidemiology of spirometric test failure. *Br J Ind Med* 1990; 47:73–74.

15. Enright PL, Johnson LR, Connett JE, et al: Spirometry in the lung health study. 1. Methods and quality control. *Am Rev Respir Dis* 1991; 143:1215–1223.

16. Knudson RJ, Lebowitz MD, Holberg CJ, et al: Changes in the normal maximal expiratory flow-volume curve with growth and aging. *Am Rev Respir Dis* 1983; 127:725–734.

17. Krowka MJ, Enright PL, Rodarte JR, et al: Effect of effort on measurement of forced expiratory volume in one second. *Am Rev Respir Dis* 1987; 136:829–833.

18. Mortan WKC, Gee JBL: A ten-year follow-up study of a group of workers exposed to isocyanate. *J Occup Med* 1985; 27:15–18.

19. Graham WGB, Ashikaga T: Pulmonary function loss in Vermont granite workers (letter). *Am Rev Respir Dis* 1983; 128:777.

20. Wegman DH, Eisen E, Peters JM: Pulmonary function loss in Vermont granite workers (letter). *Am Rev Respir Dis* 1983; 128:776–777.

21. Morgan WKC: Airborne free silica: How much?, in Gee JBL (ed): *Occupational Lung Disease*. New York, Churchill Livingstone, 1984, pp 99–109.

22. Kellie SE, Attfield MD, Hankinson JL, et al: Spirometry variability criteria—association with respiratory morbidity and mortality in a cohort of coal miners. *Am J Epidemiol* 1987; 125:437–444.

23. Gee JBL (ed): *Occupational Lung Disease*. New York, Churchill Livingstone, 1984.

24. International symposium on airway hyperreactivity. *Am Rev Respir Dis* 1991; 143:.

25. Welch L, Hertz J, Cullen MR, et al: Occupational lung disease, in Simmons DH (ed): *Current Pulmonology*. Chicago, Year Book Medical Publishers, Inc, 1985, pp 137–165.

26. Beckett WS: Calculating the response to bronchoconstrictor aerosol challenge for measurement of airway responsiveness. *J Aerosol Med* 1989; 2:329–337.

27. Boehlecke B: Medical monitoring of lung disease in the workplace, in Gee JBL (ed): *Occupational Lung Disease*. New York, Churchill Livingstone, 1984, pp 225–240.

28. Peters JM, Thomas D, Falk H, et al: Contribution of metals to respiratory cancer. *Environ Health Perspect* 1986; 70:71–83.

29. Jensen AA, Tuchsen F: Cobalt exposure and cancer risk. *Toxicology* 1990; 20:427–437.

30. Eades A, Kazantzis G: Lung cancer in a non-ferrous smelter: the role of cadmium. *Br J Ind Med* 1988; 45:435–442.

31. Tola S, Kalliomaki P-L, Pukkala E, et al: Incidence of cancer among welders, platers, machinists, and pipe fitters in shipyards and machine shops. *Br J Ind Med* 1988; 45:209–218.

32. Sorahan T: Mortality from lung cancer among a cohort of nickel cadmium battery workers: 1946–84. *Br J Ind Med* 1987; 44:803–809.

33. Davies JM, Easton DF, Bidstrup PL: Mortality from respiratory cancer and other causes in United Kingdom chromate production workers. *Br J Ind Med* 1991; 48:299–313.

34. Sferlazza SJ, Beckett WS: The respiratory health of welders. *Am Rev Respir Dis* 1991; 143:1134–1148.

35. Kalliomaki P-L, Kalliomaki K, Rahkonen E, et al: Lung retention of welding fumes and ventilatory lung functions. A follow-up study among shipyard welders. *Ann Occup Hyg* 1983; 24:449–452.

36. McMillan GHG, Health J: The health of welders in naval dockyards: Acute changes in respiratory function during standardized welding. *Ann Occup Hyg* 1979; 22:19–32.

37. Doig AT, Duguid LN: The health of welders. *Factory Department, Ministry of Labour and National Service*. London, His Majesty's Stationary Office, 1951.

38. Simonato L, Fletcher AC, Andersen A, et al: A historical prospective study of European stainless steel, mild steel, and shipyard welders. *Br J Ind Med* 1991; 48:145–154.

39. Sprince NL, Oliver LC, Eisen EA, et al: Cobalt exposure and lung disease in tungsten carbide production. *Am Rev Respir Dis* 1988; 138:1220–1226.

40. Meyer-Bisch C, Pham QT, Mur J-M, et al: Respiratory hazards in hard metal workers: A cross sectional study. *Br J Ind Med* 1989; 46:302–309.

41. Kusaka Y, Ichikawa Y, Shirakawa T, et al: Effect of hard metal dust on ventilatory function. *Br J Ind Med* 1986; 43:486–489.

42. Ohori NP, Sciurba FC, Owens GR, et al: Giant-cell interstitial pneumonia and hard-metal pneumoconiosis. *Am J Surg Pathol* 1989; 13:581–587.

43. Cugell DW, Morgan WKC, Perkins DG, et al: The respiratory effects of cobalt. *Arch Intern Med* 1990; 150:177–183.

44. Johnson NF, Haslam PL, Dewar A, at al: Identification of inorganic dust particles in bronchoalveolar lavage macrophages by energy dispersive x-ray microanalysis. *Arch Environ Health* 1986; 41:133–144.

45. Kusaka Y, Yokoyama K, Sera Y, et al: Respiratory diseases in hard metal workers: An occupational hygiene study in a factory. *Br J Ind Med* 1986; 43:474–485.

46. Demedts M, Gheysens B, Nagels J, et al: Cobalt lung in diamond polishers. *Am Rev Respir Dis* 1984; 130:130–135.

47. Kriebel D, Brain JD, Sprince NL, et al: The pulmonary toxicity of beryllium. *Am Rev Respir Dis* 1988; 137:464–473.

48. Rossman MD, Kern JA, Elias JA, et al: Proliferative response of bronchoalveolar lymphocytes to beryllium. *Ann Intern Med* 1988; 108:687–693.

49. Saltini C, Winestock K, Kirby M, et al: Maintenance of alveolitis in patients with chronic beryllium disease by beryllium-specific helper T cells. *N Engl J Med* 1989; 320:1103–1109.

50. Jones-Williams W: On the differential diagnosis of chronic beryllium disease and sarcoidosis (letter). *Am Rev Respir Dis* 1990; 142:739.

51. Newman LS, Kreiss K, King TE, et al: On the differential diagnosis of chronic beryllium disease and sarcoidosis (letter). *Am Rev Respir Dis* 1990; 142:739–740.

52. Newman LS, Reiss K, King TE Jr, et al: Pathologic and immunologic alterations in early stages of beryllium disease. Re-examination of disease definition and natural history. *Am Rev Respir Dis* 1989; 139:1479–1486.

53. Davison AG, Newman Taylor AJ, Darbyshire J, et al: Cadmium fume inhalation and emphysema. *Lancet* 1988; i:663–667.

54. Lewis GP, Juski WJ, Coughlin LL, et al: Contribution of cigarette smoking to cadmium accumulation in man. *Lancet* 1972; i:291–292.

55. Townsend MC, Sussman NB, Enterline PE, et al: Radiographic abnormalities in relation to total dust exposure at a bauxite refinery and alumina-based chemical products plant. *Am Rev Respir Dis* 1988; 138:90–95.

56. Jederlinic PJ, Abraham JL, Churg A, et al: Pulmonary fibrosis in aluminum oxide workers. Investigation of nine workers, with pathologic examination and microanalysis in three of them. *Am Rev Respir Dis* 1990; 142:1179–1184.

57. De Vuyst P, Dumortier P, Rickaert F, et al: Occupational lung fibrosis in an aluminum polisher. *Eur J Respir Dis* 1986; 68:131–140.

58. Gilks B, Churg A: Aluminum-induced pulmonary fibrosis: Do fibers play a role? *Am Rev Respir Dis* 1987; 136:176–179.

59. De Vuyst P, Dumortier P, Schandene L, et al: Sarcoidlike lung granulomatosis induced by aluminum dusts. *Am Rev Respir Dis* 1987; 135:494–497.

60. Mossman BT, Bignon J, Corn M, et al: Asbestos: Scientific developments and implications for public policy. *Science* 1990; 247:294–301.

61. Mossman BT, Gee JBL: Asbestos-related diseases. *N Engl J Med* 1989; 320:1721–1730.

62. Antman K, Aisner J (eds): *Asbestos-Related Malignancy*. Orlando, Florida, Grune & Stratton, 1986.

63. Wylie AG: Discriminating amphibole cleavage fragments from asbestos: Rationale and methodology, in Berberich J (ed): *Proceedings VIIth International Pneumoconioses Conference*. Washington, DC, US Department of Health and Human Services, DHHS (NIOSH) Publication No 90-108, 1990, pp 1065–1069.

64. Rogers AJ, Leigh J, Berry G, et al: Relationship between lung asbestos fiber type and concentration and relative risk of mesothelioma. A case-control study. *Cancer* 1991; 67:1912–1920.

65. American Thoracic Society: Health effects of tremolite. *Am Rev Respir Dis* 1990; 141:1753.

66. Smith WE, Hubert DD, Sobel HJ, et al: Biologic tests of tremolite in hamsters, in Leman R, Dement JM (eds): *Dust and Diseases*. Park Forest, Ill, Pathotox Publishers, 1979, pp 335–339.

67. Wagner JC, Chamberlain M, Brown RC, et al: Biological effects of tremolite. *Br J Cancer* 1982; 45:352–360.

68. Rom WN, Travis WD, Brody AR: Cellular and molecular basis of the asbestos-related diseases. *Am Rev Respir Dis* 1991; 143:405–422.

69. Wagner JC: The discovery of the association between blue asbestos and mesotheliomas and the aftermath. *Br J Ind Med* 1991; 48:399–403.

70. Bazas T, Oakes D, Gilson JC, et al: Pleural calcification in northwest Greece. *Environ Res* 1985; 38:239–247.

71. Hillerdal G: Pleural changes and exposure to fibrous minerals. *Scand J Work Environ Health* 1984; 10:473–479.

72. Hillerdal G: Pleura plaques in Sweden among immigrants from Finland—with an editorial note. *Eur J Respir Dis* 1983; 64:386–390.

73. Epler GR, McLoud TC, Gaensler EA: Prevalence and incidence of benign asbestos pleural effusion in a working population. *JAMA* 1982; 247:617–622.

74. Gaensler EA, Jederlinic PJ, McLoud TC: Lung function with asbestos-related circumscribed plaques, in Berberich J (ed): *Proceedings VIIth International Pneumoconioses Conference*. Washington, DC, US Department of Health and Human Services, DHHS (NIOSH) Publication No 90-108, 1990, pp 696–702.

75. Bourbeau J, Ernst P, Chrome J, et al: The relationship between respiratory impairment and asbestos-related pleural abnormality in an active work force. *Am Rev Respir Dis* 1990; 142:837–842.

76. Oliver LC, Eisen EA, Green R, et al: Asbestos-related pleural plaques and lung function. *Am J Ind Med* 1988; 14:649–656.

77. Hjortsberg U, Orbaek P, Arborelius M, et al: Railroad workers with pleural plaques: I. Spirometric and nitrogen washout investigation on smoking and nonsmoking asbestos-exposed workers. *Am J Ind Med* 1988; 14:635–641.

78. Schwartz DA, Fourtes LJ, Galvin JR, et al: Asbestos-induced pleural fibrosis and impaired lung function. *Am Rev Respir Dis* 1990; 141:321–326.

79. Harber P, Mohsenifar Z, Oren A, et al: Pleural plaques and asbestos-associated malignancy. *J Occup Med* 1987; 29:641–644.

80. Sargent EN, Boswell DB Jr, Ralls PN, et al: Subpleural fat pads in patients exposed to asbestos: Distinction from non-calcified pleural plaques. *Radiology* 1984; 152:273–277.

81. Oliver LC, Sprince NL, Greene R: Asbestos-related radiographic abnormalities in public school custodians. *Toxicol Ind Hlth* 1990; 6:629–636.

82. Oliver LC, Sprince NL, Greene R: Asbestos-related disease in public school custodians. *Am J Ind Med* 1991; 19:303–316.

83. Gaensler EA: Testimony before the Superior Court of the Commonwealth of Massachusetts: *The City of Boston, et al. versus Keene Corporation, et al., Civil Action No 82254, December 3, 1990, pp 29–30.*

84. Cordier S, Lazar P, Brochard P, et al: Epidemiologic investigation of respiratory effects related to environmental exposure to asbestos inside insulated buildings. *Arch Environ Health* 1987; 42:303–309.

85. Becklake MR, Ernst P: Asbestos exposure and airway responses, in Gee JBL (ed): *Occupational Lung Disease.* New York, Churchill Livingstone, 1984, pp 25–49.

86. Kilburn KH, Warshaw RH: Abnormal pulmonary function associated with diaphragmatic pleural plaques due to exposure to asbestos. *Br J Ind Med* 1991; 47:611–614.

87. Hjortsberg U, Orbaek P, Arborelius M Jr, et al: Railroad workers with pleural plaques: II. Small airway dysfunction among asbestos-exposed workers. *Am J Ind Med* 1988; 14:643–647.

88. Gaensler EA, Jederlinic PJ, McLoud TC: Radiographic progression of asbestosis with and without continued exposure, in Berberich J (ed): *Proceedings VIIth International Pneumoconioses Conference.* Washington DC, US Department of Health and Human Services, DHHS (NIOSH) Publication No 90-108, 1990, pp 386–392.

89. Hughes JM, Weill H: Asbestosis as a precursor of asbestos related lung cancer: Results of a prospective mortality study. *Br J Ind Med* 1991; 48:229–233.

90. Kipen HM, Lilis R, Suzuki Y, et al: Pulmonary fibrosis in asbestos insulation workers with lung cancer: A radiological and histopathological evaluation. *Br J Ind Med* 1987; 44:96–100.

91. Neuberger M, Kundi M: Individual asbestos exposure: Smoking and mortality—a cohort study in the asbestos cement industry. *Br J Ind Med* 1990; 47:615–620.

92. Hodgson JT, Jones RD: Mortality of asbestos workers in England and Wales. *Br J Ind Med* 1986; 43:158–164.

93. Turner-Warwick J, Lebowitz J, Burrows B, et al: Cryptogenic fibrosing alveolitis and lung cancer. *Thorax* 1980; 35:486–499.

94. McDonald JC, McDonald AD: Epidemiology of asbestos-related cancer, in Antman K, Aisner J (eds): *Asbestos-Related Malignancy.* Orlando, Florida, Grune & Stratton, 1987, pp 57–79.

95. Berry G, Newhouse ML, Antonis P: Combined effect of asbestos and smoking on mortality from lung cancer and mesothelioma in factory workers. *Br J Ind Med* 1985; 42:12–18.

96. Seidman H, Selikoff IJ: Decline in death rates among asbestos insulation workers 1967–1986 associated with diminution of work exposure to asbestos, in Davis DL, Hoel D (eds): *Trends in Cancer Mortality in Industrial Countries.* New York, The New York Academy of Sciences, 1990, 300–318.

97. McDonald JC, McDonald AD: Epidemiology of asbestos-related lung cancer, in Antman K, Aisner J (eds): *Asbestos-Related Malignancy.* Orlando, Florida, Grune & stratton, 1987, pp 57–79.

98. Gibbs AR: Role of asbestos and other fibres in the development of diffuse malignant mesothelioma. *Thorax* 1990; 45:649–654.

99. Corn M, Crump K, Farrar DB, et al: Airborne concentrations of asbestos in 71 school buildings. *Regul Toxicol Pharmacol* 1991;

100. Asbestos, carcinogenicity, and public policy (letters). *Science* 1990; 248:797–802.

101. Gardner MJ, Acheson ED, Winter PD: Mortality from mesothelioma of the pleura during 1968–78 in England and Wales. *Br J Cancer* 1982; 46:81–88.

102. Jones RD, Smith DM, Thomas PG: Mesothelioma in Great Britain in 1968–1983. *Br J Cancer* 1985; 51:699–705.

103. Andersson M, Olsen JH: Trend and distribution of mesothelioma in Denmark. *Scand J Work Environ Health* 1988; 14:145–152.

104. Zeckhauser RJ, Viscusi WK: Risk within reason. *Science* 1990; 248:559–564.

105. *Symposium on Health Aspects of Exposure to Asbestos in Buildings.* Harvard University, Energy and Environmental Policy Center, John F. Kennedy School of Government. Cambridge, MA, December 14–16, 1988.

106. *World Health Organization Report on Occupational Exposure Limit for Asbestos, Oxford, United Kingdom, April 10–11, 1989.* Geneva, World Health Organization, 1989.

107. *Report of the Royal Commission on Matters of Health and Safety Arising from the Use of Asbestos in Ontario.* Toronto, Ontario, Canada, Ontario Ministry of the Attorney General, 1984.

108. Asbestos-related diseases (letters). *N Engl J Med* 1990; 322:129–131.

109. Asbestos-related diseases (letters). *N Engl J Med* 1991; 324:195–197.

110. McDonald JC, McDonald AD: Asbestos and carcinogenicity (letter). *Science* 1990; 249:844.

111. Silica and silicotics, in *IARC Monographs of the Evaluation of the Carcinogenic Risk of Chemicals to Humans,* vol 42. Lyon, IARC, 1987.

112. Cullen MR, Cherniak MG, Rosenstock L: Occupational medicine. *N Engl J Med* 1990; 322:594–601.

113. McDonald JC: Silica, silicosis, and lung cancer. *Br J Ind Med* 1989; 46:289–291.

114. Brown DP, Kaplan SD, Zumwalde RD, et al: Retrospective cohort mortality study of underground gold mine workers, in Goldsmith DF, Winn DM, Shy CM (eds): *Silica, Silicosis and Cancer. Controversy in Occupational Medicine.* New York, Praeger, 1986, pp 335–350.

115. Lawler AB, Mandel JS, Schuman LM, et al: A retrospective cohort mortality study of iron ore (hematite) miners in Minnesota. *J Occup Med* 1985; 27:507–517.

116. Koskela RS, Klockars M, Jarvinen E, et al: Mortality and disability among granite workers. *Scand J Work Environ Health* 1987; 13:26–31.

117. Hessel PA, Sluis-Cremer GK, Hnizdo E: Silica exposure, silicosis, and lung cancer: A necropsy study. *Br J Ind Med* 1990; 47:4–9.

118. Hessel PA, Sluis-Cremer GK, Hnizdo E: Case control study of silicosis, silica exposure, and lung cancer in white South African gold miners. *Am J Ind Med* 1986; 10:57–62.

119. Hnizdo E, Sluis-Cremer GK: Silica exposure, silicosis, and lung cancer: A mortality study of South African gold miners. *Br J Ind Med* 1991; 48:53–60.

120. Forastiere F, Lagorio S, Michelozzi P, et al: Silica, silicosis and lung cancer among ceramic workers: A case-reference study. *Am J Ind Med* 1986; 10:363–370.

121. Neuberger M, Kundl M, Rutkowski A, et al: Silica dust, respiratory disease and lung cancer—results of a prospective study, in Berberick J (ed): *Proceedings VIIth International Pneumoconioses Conference.* Washington, DC, US Department of Health and Human Services, DHHS (NIOSH) Publication No 90-108, 1990, pp 678–682.

122. Kurppa K, Gudbergsson H, Hannunkari I, et al: Lung cancer among silicotics in Finland, in Goldsmith DF, Winn DM, Shy CM (eds): *Silica, Silicosis and Cancer.* Controversies in Occupational Medicine. New York, Praeger, 1986, pp 311–319.

123. Zambon P, Simonato L, Mastrangelo G, et al: Mortality of workers compensated for silicosis during the period 1959–1963 in the Veneto region of Italy. *Scand J Work Environ Health* 1987; 13:118–123.

124. Ng TP, Chan SL, Lee J: Mortality of a cohort of men in a silicosis register: Further evidence of an association with lung cancer. *Am J Ind Med* 1990; 17:163–171.

125. Axelson O: Confounding from smoking in occupational epidemiology. *Br J Ind Med* 1989; 46:505–507.

126. Carta P, Cocco PL, Casula D: Mortality from lung cancer among Sardinian patients with silicosis. *Br J Ind Med* 1991; 48:122–129.

127. Sherson D, Svane O, Lynge E: Cancer incidence among foundry workers in Denmark. *Arch Environ Health* 1991; 46:75–81.

128. Amandus H, Costello J: Silicosis and lung cancer in U.S. metal miners. *Arch Environ Health* 1991; 46:82–89.

129. Amandus HE, Shy C, Wing S, et al: Silicosis and lung cancer in North Carolina dusty trades workers. *Am J Ind Med* 1991; 20:57–70.

130. Parkinson DA, in Gee JBL, Morgan KWC, Brooks S (eds): *Occupational Lung Disease*. New York, Raven Press, 1984, pp

131. Autrup H, Seremet T, Sherson D: Quantitation of polycyclic aromatic hydrocarbon-serum protein and lymphocyte DNA adducts in Danish foundry workers using immunoassays, in Garner RC (ed): *Biomonitoring and carcinogen risk assessment*. Oxford, Oxford University Press, in press.

132. Perera FP, Hemminki K, Young TL, et al: Detection of polycyclic aromatic hydrocarbon-DNA adducts in white blood cells of foundry workers. *Cancer Res* 1988; 48:2288–2291.

133. Graham GB, Weaver S, Ashikaga T, et al: Radiographic abnormalities in Vermont granite workers exposed to low levels of quartz, in Berberich J (ed): *Proceedings VIIth International Pneumoconioses Conference*. Washington, DC, US Department of Health and Human Services, DHHS (NIOSH) Publication No 90-108, 1990, pp 686–687.

134. Graham GB, Weaver S, Ashigkaga T, et al: Pulmonary function changes in Vermont granite workers, in Berberich J (ed): *Proceedings VIIth International Pneumoconioses Conference*. Washington, DC, US Department of Health and Human Services, DHHS (NIOSH) Publication No 90-108, 1990, pp 870–872.

135. Cowie RL, Mabena SK: Silicosis, chronic airflow limitation, and chronic bronchitis in South African gold miners. *Am Rev Respir Dis* 1991; 143:80–84.

136. Hnizdo E, Sluis-Cremer GK, Abramowitz JA: Emphysema type in relation to silica dust exposure in South African gold miners. *Am Rev Respir Dis* 1991; 143:1241–1247.

137. White NW, Chetty R, Bateman ED: Silicosis among gemstone workers in South Africa: Tiger's-eye pneumoconiosis. *Am J Ind Med* 1991; 19:205–213.

138. Begin R, Dubois F, Cantin A, et al: Aluminum inhalation reduces silicosis in a sheep model, in Berberich J (ed): *Proceedings VIIth International Pneumoconioses Conference*. Washington, DC, US Department of Health and Human Services, DHHS (NIOSH) Publication No 90-108, 1990, pp 895–896.

139. Sharma SK, Pande JN, Verma K: Effect of prednisolone treatment in chronic silicosis. *Am Rev Respir Dis* 1991; 143:814–821.

140. Morgan WKC: Industrial bronchitis. *Br J Ind Med* 1978; 35:285–291.

141. Morgan WKC: On dust, disability and death. *Am Rev Respir Dis* 1986; 134:639–641.

142. Bates DV, Kauffman F, Annesi I, et al: Letters to editor. *Am Rev Respir Dis* 1987; 135:1215–1220.

143. Becklake MR: Occupational exposures: Evidence for a causal association with chronic obstructive pulmonary disease. *Am Rev Respir Dis* 1989; 140(suppl):S85–S91.

144. Speizer FE: Overview and summary: Prognosis of chronic obstructive pulmonary disease. *Am Rev Respir Dis* 1989; 140(suppl):S107–S107.

145. Foxman B, Higgins ITT, Oh MS: The effects of occupation and smoking on respiratory disease mortality. *Am Rev Respir Dis* 1986; 134:649–652.

146. Annesi I, Kauffman F: Is respiratory mucus hypersecretion really an innocent disorder? *Am Rev Respir Dis* 1986; 134:688–693.

147. Korn RJ, Dockery DW, Speizer FE, et al: Occupational exposures and chronic respiratory symptoms: A population based study. *Am Rev Respir Dis* 1987; 136:298–304.

148. Soutar CA, Hurley JF: Relation between dust exposure and lung function in miners and ex-miners. *Br J Ind Med* 1986; 43:307–320.

149. Morabia A, Sorenson A, Kumanyika SK, et al: Vitamin A, cigarette smoking, and airway obstruction. *Am Rev Respir Dis* 1989; 140:1312–1316.

150. Welch L, Hertz J, Cullen MR, et al: Occupational lung disease, in Simmons ED (ed): *Current Pulmonology.* Chicago, Year Book Medical Publishers, 1985, pp 137–165.

151. Cote J, Kennedy S, Chan-Yeung M: Outcome of patients with cedar asthma with continuous exposure. *Am Rev Respir Dis* 1990; 141:373–376.

152. Mapp CE, Corona PC, De Marzo N, et al: Persistent asthma due to isocyanates. A follow-up study of subjects with occupational asthma due to toluene diisocyanate (TDI). *Am Rev Respir Dis* 1988; 137:1326.

153. Bardy JD, Malo JL, Seguin P, et al: Occupational asthma and IgE sensitization in a pharmaceutical company processing psyllium. *Am Rev Respir Dis* 1987; 135:1033–1038.

154. Stenton SC, Dennis JH, Walters EH, et al: Asthmagenic properties of a newly developed detergent ingredient: Sodium iso-nonanoyl oxybenzene sulphonate. *Br J Ind Med* 1990; 47:405–410.

155. Thomas KE, Trigg CJ, Baxter PJ, et al: Factors relating to the development of respiratory symptoms in coffee process workers. *Br J Ind Med* 1991; 48:314–322.

156. Kern DG, Frumkin H: Asthma in respiratory therapists. *Ann Intern Med* 1989; 110:767–773.

157. Simon RA, Stevenson DD, Adverse NF, Yunginger JW: Adverse reaction to sulfites, in Middleton E, Reed CE, Ellis EF, et al (eds): *Allergy Principles and Practice.* St Louis, Mosby, 1988, pp 1555–1570.

158. Corrado OJ, Osman J, Davies RJ: Asthma and rhinitis after exposure to glutaraldehyde in endoscopy units. *Hum Toxicol* 1986; 5:325–328.

159. Nunn AJ, Craigen AA, Darbyshire JH, et al: Six year follow up of lung function in men occupationally exposed to formaldehyde. *Br J Ind Med* 1990; 47:747–752.

160. El-Ansary EH, Gordon DJ, Tee RD, et al: Respiratory allergy to inhaled bat guano. *Lancet* 1987; i:316–318.

161. Musk AW, Venables KM, Crook B, et al: Respiratory symptoms, lung function, and sensitisation to flour in a British bakery. *Br J Ind Med* 1989; 46:636–642.

162. Thiel H, Ulmer WT: Bakers' asthma: Development and possibility for treatment. *Chest* 1980; 78(suppl):400–405.

163. Jarvinen KAJ, Pirila V, Bjorksten F, et al: Unsuitability of bakery work for a person with atopy: A study of 234 bakery workers. *Ann Allergy* 1978; 42:192–195.

164. Brisman J, Belin L: Clinical and immunological responses to occupational exposure to x-amylase in the baking industry. *Br J Ind Med* 1991; 48:604–608.

165. Baur X, Fruhmann G, Haug B, et al: Role of aspergillus amylase in baker's asthma. *Lancet* 1986; i:43.

166. Lachance P, Cartier A, Dolovich J, et al: Occupational asthma from reactivity to an alkaline hydrolysis derivative of gluten. *J Allergy Clin Immunol* 1988; 81:385–390.

167. Chee CBE, Lee HS, Cheong TH, et al: Occupational asthma due to hexahydrophthalic anhydride. A case report. *Br J Ind Med* 1991; 48:643–645.

168. Walker CL, Grammer LC, Shaughnessey MA, et al: Diphenylmethane diisocyanate hypersensitivity pneumonitis: A serologic evaluation. *J Occup Med* 1989; 31:315–319.

169. Luo JCJ, Nelson KG, Fischbein M: Persistent reactive airway dysfunction syndrome after exposure to toluene diisocyanate. *Br J Ind Med* 1990; 47:239–241.

170. Thompson JE, Scypinski LA, Gordon T, et al: Tachykinins mediate the acute increase in airway responsiveness caused by toluene diisocyanate in guinea pigs. *Am Rev Respir Dis* 1987; 136:43–49.

171. Fabbri LM, Boschetto P, Zocca E, et al: Bronchoalveolar neutrophilia during late asthmatic reactions induced by toluene diisocyanate. *Am Rev Respir Dis* 1987; 136:36–42.

172. Newman Taylor AJ, Tee RD: Occupational lung disease. *Curr Opin Immunol* 1989; 1:684–689.

173. Nielsen J, Welinder H, Schultz A, et al: Specific serum antibodies against phthalic anhydride in occupationally exposed subjects. *J Allergy Clin Immunol* 1988; 82:126–133.

174. Shirakawa T, Kusaka Y, Fujimura N, et al: The existence of specific antibodies to cobalt in hard metal asthma. *Clin Allergy* 1988; 18:451–460.

175. Che-Huei W, Joung-Liang L: Cockroach hypersensitivity, isolation and partial characterization of major allergens. *J Allergy Clin Immunol* 1988; 82:727–735.

176. Thorpe SC, Kemeny DM, Panzani RC, et al: Allergy to castor bean. II. Identification of the major allergens in castor bean seeds. *J Allergy Clin Immunol* 1988; 82:67–72.

177. Newman-Taylor AJ, Tee RD: Occupational lung disease. *Curr Opin Immunol* 1989; 1:684–689.

178. Newman-Taylor A, Tee RD: Environmental and occupational asthma. Exposure assessment. *Chest* 1990; 98:209A–211S.

179. Venables KM, Topping MD, Howe W, et al: Interaction of smoking and atopy in producing specific IgE antibody against a hapten protein conjugate. *BMJ* 1985; 290:201–204.

180. Mitchell CA, Gandevia G: Respiratory symptoms and skin reactivity in workers exposed to proteolytic enzymes in the detergent industry. *Am Rev Respir Dis* 1771; 104:102–104.

181. Greenberg M, Milne JF, Watt A: A survey of workers exposed to dusts containing derivatives of Bacillus subtilis. *BMJ* 1970; ii:629–633.

182. Zetterstrom O, Nordvall SL, Bjorksten B, et al: Increased IgE antibody responses in rats exposed to tobacco smoke. *J Allergy Clin Immunol* 1985; 75:594.

183. Editorial: Smoking, occupation, and allergic lung disease. *Lancet* 1985; i:965.

184. doPico GA: Occupational lung disease in the rural environment, in Gee JBL (ed): *Occupational Lung Disease*. New York, Churchill Livingstone, 1984, pp 141–181.

185. Donham KJ: Introduction to Conference on Agricultural Occupational Health: Policy strategy for the future. *Am J Ind Med* 1990; 18:239–240.

186. Enarson DA*Clin Invest Med* 1988; 11:193–197.

187. James AL, Zimmerman MJ, Ee H, et al: Exposure to grain dust and changes in lung function. *Br J Ind Med* 1990; 47:466–472.

188. Dosman JA, Cotton DJ (eds): *Occupational Pulmonary Disease. Focus on Grain Dust and Health*. New York, Academic Press, 1980.

189. Enarson DA, Chan-Yeung M: Characterization of health effects of wood dust exposures. *Am J Ind Med* 1990; 17:33–38.

190. Richerson HB, Bernstein IL, Fink JN, et al: Guidelines for the clinical evaluation of hypersensitivity pneumonitis. Report of the subcommittee on hypersensitivity pneumonitis. *J Allergy Clin Immunol* 1989; 84:839–844.

191. Cormier Y, Belanger J: The fluctuant nature of precipitating antibodies in dairy farmers. *Thorax* 1989; 44:469–473.

192. Marx JJ Jr, Guernsey J, Emanuel DA, et al: Cohort studies of immunologic lung disease among Wisconsin dairy farmers. *Am J Ind Med* 1990; 18:263–268.

193. Bourke SJ, Banham SW, Carter R, et al: Longitudinal course of extrinsic allergic alveolitis in pigeon breeders. *Thorax* 1989; 44:415–418.

194. Gee JBL, Lwebuga-Mukasa J: Cellular and matrix mechanisms in occupational lung disease, in Mortan WKC, Seaton A (eds): *Occupational Lung Diseases,* 2nd ed. Philadelphia, WB Saunders Company, 1984, pp 184–185.

195. Pesci A, Bertorelli G, Dall'Aglia PP, et al: Evidence in bronchoalveolar lavage for third type immune reactions in hypersensitivity pneumonitis. *Eur Respir J* 1990; 3:359–361.

196. Pforte A, Breyer G, Prinz JC, et al: Expression of the Fc-receptor for IgE (Fc$_e$RII, CD23) on alveolar macrophages in extrinsic allergic alveolitis. *J Exp Med* 1990; 171:1163–1169.

197. Marx JJ, Guernsey J, Emanual DA, et al: Cohort studies of immunologic lung disease among Wisconsin dairy workers. *Am J Ind Med* 1990; 18:263–268.

198. Anderson K, Watt AD, Sinclair D, et al: Climate, intermittent humidification, and humidifier fever. *Br J Ind Med* 1989; 46:671–674.

199. McSharry C, Anderson K, Boyd G: Serological and clinical investigation of humidifier fever. *Clin Allergy* 1987; 17:15–22.

200. Morris PD, Lenhart SW, Service WS: Respiratory symptoms and pulmonary function in chicken catchers in poultry confinement units. *Am J Ind Med* 1991; 19:195–204.

201. Murphy RL, Becklake MR, Brooks SM, et al: The diagnosis of nonmalignant diseases related to asbestos. *Am Rev Respir Dis* 1986; 134:363–368.

CHAPTER 9

Fungal Diseases

George A. Sarosi, M.D.

Clinical Professor of Medicine, University of Arizona College of Medicine; Chairman, Department of Internal Medicine, Maricopa Medical Center, Phoenix, Arizona

Scott F. Davies, M.D.

Associate Professor of Medicine, University of Minnesota Medical School—Minneapolis; Director, Pulmonary Division, Hennepin County Medical Center, Minneapolis, Minnesota

The endemic fungal diseases, histoplasmosis, blastomycosis, and coccidioidomycosis, continue to be major hazards in large parts of North America. While all three occur on other continents as well, and most likely will increase in significance outside of North America, for practical purposes, all new information pertaining to these rather common infections originates in the United States and other parts of North America. All these fungi are soil-dwelling organisms, found in fairly well-defined areas where soil, moisture, and climatic conditions favor their growth. Man and other mammals become infected when the fragile mycelia are disturbed and the small infective particles become airborne. Following inhalation, the particles elude the nonspecific defenses of the airways and reach the alveolar spaces, where each will begin multiplying in its own way. Both *Histoplasma* and *Blastomyces* species convert to the yeast form and multiply by binary fission. The arthrospores of *Coccidioides immitis* form giant spherules; within these giant spherules septations appear, leading to the formation of endospores, which are released when the giant spherule matures and ruptures. Each endospore then gives rise to a new giant spherule and the process repeats itself.

HISTOPLASMOSIS

The history of histoplasmosis is fascinating because it took so long for the true nature of this very common disease to emerge. Briefly, Dr.Samuel T. Darling, a young U.S. Army pathologist assigned to the Panama Canal Zone, described in 2 years three patients with a fatal infection.[1, 2] At autopsy he saw a small microorganism in the organs of the reticuloendothelial (RE) system. Even though he mistakenly thought that the organism was a protozoan and had a capsule (both subsequently proven to be incorrect), he clearly described a new disease. His seminal observation was nearly lost when no further cases of this illness were noted. Fortunately, in 1926, a young pathology resident in Minneapolis, Cecil J. Watson (subsequently to become chairman of medicine at the University of Minnesota), recognized the same parasite in postmortem tissues of a lifelong resident of Minnesota.[3] Through diligent search of the literature, he rediscovered Darling's original work and rescued it from obscurity.

The first case of histoplasmosis diagnosed during life was at Vanderbilt University, where in 1934 Dr. Edna Tompkins recognized the same organism in peripheral blood phagocytes from an infant dying of a febrile wasting illness with hepatosplenomegaly.[4] Following the death of the infant, DeMonbreun, in the department of pathology of the same university, was able to grow the organism; he also infected experimental animals and proved that the "protozoan" was a thermal dimorphic fungus.[5] When the first large review was published in 1945, its authors reported seven of their own cases and collected 71 cases from the literature, most of them fatal.[6]

The next major step occurred during World War II, when investigators, also from Vanderbilt University, showed that most patients with pulmonary calcification and negative tuberculin skin tests reacted to a skin test antigen prepared from *Histoplasma capsulatum*.[7] These observations were confirmed by Palmer of the United States Public Health Service.[8] Large-scale skin test surveys then quickly identified the endemic areas in the south-central United States. Thus, in a short time, histoplasmosis moved from a uniformly fatal and rare disease to a common and seldom severe infection.

In rapid succession, the fungus was isolated from soil (enriched by bird or animal excreta)[9] and a chronic tuberculosis-like pulmonary infection was identified in tuberculosis sanitoriums in the endemic area.[10] Thus, by the end of the 1940s, most of histoplasmosis had been described—at least the part that was apparent to hospital-based infectious disease specialists, pathologists, and public health epidemiologists. What was not yet known was how the fungus spread from its microenvironment in the soil to man—no one knew the features of the acute disease that was recognized years later associated with a positive histoplasmin skin test and multiple calcifications on the chest radiograph. In a remarkable paper, Amos Christie described the wide spectrum of histoplasmosis,[11] and shortly after, Loosli and his associates described the first point-source epidemic.[12]

Encouraged by this work, Furcolow then postulated that a series of unusual outbreaks of uncharacterized pulmonary infections, published earlier, were in fact epidemics of histoplasmosis. With the help of Grayston, he was able to track down six previously reported outbreaks of "disseminated pulmonary infection" and prove retrospectively that they all were caused by *H. capsulatum*. All the outbreaks had a "point source," a single place where all involved individuals were exposed.[13]

During the retrospective evaluation, Grayston and Furcolow recovered the fungus from contaminated soil at most of the "point sources" and showed that most patients who had an acute pulmonary syndrome during the outbreaks had a positive histoplasmin skin test. Many still had serologic evidence of previous *Histoplasma* infection.[13] The acute illness reported in these outbreaks was a febrile respiratory syndrome with a dry, hacking cough, frequently accompanied by central anterior retrosternal pain and severe myalgias.

Most of the original outbreaks were small. Exposure occurred in closed spaces such as storm cellars, chicken coops, and caves (in which bat droppings provided the nitrogen-rich soil for fungal growth). An entire new dimension was added in 1961 when Furcolow investigated an outbreak and traced it back to a blackbird-starling roost in an urban park.[14] Subsequently, many other similar outbreaks were traced back to blackbird roosts, which rapidly overtook in importance outbreaks traced back to chicken coops.

Two large outbreaks in Mason City, Iowa[15, 16] and the incompletely investigated but presumably much larger outbreak in Montreal[17] introduced yet another, potentially highly dangerous manifestation of histoplasmosis — the community-wide outbreak. These outbreaks occurred in areas of low background histoplasmin activity, where large numbers of nonimmune individuals could be exposed to a "point-source," thus exposing a significant number of potentially vulnerable hosts to a large, infective aerosol.

To emphasize the potential for a large-scale public health hazard, let us look at the two outbreaks in Mason City, Iowa. During August and early September of 1962, a community-wide outbreak occurred in this town of 30,000 associated with bulldozing of a stand of trees, which also served as a blackbird roost.[15] During the ensuing investigation, over 3,000 children between the ages of 5 and 15 years were skin tested and, on the basis of these data, it was estimated that 30% of the town's poulation became infected. Even though the loss of life was minimal, the economic impact of this outbreak was staggering. While less than 40% of infected individuals were symptomatic, this still represented a formidable number of sick people in a small town. If the first outbreak in Mason City was a serious problem, the second outbreak was even worse.

Because the first outbreak clearly was related to bulldozing the starling roost, all work at the site was suspended once the extent of the epidemic became known. After much debate, it was decided that the site should be cleared only when the likelihood of aerosol formation was reduced to a minimum. Thus, work began during January 1964, when the ground was frozen. Even though all reasonable precautions were made, a second outbreak occurred.[16]

Since the skin test status of children in 1962 was established, investigations of the nonreactors showed that 49% of previously noninfected children converted their formerly negative histoplasmin skin test to positive. Assuming that adults in the community became infected at the same rate, the second outbreak involved over 10,000 people! Put another way, at the end of the second outbreak, 63% to 64% of *all* Mason City residents had a positive histoplasmin skin test. Even though the pre-outbreak skin test status of this town cannot be established with certainty, in an adjacent town, 15% of the adults and 1.4% of the children had a positive histoplasmin skin test. Assuming that baseline skin test reactivity in Mason City was similar, about one half of the entire town was infected by one interrupted construction project.[16]

In addition to showing the explosive potential of a community-wide outbreak, the second Mason City outbreak also confirmed the association of erythema nodosum-erythema multiforme complex with associated arthralgias as one of the main manifestations of acute histoplasmosis. This association was pointed out first during the investigation of an outbreak in Greenwood, South Carolina,[18] and was observed during the incompletely studied outbreak in Montreal as well.[17] The striking feature of all reported large outbreaks of histoplasmosis complicated by erythema nodosum-erythema multiforme was that these dramatic skin lesions occurred predominantly in young to middle-aged white women; in fact, females outnumbered males 7 to 8:1.[19]

Outbreaks of histoplasmosis undoubtedly continue throughout the endemic areas, but unless something extraordinary occurs, they are no longer considered newsworthy and do not get reported. Two outbreaks were extraordinary and were reported in detail because both occurred in highly endemic areas where the vast majority of adults already should have had histoplasmosis.[20, 21] Using the data from the large skin test survey of naval recruits who were lifetime residents of one county, one would have expected most of the involved individuals to have been infected years before, and thus to be immune.[22] Yet, most individuals developed acute histoplasmosis. While the reason for this discrepancy is not clear, it is possible that previous data obtained in the 1950s no longer apply. The long and the short of it is that, even in highly endemic areas, epidemics can and do occur.

This was underscored by a massive, community-wide outbreak in Indianapolis, which was thought by most to be in a heavily endemic area. The skin test survey of naval recruits showed that by 21 years of age, 55% of white males tested were histoplasmin-positive.[22] Yet, a huge outbreak occurred, infecting as many as 100,000 people during its first phase[23] (it is estimated that the outbreak ultimately involved 200,000 people).[24] The highest attack rate was in adolescents and young adults between the ages of 15 and 34 years. This may not be the entire story, however, since younger children were not studied in detail. The investigators relied on serologic studies to estimate the number of individuals involved, different from the previous studies, which used skin test sensitivity. Comparison of seropositivity from sera collected before the first outbreak and that collected during the outbreak showed that, in some inner-city schools, 80% of the sudents were infected during the first outbreak, rather than the 45% one would have predicted on the basis of previous skin test surveys (55% skin test–positive before). The authors advanced the hypothesis that, due to the increasing tempo of urbanization in the recent past, fewer and fewer young adults have been exposed to the fungus. This argument, while unproven, is attractive, since urban residents are less likely to be exposed to contaminated soil than are rural dwellers. Alternatively, since the majority of young people involved in these inner-city schools were black, these individuals may well have had lower previous skin test positivity rates than the 55% that was found among white naval recruits.[22]

Case finding was limited to sicker patients, since most cases were found during searches of hospital records. While this method undoubtedly underestimated the number of the clinically ill, some observations were truly startling. Before this outbreak, pericarditis had been reported only once during an outbreak, even though many other isolated cases had been reported. During the first Indianapolis outbreak, investigators noted 24 patients with acute pericarditis. With the second Indianapolis outbreak, a total of 45 patients with this complication were recognized.[24]

The picture of pericarditis that emerges is noteworthy. First of all, pericarditis was a late complication. Most patients involved were young, between 20 and 39 years of age, similar in age to other infected patients. Even though 9 patients presented with pericardial tamponade, fluid obtained during pericardiocentesis and pericardial tissue obtained during open drainage failed to yield the fungus. Thus, the diagnosis was established purely on serologic grounds, since clinical suspicion was extremely high during both outbreaks. Therefore, it is easy to see why so few patients had been diagnosed before; doctors investigating patients with sporadically occurring pericarditis seldom considered histoplasmosis. Since the fungus never was recovered from either fluid or pericardium, it is likely that the etiology was immunologic, rather than direct infection, especially since most patients responded well to the administration of anti-inflammatory agents.[24]

The careful study of epidemics of histoplasmosis has helped develop our understanding of the entire spectrum of human infection caused by this fungus. Observations during the second of two outbreaks in Mason City have helped understanding of another manifestation of histoplasmosis, the development of chronic cavitary histoplasmosis, usually in the upper lobes.[16] That *Histoplasma* species could produce a tuberculosis-type illness had been recognized since 1948. Large numbers of such patients were identified in tuberculosis sanatoriums in the endemic area.[10] They originally were thought to have tuberculosis on the basis of symptoms and radiographic appearance. However, sputum cultures were negative for tuberculosis and repeatedly positive for histoplasmosis. These patients had a chronic, slowly progressive wasting illness with low-grade fever, anorexia, and weight loss, and chest radiographs uniformly showed unilateral or bilateral fibrocavitary disease that progressed relentlessly. Similar patients were seen in Veterans Administration hospitals throughout the endemic area as well.

Careful studies by Furcolow and his associates showed that this illness had an extremely poor prognosis,[25] leading to death from pulmonary failure in 50% of patients in 5 years.[26] This dismal outlook was improved significantly when specific antifungal therapy, amphotericin B (AMB), became available.[26, 27] Although the chronic progressive form of upper lobe histoplasmosis, as seen in tuberculosis sanatoriums or Veterans Administration hospitals, seems simple enough, considerable controversy existed in the literature as to how these patients acquired their illness. Once again, careful study of histoplasmosis outbreaks has provided the best insight into the pathogenesis.

Very early during the study of chronic cavitary histoplasmosis, it became obvious that certain demographic features were present. The vast majority of affected individuals were middle-aged white males, and blacks were markedly underrepresented. Moreover, white women seldom were involved and the disease practically never was seen in black women, even if one discounted the patients reported from Veterans Administration hospitals. Additionally, most patients were heavy cigarette smokers. When lung specimens were examined following either pulmonary resection or at the time of a postmortem examination, virtually all showed evidence of centrilobular emphysema.[28]

Not all investigators agreed that this form of histoplasmosis was uniformly progressive and that the prognosis of the infected patients was as dismal as reported by the Centers for Disease Control Cooperative Mycosis Study. Goodwin, on the basis of careful observations, reported that, in the majority of his patients, this illness, far from being a severe destructive process, frequently was self-limited. Borrowing a term and a technique from tuberculosis, he reported that activity management (i.e., bed rest) in fact was curative in many of his patients.[29] In his monumental study of 228 patients, he was able to show that 80% of his patients eventually recovered, and that progressive, destructive disease occurred in only the remaining 20%.[28] His careful study, therefore, established that most patients, rather than going on to a progressive and inevitably incapacitating illness, slowly improved and usually resolved their pulmonary infiltrate. While his work established the varying clinical picture of the illness, he could not say for certain how the illness began.

Because of the radiographic similarity to reinfection tuberculosis, and because most physicians caring for these patients initially were physicians who took care of patients with tuberculosis, the consensus that chronic cavitary histoplasmosis was due to reinfection, whether exogenous or endogenous, was questionable. Since most patients had low-grade chronic symptoms, there was no clear evidence for an acute infection antedating the onset of the chronic illness.

During investigation of the second Mason City epidemic, a total of 270 patients were recognized with a clinical illness that could be attributed to work on a starling roost. Eighty-seven of these patients were investigated in detail; 5 were found to have extensive upper lobe cavitary histoplasmosis. Since none of these patients had an antecedent acute infection, the consensus was that these cases represented reinfection, most likely exogenous in origin.[16] Although it is virtually impossible to reinfect experimental animals with spores of *H. capsulatum*,[30] exogenous infection best fitted the epidemiologic circumstances and the biases of the investigators. A small outbreak of chronic cavitary histoplasmosis during 1976 to 1977 (reported in 1980) first cast doubt on the exogenous reinfection hypothesis.[31] This epidemic occurred in Hopkinsville, Kentucky, a town of 26,000 in an area considered to be endemic for histoplasmosis. In a relatively short period, five patients with chronic pulmonary histoplasmosis were recognized; in four, the diagnosis was established by open lung biopsy. Perhaps the most instructive individual was the fifth patient (the index case). This man was a bulldozer operator who worked at the site of the outbreak. An illness compatible with acute pulmonary histoplasmosis developed 2 weeks after his work on the epidemic site. He failed to improve under observation and in 2 months progressed to pulmonary insufficiency and was shown to have sputum culture–positive chronic pulmonary histoplasmosis. During the ensuing epidemiologic investigation, in addition to the five very sick individuals, ten more patients with the clinical and radiographic picture of chronic pulmonary histoplasmosis were identified. It is of note that seven of these ten patients, all with mild illness, proceeded to recover rapidly and, by the end of the 3 months, their pulmonary infiltrates resolved completely.[31]

This small outbreak clearly established that the syndrome recognized as chronic pulmonary histoplasmosis actually is another variant of acute pulmonary histoplasmosis, occurring in patients with established centrilobular emphysema. It further demonstrated that, while occasional patients will go on to develop severe progressive pulmonary insufficiency, the majority will behave quite similar to those who develop the more common form of acute pulmonary histoplasmosis; they will recover completely (although more slowly), with disappearance of the upper lobe infiltrates. Moreover, the source of the infected organism is exogenous, rather than endogenous.

A single patient, seen by us in 1976, further confirmed that acute *Histoplasma* infection in a patient with established, smoking-related, centrilobular emphysema may result in the clinical picture of chronic pulmonary histoplasmosis. Two weeks after our patient was heavily exposed to bat droppings at a construction site, he suffered an unrelated rib injury. Even though he had no symptoms except rib pain, serial chest radiographs progressed from normal 2 weeks after his exposure to bilateral upper lobe fibrocavitary infiltrates just 2 weeks later. Although *H. capsulatum* was not recovered from his sputum or from material at transbronchial biopsy (even though noncaseating granulomas were seen), the patient had diagnostic *Histoplasma* serologies showing a fourfold decrease over the period of observation, coinciding with clearing of his chest radiographic infiltrates.[32]

Thus, it is now clear that chronic pulmonary histoplasmosis is the result of an acute, exogenous infection in middle-aged, usually white, male smokers. Similar to the more common lower lobe infection seen in young patients, upper lobe disease slowly resolves in most cases. Only rarely does the disease progress to the severe illness that was described originally from tuberculosis sanatoriums, and Veterans Administration hospitals in the endemic area. Therefore, it is clear that Goodwin was correct when he first proposed that chronic pulmonary histoplasmosis was an opportunistic infection in patients with severe structural pulmonary abnormalities (i.e., centrilobular emphysema).[28]

Following inhalation of infecting particles, the organism multiplies in alveoli. During the preimmune phase of the illness organisms gain access to the lymphatics, reach the hilar nodes, and then reach the blood stream. As they disseminate throughout the body, cells of the RE system phagocytose the yeasts, but are unable to destroy them. Within the macrophages, multiplication continues until the development of cell-mediated immunity (CMI), when the now "armed" macrophages finally can kill the fungus. These healed foci eventually may undergo calcification and are found as silent witnesses to previous *Histoplasma* infections.[33] Multiple lines of evidence confirm this hypothesis. In occasional patients, routine blood cultures are positive for *Histoplasma* capsulatum, yet the patient recovers completely.[34] This indicates that blood-borne dissemination is not synonymous with established disseminated histoplasmosis. Furthermore, in occasional patients, *Histoplasma* is either seen in biopsies of the RE system (liver or bone marrow) or is cultured successfully from these biopsies, yet these patients recover from the infection without treatment.[35] Finally, many patients have multiple calcified granulomas in their liver and spleen as incidental findings during postmortem examination.[36] Therefore, it is clear that probably all individuals have extrapulmonary dissemination during the acute phase of the illness, but only those patients who are unable to mount an effective CMI response will develop progression of this dissemination.

This type of histoplasmosis, progressive disseminated histoplasmosis (PDH), was the form best described before the more benign forms of the disease were appreciated. Two main forms were recognized: a rapidly fatal, febrile and wasting illness with hepatosplenomegaly, seen primarily in young infants and called the "infantile" form of the disease; and a less rapidly progressive, chronic illness, involving the lungs and presenting with mucocutaneous junction ulcers. Since the latter form usually occurred in older patients, it was referred to as the "adult" form. Histopathologically, these two forms were different, with the adult form showing well-formed granulomas and a paucity of organisms, and the infantile form exhibiting either no or usually poorly formed granulomas, with many organisms clearly visible.[37]

Early during the history of histoplasmosis, many authors reported a clear-cut association of PDH with illnesses known to be characterized by immune suppression, such as lymphomas.[6] Even though many similar cases were reported, it was not until Tompsett and Portera reported the frequent association between PDH on the one hand and several immunosuppressing conditions on the other[38] that the concept emerged that PDH was an opportunistic infection. Goodwin has popularized this concept and pointed out that, while PDH clearly develops in patients known to be immunosuppressed, in a few instances it occurred in patients who, upon recovery, had no evidence of immunosuppression. Goodwin felt that these patients may have had transient suppression of their immune systems, perhaps as a consequence of a viral infection.[33, 37] While this concept is attractive, it is only a hypothesis.

In rapid sequence, we and others reported series of patients who clearly were immunocompromised prior to the clinical onset of PDH.[39, 40] In a small study of eight patients, we suggested that initiation of immunosuppressive therapy with either glucocorticoids or cytotoxic agents reactivated dormant foci of histoplasmosis, leading to dissemination. We based this hypothesis on a series of observations: (1) all of our patients had, in the remote past, resided in areas endemic for the fungus, so they easily could have been infected previously; (2) they now resided in areas of very low background endemicity; and (3) they were all ill, thus not likely to have been engaged in activities that could bring them into intimate contact with environmental sources of the fungus. In addition, several of these patients had normal chest radiographs, so there was no evidence of a recent primary pulmonary infection.[39]

While our description was consistent with the reactivation hypothesis, it certainly did not exclude the possibility that a primary infection may lead to rapid progression in an immunocompromised host. The previously mentioned massive outbreak in Indianapolis clearly established that the immunosuppressed state was the most significant risk factor for the development of PDH.[35] Other risk factors were white race and age over 54 years. While this outbreak did answer some questions about the role of the immunosuppressed state in the development of PDH, it also raised several questions that remain unanswered. There were 42 patients who were immunosuppressed and developed histoplasmosis, yet only 31 (74%) developed PDH. Moreover, there were an additional 29 patients who developed PDH and were not immunosuppressed.[35] Why these individuals developed PDH is unclear as yet; it is clear that being immunosuppressed is but one of the predisposing factors leading to PDH!

Still, inadequate CMI clearly is the most important risk factor leading to the development of PDH. With the advent of the pandemic of the acquired immunodeficiency syndrome (AIDS), the number of profoundly immunocompromised individuals increased tremendously. Since infection by the human immunodeficiency virus (HIV) leads to a profound suppression of CMI, it was predictable that PDH should occur among these patients. Therefore, it was surprising that it took several years before PDH clearly emerged as one of the AIDS-defining opportunistic infections. Even though a single instance of PDH appeared among the various forms of opportunistic infections complicating AIDS as early as 1981,[41] and multiple cases and small series were published beginning in 1983,[42] the Centers for Disease Control did not accept PDH as an AIDS-defining condition until 1987.[43] By the end of 1990, over 230 such patients had been reported[44] and, in some parts of the United States, PDH became the second most common form of opportunistic infection behind *Pneumocystis carinii* pneumonia.

The occurrence of PDH complicating HIV infection furthered our understanding of the disease in a number of ways. Once again, a community-wide outbreak provided added insight into the pathophysiology of the disease. Beginning in the fall of 1988, Indianapolis was experiencing yet another epidemic of histoplasmosis. During the ensuing months, 64 of 239 patients residing in Indianapolis with known HIV infection developed PDH, an astonishingly high 27%! During the same time, among the 341 known HIV-infected patients residing outside Indianapolis in the state of Indiana, only 7 (2%) developed PDH. This observation clearly confirmed the previously stated hypothesis, showing that the immunosuppressed state is the most powerful risk factor for the development of PDH; that is, acute infection while immunosuppressed leads to PDH.[45]

At the same time, the alternative hypothesis first proposed by us also received support as several series of HIV-infected patients with PDH were reported from nonendemic areas of the United States. Careful analysis of these reports shows that most of these patients were previous residents of endemic areas, usually in the Caribbean basin.[46, 47] Therefore, it is likely that these patients were exposed to the fungus early in life and that endogenous reactivation occurred when their previously normal CMI diminished due to the infection with HIV. From the study of reported cases, it is clear that PDH may complicate HIV-infected patients both ways, by endogenous reactivation or by progression of the primary infection.

Diagnosis of Histoplasmosis

The gold standard for the diagnosis of histoplasmosis, as for other fungal diseases, is the cultural or histopathologic identification of the fungus. Unfortunately, cultural identification is slow and patients have no or minimal respiratory secretions. Histopathologic examination also is not easy. Invasive procedures usually are needed to obtain appropriate specimens.

Since both cultural and histopathologic methods have limitations, many attempts have been made to develop less costly and less difficult methods of diagnosis. The two most frequently used methods are serologic tests to identify humoral antibody response to the invading fungus and the application of the histoplasmin skin test, which documents evidence of delayed hypersensitivity against antigens derived from the fungus in question.

The histoplasmin skin test is well developed and standardized. Unfortunately, it plays essentially no role in diagnosing the disease in individual patients. Since, in endemic areas, histoplasmin reactivity is nearly universal, a positive skin test in association with a clinical illness is most likely to represent previous rather than recent exposure. Alternatively, a negative histoplasmin skin test does not rule out histoplasmosis, especially early during the illness or at any time during the investigation of a seriously ill patient, when anergy is expected. At present, skin testing for histoplasmosis remains an excellent epidemiologic tool, but can offer only confusion for the diagnosis of an individual patient.[48]

Serologic diagnosis of histoplasmosis is well developed and readily available. Unfortunately, it is seldom timely and, because of its limited role, it has developed a negative image. The time-honored complement-fixation (CF) test is quite sensitive, but not very specific. In addition, it frequently takes 4 weeks into the

TABLE 1.
Approximate Sensitivity of Various Serologic Tests in the Different Forms of Histoplasmosis*†

	Sensitivity, %	
Clinical Form of Histoplasmosis	Immunodiffusion	Complement Fixation
Acute pulmonary		
1 week after onset	<1	20
4 weeks after onset	50	80
Chronic cavitary histoplasmosis	75	90
Progressive disseminated	60	80
histoplasmosis (PDH)		
PDH in immunocompromised	30	50
patients		

*Adapted from Davies SF, Sarosi GA: *Clin Chest Med* 1987; 8:135–146.
†Estimates based on published reports.

course of the illness to develop diagnostic titers. Most laboratories will perform two CF tests, one for the yeast (CFY) and one for the mycelial (CFM) antigen. For all practical purposes, the CFM adds nothing to the CFY and should be eliminated. A more recent development has been the immunodiffusion test. This is more specific than the CFY, but far less sensitive. A positive M band can be expected in about 50% of the patients, and about 20% of these also will have an H band (or 10% overall). The two occurring together are 100% specific. The H band probably never occurs alone. Peak activities can be expected to occur 4 weeks after the onset of symptoms (Table 1).[48]

Two experimental tests deserve mention. Radioimmunoassay measures both IgM and IgG antibodies. Unfortunately, increased sensitivity is offset by decreased specificity.[49] Potentially more important is Wheat's recent report on measurement of *Histoplasma* antigen in urine or blood. In his laboratory, this test is both highly specific and sensitive in severe infections, particularly in immunosuppressed patients.[50]

In summary, while immunologic tests exist, currently available tests lack either specificity (as the skin test) or are not timely (CF and immunodiffusion). Once the radioimmunoassay or urinary antigen becomes commercially available, immunologic tests are likely to assume a more important place in our diagnostic armamentarium.

Treatment of Histoplasmosis

Since the vast majority of patients with acute histoplasmosis recover rapidly and spontaneously, no treatment is needed (Table 2). Occasionally, a patient develops severe pulmonary histoplasmosis with widesread infiltrates. These rare patients may develop gas exchange abnormalities rapidly and may even progress to the

TABLE 2.
Recommended Therapy for Histoplasmosis*

Acute	Observation
Acute, with gas exchange problems	AMB 500 mg or more as indicated
Upper lobe fibrocavitary	Observation
Progressive upper lobe disease	Ketoconazole 400 mg to 800 mg
	AMB 35 mg/kg if ketoconazole fails
PDH, slowly progressive	Ketoconazole 400 to 800 mg/day
PDH, rapidly progressive	AMB 40 mg/kg
PDH complicating HIV infection	AMB 2,000 mg total, followed by biweekly AMB 50 to 80 mg per dose
	Itraconazole 200 to 400 mg/day

*AMB = amphotericin B; HIV = human immunodeficiency virus; PDH = progressive disseminated histoplasmosis.

adult respiratory distress syndrome (ARDS). With such patients, invasive diagnostic tests usually are needed to establish the etiology of the illness. Once the etiology is clear and the patient continues to deteriorate, AMB is needed urgently. The usually recommended dose is around 500 mg, but more may be needed if gas exchange abnormalities are slow to improve.

Treatment of the upper lobe fibrocavitary form of histoplasmosis is more complex. Since most of these patients likely will improve spontaneously, careful follow-up is required before treatment is started. Once the progressive nature of this illness is established, ketoconazole in doses of 400 mg/day is likely to be helpful. In patients slow to respond, this may be increased to 800 mg/day, provided the patient is able to tolerate its considerable gastrointestinal toxicity. There is no evidence that increasing the dose of ketoconazole to above 800 mg/day has anything further to offer.[51] In the event the disease fails to improve or relapses after ketoconazole therapy is completed, AMB is highly effective. On the basis of a large retrospective study, a total dose of 35 mg/kg of body weight of AMB has been associated with good results and a low rate of relapse.[26]

PDH also may be treated with ketoconazole, provided the patient is not critically ill and the tempo of the disease is leisurely.[51] In more critically ill patients, an AMB dose of 40 mg/kg has been associated with excellent results and a low rate of relapse. Since some patients with the "adult" type of PDH may have adrenal gland destruction, symptomatic hypoadrenalism must be looked for before potentially stressful therapy with AMB is initiated.[52]

PDH complicating HIV infection usually responds well to AMB. Best results have been associated with the administration of about 2 g of AMB. Following the initial therapy, suppressive therapy is indicated, since relapses are so common as to be nearly universal. Continued weekly or biweekly AMB in doses of 50 to 80 mg has produced excellent results with a low rate of relapse.[53] Itraconazole, a new triazole, is emerging as an excellent agent for suppression. Itraconazole also is promising as the agent for primary therapy of PDH complicating HIV infection.

BLASTOMYCOSIS

Blastomycosis, the least common and least understood endemic mycosis of the "big three" (the other two being histoplasmosis and coccidioidomycosis) was the only one first described in North America. T. Caspar Gilchrist, a pathologist at Johns Hopkins University, first described the disease in 1894.[54] The patient was from Philadelphia; the original tissue was a skin biopsy. In this small piece of tissue, he identified "peculiar parasitic bodies." When he published a full report of the case in 1895, he referred to the organism as a blastomycete. When a second case came to his attention in 1896, he was ready to proceed further and identify the causative organism. He was able to grow the fungus both as a yeast, where propagation is by binary fission, and as a mycelium, thus recognizing the dimorphic nature of the fungus. He then proceeded to prove Koch's postulates and was able to infect a number of dogs.[55] Thus, by 1898, much of the preliminary work on this fungus was done, establishing the thermal dimorphic nature of the fungus and identifying the dog as a species uniquely susceptible to the newly named fungus, *Blastomyces dermatitidis*. Following Gilchrist's elegant studies, a large number of patients were reported from many parts of the United States and Canada. Since many subsequent reports came from Cook County Hospital in Chicago, the disease became known as the "Chicago disease." By 1939, Martin and Smith of Duke University were able to collect 347 reported cases. They accepted only 80 cases as definite, since documentation was inadequate in the others. On the basis of these 80 patients, they described two main forms of the infection: a slowly progressive and indolent cutaneous form with a good prognosis, and a more aggressive pulmonary and disseminated form with a much poorer prognosis.[56] Although inadvertent, the net result of their monumental effort was to inject an artificial separation between the various forms of blastomycosis, which for almost 15 years hindered further progress in understanding the disease.

In 1951, Schwarz and Baum finally ended this artificial separation when they showed that, in the vast majority of cases, the common cutaneous form of the disease was preceded by pulmonary lesions.[57] As a result of their work, it is now accepted universally (and subsequently proven by many others) that the portal of entry is the lung. While there are indeed a few instances of cutaneous entry, these were linked invariably to inoculation of the organism from pus during either postmortem examination or work in the laboratory.[58]

Similar to histoplasmosis, much was known about blastomycosis by the middle 1950s, but only about the severe forms of the illness seen by hospital-based internists and dermatologists. Following the highly successful epidemiologic work on histoplasmosis, attempts were made to perform community-wide surveys with the blastomycin skin test, looking for the less seriously ill patients. Unfortunately, these attempts have met with complete failure. The crude skin test preparations available for testing in blastomycosis were neither sensitive nor specific. To this date, large-scale epidemiologic work has not been done successfully.

The first outbreak, or more correctly termed, the first cluster of cases, was recognized in 1953 to 1954 in Grifton, North Carolina, a town of 1,000.[59] During a period of a few months, 10 patients were identified; subsequently 6 more cases were seen, for a total of 16 cases in one small town. All of the original group of 10 had pulmonary disease, and only 1 had a cutaneous lesion in addition to the pulmonary involvement. Several noteworthy events were recorded in this cluster, even if no "point source" was ever identified. Perhaps most important, the authors were the first to describe an apparently self-limited case of blastomycosis. The patient, a 3-year-old child, had pulmonary disease, but by the time the diagnosis was established, he had improved. No further therapy was given and he remained well. In addition to describing the first self-limited case, the authors also described erythema nodosum in 3 of the children involved.[59] While, strictly speaking, this cluster does not qualify as a "point source" outbreak, it nevertheless supported the concept that the portal of entry was the lung. Furthermore, it also documented that self-limited blastomycosis exists and that not all patients necessarily progress to a life-threatening illness.

Following the description of this cluster of cases, the entire subject of blastomycosis sank back into its previous torpor. Cases continued to be reported; indeed, large series appeared without shedding any additional light on how individual patients acquired the infection. Epidemiologic studies were stymied by the lack of a sensitive skin test antigen and the only available serologic test, the CF test, was better at picking up histoplasmosis than blastomycosis.

Furcolow et al. compiled all published cases of human and canine blastomycosis up to 1968.[60] Their careful, indeed compulsive, compilation of cases outlined the endemic area, which appeared largely to overlap the endemic area of histoplasmosis, except that blastomycosis extended further north along the eastern shore of Lake Michigan and then westward across northern Wisconsin and northern Minnesota. Soon afterward, cases were reported from Winnepeg, Manitoba, extending the area of known endemicity north of the 49th parallel into the middle Canadian provinces.[61]

During the fall of 1972, a large outbreak occurred in the tiny hamlet of Big Fork, Minnesota, population 396.[62] Twenty-one individuals from four families built a lake cabin together. Four of these 21 subjects developed pulmonary blastomycosis. All had fever and were systemically ill. All had multiple nodules on the chest radiograph and positive cultures from sputum. Although 3 of these patients were sick enough to warrant hospitalization, by the time the diagnosis of blastomycosis was established they all were markedly improved. Because of their improved clinical state, AMB treatment was withheld and all recovered completely.[63]

During the ensuing epidemiologic investigation, 14 additional individuals were identified with evidence of a recent infection but no cultural proof of blastomycosis. Three of these patients had brief, self-limited symptoms, which were mild enough that they initially did not seek medical attention. Chest radiographs showed multiple nodules and they all had a positive blastomycin skin test. Under observation, their radiographs cleared and they remained well. In addition, five totally asymptomatic patients had abnormal chest radiographs that cleared under observation. For the other seven patients, the only evidence of blastomycosis was a positive blastomycin skin test.[63] Although the skin test antigen for blastomycosis is suspect, Big Fork is beyond the limit of the endemic zone for histoplasmosis, making the skin test perhaps more useful than in an area coendemic for both diseases.

Analysis of this outbreak showed that, like histoplasmosis and coccidioidomycosis, blastomycosis also can cause self-limited pulmonary infections as well as totally asymptomatic skin test conversions. Although this sequence of events was predicted previously, the outbreak proved the wide clinical spectrum of primary blastomycotic infection. Unfortunately, in spite of extensive investigation of the site of this "point source" outbreak, the fungus was not recovered from soil near the building site. Isolation of the fungus from nature has proven to be extremely difficult. Even though the organism has been recovered from enriched soil on rare occasions,[64, 65] most epidemiologic investigations have been stymied by inability to culture the fungus from the suspected site of the outbreak.

Finally, investigation of the largest outbreak to date succeeded where others have failed. This epidemic occurred at an environmental camp at Eagle River in northern Wisconsin. Of the 99 individuals exposed at the site, 95 were studied; 48 of them had evidence of blastomycosis. At the "point source" was a beaver lodge; several soil samples on or near this beaver lodge yielded the fungus. While the initial 9 patients (all culturally proven) were treated, an additional 39 probable cases were not treated and all recovered completely.[66] Klein, in addition to describing this large outbreak, also studied two smaller outbreaks in northern Wisconsin and was able to isolate the fungus once more from soil with a high organic content.[67]

These observations unequivocally established that blastomycosis can produce an acute illness that may clear spontaneously without sequelae. Repeated isolation of the fungus in association with outbreaks highlighted the ecologic niche of the fungus: shaded areas, rich in organic material, near to rivers, streams, or ponds. Under optimal conditions for growth, mycelia form; when disturbed, the infectious particles become airborne, are inhaled by the patient, and pneumonitis occurs. Growth is favored by rapidly rising soil temperatures. Rain on the day of exposure enhances aerosolization of spores.

Humans are not the only mammals involved. During his inoculation experiments, Gilchrist realized that dogs were susceptible, while rodents were not.[55] Parallel to published cases in humans, canine blastomycosis emerged as a common infection of dogs in endemic areas.[60] In fact, practitioners of veterinary medicine in the endemic area are well versed in the diagnosis and treatment of canine blastomycosis. The presence of large numbers of canine cases of blastomycosis should suggest that human cases must exist also and should be looked for.[68]

Diagnosis of Blastomycosis

As with all three endemic mycoses, isolation or visualization of the fungus from biologic material is the gold standard. Cultural isolation of the organism is not difficult but is time-consuming. With a large inoculum, growth may occur within 3 to 5 days; an experienced laboratory technician can give a preliminary reading then. For this reason, it is important that the clinician communicate his diagnostic suspicion, which helps early diagnosis. With a small inoculum, growth is much slower and may take up to 30 days for positive identification.

Fortunately, rapid diagnosis may be made with a 10% potassium hydroxide (KOH) digestion of sputum or pus. When these are mixed with fresh KOH and allowed to digest for 30 minutes, the characteristic large, single budding yeast of *B. dermatitidis* may be seen under the microscope. This method is extremely sensitive and, because of its speed, is the mainstay of diagnosis.[58] In addition, the characteristic large yeasts may be seen on standard cytologic preparations.[69]

Even though clinical cases may be diagnosed promptly with KOH digest of sputum or pus, less difficult and less invasive tests would be helpful. Early attempts to use the blastomycin skin test failed and there now is no commercially available blastomycin skin test. Yet, the terrible reputation of the blastomycin skin test probably is not fully deserved. When patients with acute epidemic blastomycosis were tested in Big Fork, Minnesota, 16 of 18 were positive[62] and, in the epidemic described by Klein in northern Wisconsin, 19 of 46 were positive![66]

Review of previous series where the lack of sensitivity of the blastomycin skin test was documented shows that the majority of patients tested had either disseminated blastomycosis or long-standing chronic pulmonary disease. Patients with disseminated disease would not be expected to show delayed cutaneous hypersensitivity, while patients with chronic disease may have lost their ability to exhibit a positive skin test. That the blastomycin skin test sensitivity may diminish with time is suggested by our follow-up studies of the Big Fork outbreak. When retested 3 years after the original outbreak (35 months after the first set of skin tests was applied), only 5 of the 16 available patients showed at least 5 mm induration.[70] Thus, the blastomycin skin test actually may be better than generally believed.

Serologic tests have been used also; three separate tests are currently available. The CF is the least sensitive (7% at Eagle River) and also lacks specificity. The immunodiffusion test is more specific, but also has poor sensitivity (28% at Eagle River). The recently developed enzyme immunoassay for antibody to the A antigen of *B. dermatitidis* appears to be the most sensitive test (77% at Eagle River), but high specificity is still unproven and more experience is needed (Table 3).[71]

Bradsher recently developed another in vitro test for infection.[72] He measured [^{3}H] thymidine uptake by lymphocytes in response to a *Blastomyces* alkali and water-soluble antigen. This test was the single most useful one during investigation of the Eagle River outbreak[66]; recently it was used successfully in another

TABLE 3.
Expected Sensitivity of Serologic Tests in the Various Clinical Forms of Blastomycosis*†

Clinical Form of Blastomycosis	Sensitivity (%)		
	Immunodiffusion	Complement Fixation	Enzyme Immunoassay
Acute pulmonary	30	10	80
Chronic pulmonary	60	40	90
Disseminated	80	50	90

*Adapted from Davies SF, Sarosi GA: *Clin Chest Med* 1987; 8:135–146.
†Estimates drived from various published reports.

epidemiologic study as well.[73] It is extremely efficient for documenting previous exposure to the fungus. Unfortunately, the test is available only in Bradsher's laboratory and its commercial availability is not expected.

Treatment of Blastomycosis

Before the description of the Big Fork, Minnesota outbreak,[63] the orthodox widsom was that all patients with proven blastomycosis should be treated. Yet, even before the observation of self-limited cases during this outbreak, there were tantalizing clues that spontaneous recovery could occur. In addition to the single case reported from the Grifton cluster,[59] Baum and Lerner reported a single patient in whom laboratory-acquired infection resolved spontaneously.[74] We have collected and followed a total of 39 patients with apparent self-limited blastomycosis, with only 1 late relapse.[75]

That self-limited illness (and asymptomatic infections as well) occur is well established. One could argue that had we had an acceptable, well-tolerated, and safe oral alternative to AMB, we would not have followed our patients, but would have treated them. While this is likely, when we diagnosed the 39 patients, the option did not exist, and thus we now know that self-limited blastomycosis is a reality. Our practice has been to follow stable patients without evidence of extrapulmonary spread closely for 2 weeks. This is usually adequate to see which patient will go on to healing and which will progress.[75] There are other investigators who treat all diagnosed patients and dismiss a period of observation as unnecessary and inadequate (Table 4).

AMB remains the treatment of choice for patients with rapidly progressive disease, especially when gas exchange problems occur, and for patients with meningeal involvement. A total dose of 2.0 g usually is curative.[58] Ketoconazole is an excellent drug for treating both progressive pulmonary or extrapulmonary blastomycosis when gas exchange abnormalities are not present. Both the Mycosis Study Group[51] and Bradsher[76] reported an approximately 90% success rate with ketoconazole in 400 to 800 mg/day doses. Ketoconazole should be started at 400

TABLE 4.
Recommended Therapy for Blastomycosis*

Acute pulmonary	Observation
Acute pulmonary, progressing	Ketoconazole, 400 mg/day for 6 months
Acute pulmonary, with gas-exchange problems	AMB, up to 2 g total dose
Chronic pulmonary	Ketoconazole, 400 mg/day for 6 months
Nonmeningeal disseminated	May advance to 800 mg/day
Meningitis	AMB, 2 g total dose
	Indications for intrathecal therapy are unclear
Complicating HIV infection	AMB, 2 g total dose, followed by ketoconazole suppression

*AMB = amphotericin B; HIV = human immunodeficiency virus.

mg and advanced slowly to 800 mg if clearing is slow or progression occurs. There is no evidence that anything may be gained by increasing the dose of ketoconazole above 800 mg/day. Itraconazole in all likelihood will replace ketoconazole; it is equally as effective but appears to be better tolerated.[77]

COCCIDIOIDOMYCOSIS

As with the other two endemic mycoses, the original description of coccidioidomycosis referred to the pathogen as a protozoan.[78, 79] However, Ophüls cultured the organism in short order and proved it was a fungus.[80] As with the other endemic mycoses, attention focused on the disseminated form of the disease, referred to as "coccidioidal granuloma."[81]

Although it was quickly apparent that the disease was not acquired from either man or animals, the exact method of acquisition was not clear. Strong support for a respiratory route of infection came from chance occurrences, breaks in laboratory technique. A student working in Dr. Dickson's laboratory opened a petri dish containing a mature culture of the fungus.[82] Nine days later the student developed a symptom complex that included a "flulike" illness along with fever and cough. He also developed painful erythema nodosum over his shins. His sputum grew the fungus and he recovered without any noticeable sequelae. Shortly after, in a different setting, another young man developed a similar respiratory illness. Unlike the previous case, he did not have erythema nodosum. Similar to the first case, his sputum culture was positive and the illness was self-limited.[83]

Although these two patients clearly had self-limited disease, the exact nature of the primary infection remained elusive. At about that time it became clear that the San Joaquin Valley seemed to be the most heavily endemic area in the United States. Over 80% of North American cases came from within the four counties that comprise this valley. It also became obvious that an acute febrile illness, usually with some cough, was extremely common in these four counties. This illness was referred to as "valley fever" and its cardinal manifestation was the appearance of erythema nodosum and a febrile state. Since no specific etiology was known, the patient was diagnosed as having "valley fever" only after the erythema nodosum became obvious. Many patients had minimal or no symptoms except erythema nodosum. Until these characteristic skin manifestations became obvious, patients did not seek medical attention. Obversely, there were many patients who had a nonspecific febrile illness without the appearance of erythema nodosum. Despite the great likelihood they also represented "valley fever," they were not fully recognized as such.[84]

Since many patients with cough and fever also had a positive sputum culture for *C. immitis*, it was clear that this illness was not as formidable as the "coccidioidal granuloma" cases described in the early reports. In fact, 75 physicians from the San Joaquin Valley responding to a survey reported that they recognized a total of 354 patients with "valley fever" during a 17-month period. All but 1 patient recovered. The exception developed coccidioidal meningitis and died.[84]

Following the widespread recognition of "valley fever" as the acute, self-limited form of the highly fatal coccidioidal granuloma, an unparalleled opportunity arose to study the acquisition of the illness. When the clouds of war began to gather in 1940, the United States Army Air Corps began building a series of airfields in the San Joaquin Valley. Even though the risk of acquiring coccidioidomycosis was recognized, large numbers of favorable flying days and the availability of multiple landing sites had been persuasive in the site selection.

Under the leadership of Dr. Charles E. Smith, an outstanding group of epidemiologists was assembled. Even though no ground maneuvers were held in the San Joaquin Valley, large numbers of troops were rotated in at regular intervals. All these were carefully skin-tested on arrival and once again when they departed the endemic area. In addition, provisions were made to study in depth all soldiers who became ill and arrangements were made to do careful postmortem examinations on those who died of coccidioidomycosis. These studies documented a number of critical points.[85]

First of all, a positive coccidioidin skin test was protective against subsequent infection in the endemic area. On the other extreme, soldiers with a negative skin test on arrival were highly susceptible to acute pulmonary coccidioidomycosis. In the majority of instances, skin test conversion was asymptomatic. Even amongst symptomatic patients, the illness was usually mild, frequently leading to hospitalization, but seldom fatal.[85]

A strong seasonal variation was noted also. The risk of an acute infection (and of the skin test conversion) was greatest during the hot and dry summer months and lowest during the cold and wet winter and spring months. It was suggested that the wet weather allowed rapid growth of the fungus. The infected particles then became airborne when the dry weather started. Furthermore, even in the highly endemic area, there were great differences in the rate of infection at different sites, suggesting that the fungus was distributed in a nonuniform manner. Once the role of dry, dusty conditions was appreciated, efforts were made to hold down dust. Large areas were paved and lawns were established. To reduce the risk for the troops further, field recreation was discouraged. All these measures successfully reduced the risk of infection.[86]

Since the San Joaquin Valley was not the only area of increased military activity, it soon became obvious that the entire contiguous area extending to west Texas was highly endemic for coccidioidomycosis. During these investigations it was found that southern Arizona, along the Yuma-Phoenix-Tucson axis, was actually the most highly endemic area known.[85] This area received less attention than the San Joaquin Valley at that time because of the smaller population.

Finally, the role of race also emerged as an important predictor of outcome. While the rate of infection among black soldiers was not different from that among white soldiers, progression to disseminated disease was more common among blacks.[85]

The movement of a large number of coccidioidin skin test–negative soldiers into the endemic area during a 5-year period can be viewed as a huge, ongoing, controlled epidemic. Meticulous studies were done that described the many facets of this infection. The clinical picture observed is still the best description of acute coccidioidomycosis. Most patients had a cough, which usually was productive. Fever and pleuritic chest pain accompanied the illness. Erythema nodosum occurred in about 20% of the patients. Erythema multiforme was noted also, but much less often. In addition, very early during the course of the illness a fine morbilliform rash might appear. In about one quarter of the cases arthralgias were noted, but frank arthritis was not recognized. Laboratory evaluation was nonspecific. Eosinophilia was noted in many, but the percent of eosinophils was highly variable, ranging from 0% to 22%, with the average about 6% to 8%.[87]

Chest roentgenograms also were highly variable. Hilar adenopathy was the most common manifestation, while pleural effusions and cavity formation were much less frequent. Infiltrates were noted in many chest radiographs, but there was nothing characteristic or diagnostic. All infiltrates resolved slowly. Only one of the cavities failed to close at 6 months, even though the patient remained clinically well.[87]

Thus, by the end of World War II, the entire clinical story of primary coccidioidomycosis was complete. The disease, like histoplasmosis and blastomycosis, is most commonly an asymptomatic skin test conversion. Even when the patient is symptomatic, recovery usually follows and disseminated, life-threatening illness is quite uncommon. While chest radiographs frequently are abnormal and resolve slowly, persistent pulmonary abnormalities (such as thin-walled cavities) also are compatible with the return to good health. In occasional patients, however, persistent pulmonary lesions remain symptomatic and occasionally may progress while under observation.[88]

Not a great deal has been added to the corpus of knowledge on acute coccidioidomycosis since these careful studies. While the close association of erythema nodosum with primary coccidioidomycosis now is entrenched firmly in most medical students' minds, the so-called early rash or "toxic erythema" is less well understood. For this reason, a well-studied outbreak of coccidioidomycosis among archeology students in northern California is quite noteworthy. Of the total of 103 individuals at the epidemic site, 94 returned a subsequent questionnaire; 61 reported an acute illness compatible with coccidioidomycosis. Thirty of these 61 patients reported the rash (49%); even when one considers only patients with a laboratory-confirmed diagnosis or coccidioidomycosis, 14 of 27 (52%) had the same rash. Thus, it appears that the "rash" is actually the single most common visual clue that leads one to consider coccidioidomycosis as the etiology of an illness. By comparison, erythema nodosum was noted in only 10 of the patients (16%).[89]

The true economic and human cost of coccidioidomycosis is difficult to estimate. Relatively few patients die of the disease. Since infections, even when symptomatic, are seldom serious, it is easy to be complacent about this disease. Yet, coccidioidomycosis remains an enormous and potentially highly dangerous public health hazard.

Early during the morning of Dec 20, 1977, a huge windstorm, originating in the extreme southern end of the San Joaquin Valley, tore into northern California. The dust storm raised by the high winds deposited dusty material containing infecting spores of *C. immitis* in most of the near-northern counties of California, especially in the Sacramento area. The result of this unprecedented dust storm was a marked increase in clinically recognized cases of coccidioidomycosis in northern California, outside the recognized endemic area for the disease.[90]

Even though no formal population-based epidemiologic investigation was conducted, the dramatic increase in recognized cases of coccidioidomycosis afforded many opportunities to study the biology of this infection. Since most data were collected from reviews of hospitalized or clinically ill patients, the data significantly overestimated the frequency of life-threatening coccidioidomycosis. Nevertheless, it provided highly useful information.

Previously, it had been clear that there was a significant racial factor predicting the development of life-threatening disease.[91] This, however, was questioned by some, who felt that the apparent increase of life-threatening coccidioidomycosis (both the disseminated and the severe pulmonary form) in blacks and other dark-skinned races would be explained by this group's increased and intimate contact with soil.[92] Since this dust storm involved all without regard to occupation or any other factor that might have discriminated for or against any racial group, the data are highly significant. Results confirmed the greatly increased risk of dissemination in blacks, in whom disseminated disease occurred five times as frequently as in whites. Similarly, increased risk for dissemination was observed among patients with Hispanic surnames and in Orientals; the previously noted marked increase in risk among Filipinos was noted also, but the total number of Filipinos was so small that its significance was uncertian.[93]

Persistent Pulmonary Coccidioidomycosis

Recognition of acute pulmonary coccidioidomycosis is seldom difficult if the patient is symptomatic and seeks medical attention. From population-based studies it is clear that most patients are not symptomatic enough to do so. Thus, they may present with either a complication of the acute pulmonary syndrome or progressive pulmonary disease.

The primary infection, besides involving the parenchyma and hilar lymph nodes, frequently involves the pleura. Pleuritic chest pain is noted in about 70% of the cases. If pleural disease is defined by a large accumulation of pleural fluid, however, the incidence is much lower. Unlike tuberculosis, coccidioidal pleural effusion usually is accompanied by a small parenchymal infiltrate.[94]

The most common form of pulmonary coccidioidomycotic syndrome is persistent pulmonary disease. Most pulmonary symptoms clear by 3 weeks. When they persist 6 to 8 weeks, patients are considered to have persistent pulmonary coccidioidomycosis. These ptients tend to be sick, with continuing fever, cough, and shortness of breath. Chest radiographs show extensive disease that fails to clear under observation.[95]

In immunosuppressed patients, the course is rapid, with relentlessly progressive illness. Even with prompt therapy, prognosis is poor. Interestingly, even in fatal cases, this form of coccidioidomycosis usually is restricted to the lung.[96] In non-immunocompromised patients, the disease progresses slowly, with low-grade symptoms including weight loss and hemoptysis. Chest radiographs frequently show bilateral apical fibrocavitary disease, looking very much like reactivation tuberculosis.[97]

Residual Pulmonary Lesions

Following the initial episode of pneumonitis, the radiograph evolves from an indistinctly bordered lesion to a more sharply defined nodule without a surrounding infiltrate. When biopsied or resected, viable endospores and spherules are identified readily in the material. These nodules may persist for years and can continue to shed viable spores of *C. immitis* in the sputum.[98] These lesions are similar to histoplasmomas, except that calcification is far less common in coccidioidomycosis.

Alternatively, the pneumonic lesion may undergo necrosis and subsequent cavitation. These cavities are originally thick-walled and "shaggy" and only later, when most of the cavity is "shelled out," will the characteristic thin-walled cavity appear. These cavities may persist for a long time or they may close spontaneously.[99, 100] In some cases, the cavities fill up with necrotic debris from time to time, and may "shell out" repeatedly. These lesions then may be thought of as coccidioidomycotic abscesses. In some patients, the cavities evolve from symptomatic pulmonary infections, while in many others, they are discovered as incidental findings when chest radiographs are obtained for other reasons. Finally, some cavities may present first when they rupture during the early part of the infection or later after many months of stability.[101] Hemoptysis is the most common clinical finding and occasionally it may be severe.

Disseminated Coccidioidomycosis

Unlike histoplasmosis, where dissemination throughout the body is universal during the preimmune phase of the infection, the true incidence of subclinical dissemination in coccidioidomycosis is unknown. Clinically recognized disseminated coccidioidomycosis is uncommon; its incidence also is not known. In extensive studies during World War II, 1.1% of symptomatic cases proceeded to dissemination. If one counted all diagnosed patients, including asymptomatic skin tests and seroconversions, the incidence of dissemination dropped to 0.26%.[91] These figures apply only to otherwise healthy young adults—similar data do not exist for children or for older, otherwise unwell adults. Dissemination is more common in patients with underlying immunocompromise.[102, 103] It also is more common in blacks, Filipinos, and Mexican-Americans.[91, 93] Early data implicated pregnancy, especially the third trimester, as a major risk factor.[94] Subsequent studies have cast some doubt on pregnancy as a serious risk factor for dissemination. While diabetes mellitus is a risk factor for the development of residual pulmonary cavities, it does not appear to be a risk factor for the development of disseminated disease.

Dissemination in coccidioidomycosis generally occurs early during the course of the acute infection.[91] Evidence of pulmonary disease may be totally lacking when extrapulmonary dissemination is recognized for the first time. Considerable debate centers on the question whether "late" dissemination occurs or not. It is more likely that the appearance of disseminated coccidioidomycosis long after the primary infection just represents a biologically more indolent infection.

Since residual coccidioidomycotic lesions may persist in patients for years, it is not surprising that such persistent foci may be reactivated when an immunosuppressed state develops. Immunosuppression may be secondary to an illness such as HIV infection or Hodgkin's disease, or it may result from the administration of glucocorticoids or cytotoxic agents for the treatment of other illnesses. Any organ may be involved in dissemination. Ultimately, the skin is involved in nearly all patients unless they die early secondary to meningeal involvement. Bones and joints also are involved frequently. The most feared complication of disseminated coccidioidomycosis is meningitis, which often is the only evidence of extrapulmonary spread.

Diagnosis of Coccidioidomycosis

As is the case with the other endemic mycoses, cultural isolation or histopathologic identification of the fungus is the gold standard. While the fungus is not difficult to grow, it may take up to 3 weeks to identify it. Since the mycelia of *C. immitis* are very fragile, and it takes as little as ten arthroconidia to produce an infection, extraordinary care must be exercised to prevent laboratory contamination. Recently, new techniques have been introduced for identifying a specific fungal exoantigen in as few as 5 days. In addition to its speed, this method clearly is advantageous, because it reduces the risk of laboratory-acquired infections.[105]

An often neglected but very helpful test is looking for spherules or endospores in expectorated sputum or other biologic material. While the standard KOH digested sputum occasionally may yield the fungus, the best method appears to be the standard cytologic preparation (Papanicolaou stain). From limited published data, it appears that the cytologic preparation is at least twice as sensitive as the KOH digest. Because of its simplicity, speed, and safety, this stain should be applied to all suitable biologic material to expedite diagnosis.[106]

Since direct visualization of the fungus is not a sensitive test and culture recovery is both dangerous and time-consuming, immunologic tests have assumed considerable importance. Skin testing is well standardized; there are two excellent commercially available antigens. Coccidioidin is prepared from the mycelial growth, while spherulin is prepared from the spherules. In early comparative trials, spherulin appeared to be somewhat more sensitive than coccidioidin, but it is doubtful whether this is clinically significant.[107] Unfortunately, just as in histoplasmosis, the clinical utility of a positive coccidioidin skin test is limited. A positive skin test does not establish the clinical illness as coccidioidomycosis, while a negative skin test does not rule out coccidioidomycosis.

Serologic tests are well developed and standardized in coccidioidomycosis and they are readily available (Table 5). Two main types of tests exist: measurements of IgM and IgG antibodies. For measurement of IgM antibodies, the original tube precipitin assay has been replaced by the latex agglutination test. The test measures IgM; therefore, it is positive during the early phase of the acute infection and disappears quickly. Symptomatic patients usually will show a positive test, while in asymptomatic skin test converters, the test frequently is negative. Neither the tube precipitin nor the latex agglutination test is performed on cerebrospinal fluid.

The CF serologic test is the mainstay of diagnosis, largely due to the monumen-

TABLE 5.
Expected Sensitivity of Various Serologic Tests for the Different Clinical Forms of
Coccidioidomycosis*†

Clinical Forms of Coccidioidomycosis	Sensitivity, %		
	Tube Precipitin	Complement Fixation	Complement Fixation ($>$1:32 titer)
Skin test conversion	80	30	$<$1
Acute pulmonary	90	70	5
Disseminated	40	80	60
Meningitis (tested on cerebrospinal fluid)	$<$5	65	?

*Adapted From Davies SF, Sarosi GA: *Clin Chest Med* 1987; 8:135–146.
†Estimates based on published reports.

tal work of Dr. Charles E. Smith. The test is not only diagnostic, but may have prognostic value also. High, and especially rising, titers usually are associated with severe and/or disseminated coccidioidomycosis, while a diminishing titer implies a favorable outcome. In Smith's laboratory, a titer between 1:16 and 1:32 had a greater than 95% chance of being associated with disseminated disease.[108] Perhaps in all of clinical medicine, no set of data has been misinterpreted as often as Dr. Smith's. It is extremely important to realize that *no* single titer is diagnostic of disseminated disease. Smith *never* suggested that a titer 1:16 or 1:32 *meant* dissemination; he merely stated that, given this titer, one should worry about dissemination. Moreover, his technique is not used by most laboratories today. To put it in perspective, CF titers are extremely helpful in diagnosing coccidioidomycosis. They also are useful indicators of progression or regression of the illness, but no set height of a titer may be used to determine whether the illness is disseminated or not. It is important to realize that the CF test is difficult to perform and fraught with many technical problems. To avoid batch-to-batch variation, *all* samples from the same patient should be run concurrently, to better evaluate progression or regression. CF activity may be measured in cerebrospinal fluid as well. Except when there is a bony parameningeal focus due to coccidioidomycosis, any CF activity in cerebrospinal fluid is diagnostic of coccidioidal meningtiis.

Treatment of Coccidioidomycosis

Over 60% of coccidioidomycotic infections are asymptomatic. The disease is self-limited even in most of the 40% of symptomatic patients (Table 6). On the other hand, treatment usually is indicated for patients who are quite ill, develop air

TABLE 6.
Recommended Therapy for Coccidioidomycosis*

Acute pulmonary	Observation
Acute pulmonary in high-risk patients	AMB, 1.5 to 2.5 g total dose
Persistent pulmonary disease	AMB, 2.5 g total dose
	Ketoconazole, 400 to 800 mg/day for
	minimum 6 months in indolent disease
Disseminated	AMB, 2.5 to 4.0 g total dose
Disseminated complicating HIV infection	AMB, 2.5 to 4.0 g total, followed by
	suppression with either AMB or fluconazole
Meningitis	AMB, 2.5 to 4.0 g total dose *plus* intrathecal
	AMB
Meningitis complicating HIV infection	AMB 2.5 to 4.0 g total *plus* intrathecal AMB
	The role of fluconazole as either primary or
	suppressive therapy is not firmly established

*AMB = amphotericin B; HIV = human immunodeficiency virus.

exchange problems due to fulminant pneumonia, or are at increased risk of dissemination because of race or an immunosuppressed state. In this setting, AMB is the treatment of choice; a dose of 1,500 to 2,500 mg usually is given.[109] This dose should be individualized for the rate of progression or regression. It is important to realize that there is no such thing as a "curative" dose. In endemic areas, practitioners frequently will treat mild coccidioidal illness with either ketoconazole or now with the newly available triazole, fluconazole. While this practice is widespread, evidence of its efficacy is totally lacking.

AMB also is the treatment of choice for disseminated coccidioidomycosis. It is customary to deliver a total dose of 2,500 to 4,000 mg, depending on the severity of the illness. Even in higher doses, therapeutic failures occur and relapses are quite common.[109] Ketoconazole has been used extensively in the more stable forms of dissemination not involving the meninges. While early reports were highly favorable, the Mycosis Study Group results reported by Galgiani showed that only about one third of the patients responded favorably and stayed well. It is reasonable to start ketoconazole in patients whose illness is indolent and who are not acutely ill. It is started at a daily dose of 400 mg, which may be increased to 800 mg if necessary. There is no evidence that higher doses provide further therapeutic benefit.[110] Relapse is common, even after prolonged therapy.

Meningeal coccidioidomycosis should be treated with both intravenous and intrathecal AMB. A total of 2,500 to 4,000 mg is given intravenously and intrathecal therapy is continued until the cerebrospinal fluid CF antibodies either stabilize at a low level or disappear completely. Most authorities suggest continuing intrathecal therapy weekly or twice a month for the remainder of the patient's life. Although a "cure" is difficult to achieve, long-term functional life may be achieved.[109]

A lengthy discussion of intrathecal therapy is beyond the scope of this paper. A few words on the various methods of administration are in order, however. Since the meningeal inflammation is primarily over the base of the brain, high intracisternal drug levels are the goal. In experienced hands, cisternal puncture may be used or, alternatively, an Ommaya reservoir may be placed in the cisterna. To reduce the high risk of bacterial meningitis, we prefer to place the reservoir below the hairline.

The recently released triazole, fluconazole, rapidly is becoming the treatment most practitioners prefer. While it is clear that the drug is effective, its exact role in the treatment of coccidioidomycosis is unclear as yet. It is likely that it will have a major role to play in the treatment of meningeal and nonmeningeal disseminated coccidioidomycosis in the future.

Treatment of HIV-infected patients with coccidioidomycosis is best started with AMB. Because of the ease of administration, once a patient's condition has stabilized, it is reasonable to switch him or her over to fluconazole, since long-term maintennce therapy will be necessary.[111]

REFERENCES

1. Darling ST: Protozoan general infection producing pseudotubercles in the lungs and focal necrosis in liver, spleen and lymph nodes. *JAMA* 1906; 46:1283–1285.

2. Darling ST: Histoplasmosis: A fatal infectious disease resembling kala-azar found among natives of tropical America. *Arch Intern Med* 1980; 2:107–112.

3. Riley WA, Watson CJ: Histoplasmosis of Darling with report of a case originating in Minnesota. *Am J Trop Med Hyg* 1926; 6:271–282.

4. Dodd K, Tompkins EH: Case of histoplasmosis of Darling in an infant. *Am J Trop Health* 1934; 14:127–134.

5. DeMonbreun WA: The cultivation and cultural characteristics of Darling's *Histoplasma capsulatum*. *Am J Trop Med Hyg* 1934; 14:93–126.

6. Parsons RJ, Zarafonetis CJD: Histoplasmosis in man: Report of 7 cases and a review of 71 cases. *Arch Intern Med* 1945; 75:1–23.

7. Christie A, Peterson JC: Pulmonary calcification in negative reactors to tuberculin. *Am J Public Health* 1945; 35:1131–1147.

8. Palmer CE: Nontuberculous pulmonary calcification. *Public Health Rep* 1945; 60:513–521.

9. Emmons CW: Isolation of *Histoplasma capsulatum* from soil. *Public Health Rep* 1949; 64:892–896.

10. Bunnell IL, Furcolow ML: A report of 10 proven cases of histoplasmosis. *Public Health Rep* 1948; 63:299–316.

11. Christie A: The disease spectrum of human histoplasmosis. *Trans Assoc Am Physicians* 1951; 64:147–154.

12. Loosli CG, Grayston JT, Alexander ER, et al: Epidemiological studies of pulmonary histoplasmosis in a farm family. *Am J Hyg* 1954; 55:392–401.

13. Grayston JT, Furcolow ML: The occurrence of histoplasmosis in epidemics—epidemiological studies. *Am J Public Health* 1953; 45:665–676.

14. Furcolow ML, Tosh FE, Larsh HW, et al: The emerging pattern of urban histoplasmosis. *N Engl J Med* 1961; 264:1226–1230.

15. D'Alessio DJ, Heeren RH, Hendricks SL, et al: A starling roost as the source of urban epidemic histoplasmosis in an area of low incidence. *Am Rev Respir Dis* 1965; 92:725–731.

16. Tosh FE, Doto IL, D'Alessio DJ, et al: The second of two epidemics of histoplasmosis resulting from work on the same starling roost. *Am Rev Respir Dis* 1966; 94:406–413.

17. Leznoff A, Frank H, Telner P, et al: Histoplasmosis in Montreal during the fall of 1963, with observations on *erythema multiforme*. *Can Med Assoc J* 1964; 91:1154–1160.

18. Sellers TF Jr, Price WN Jr, Newberry WM Jr: An epidemic of *erythema multiforme* and *erythema nodosum* caused by histoplasmosis. *Ann Intern Med* 1965; 62:11244–11262.

19. Sarosi GA, Parker JD, Tosh FE: Histoplasmosis outbreaks: Their patterns, in Balows A (ed): *Histoplasmosis. Proceedings of the Second National Conference* 1969. Atlanta, Charles C Thomas, 1971, pp 123–128.

20. Brodsky AL, Gregg MB, Loewenstein MS, et al: Outbreak of histoplasmosis associated with the 1970 Earth Day activities. *Am J Med* 1973; 54:333–342.

21. Ward JI, Weeks M, Allen D, et al: Acute histoplasmosis: Clinical, epidemiologic and serologic findings of an outbreak associated with exposure to a fallen tree. *Am J Med* 1979; 66:587–595.

22. Edwards LB, Acquaviva FA, Livesay VT, et al: An atlas of sensitivity to tuberculin, PPD-B and histoplasmin in the U.S. *Am Rev Respir Dis* 1969; 99(suppl):1–18.

23. Wheat LJ, Slama TG, Eitzen HA, et al: A large urban outbreak of histoplasmosis: Clinical features. *Ann Intern Med* 1981; 94:331–337.

24. Wheat LJ, Stein L, Corya BC, et al: Pericarditis as a manifestation of histoplasmosis during two large urban outbreaks. *Medicine (Baltimore)* 1983; 62:110–119.

25. Furcolow ML, Doto IL, Tosh FE, et al: Course and prognosis of untreated histoplasmosis. A United States Public Health Service Cooperative Mycoses Study. *JAMA* 1961; 177:292–296.

26. Parker JD, Sarosi GA, Doto IL, et al: Treatment of chronic pulmonary histoplasmosis. *N Engl J Med* 1970; 283:225–229.

27. Doto IL, Furcolow ML, Tosh FE: Comparison of treated and untreated severe histoplasmosis. A Communicable Disease Center Cooperative Mycoses Study. *JAMA* 1963; 183:823–829.

28. Goodwin RA Jr, Owens FT, Snell JD, et al: Chronic pulmonary histoplasmosis. *Medicine (Baltimore)* 1976; 55:413–452.

29. Goodwin RA Jr, Snell JD, Hubbard WW, et al: Early chronic pulmonary histoplasmosis. *Am Rev Respir Dis* 1966; 93:47–51.

30. Procknow JJ: Reinfection histoplasmosis, in Balows A (ed): *Histoplasmosis. Proceedings of the Second National Conference 1969.* Atlanta, Charles C Thomas, 1971, pp 252–259.

31. Latham RH, Kaiser AB, DuPont WD, et al: Chronic pulmonary histoplasmosis following excavation of a bird roost. *Am J Med* 1980; 68:504–508.

32. Davies SF, Sarosi GA: Acute cavitary histoplasmosis. *Chest* 1978; 73:103–105.

33. Goodwin RA Jr, DesPrez RM: Histoplasmosis: State of the art. *Am Rev Respir Dis* 1978; 117:929–956.

34. Paya CU, Robert GN, Cockerill FR III: Transient fungemia in acute pulmonary histoplasmosis: Detection by new blood-culturing techniques. *J Infect Dis* 1987; 156:313–315.

35. Wheat LJ, Slama TG, Norton JA, et al: Risk factors for disseminated or fatal histoplasmosis: Analysis of a large urban outbreak. *Ann Intern Med* 1982; 96:159–163.

36. Straub M, Schwarz J: Healed primary complex in histoplasmosis. *Am J Clin Pathol* 1955; 25:727–738.

37. Goodwin RA Jr, Shapiro JL, Thurman GH, et al: Disseminated histoplasmosis: Clinical and pathological correlations. *Medicine (Baltimore)* 1980; 59:1–33.

38. Tompsett R, Portera LA: Histoplasmosis: Twenty year experience in a general hospital. *Trans Am Clin Climatol Assoc* 1975; 87:214–223.

39. Davies SF, Khan M, Sarosi GA: Disseminated histoplasmosis in immunologically suppressed patients: Occurrence in a non-endemic area. *Am J Med* 1978; 64:94–100.

40. Kaufman CA, Israel KS, Smith JW, et al: Histoplasmosis in immunosuppressed patients. *Am J Med* 1978; 64:923–932.

41. Centers for Disease Control: Update on acquired immunodeficiency syndrome (AIDS) among patients with hemophilia A. *MMWR* 1981; 31:646–652.

42. Jones PE, Cohen RL, Batts DH, et al: Disseminated histoplasmosis, invasive pulmonary aspergillosis and other opportunistic infections in a homosexual patient with acquired immune deficiency syndrome. *Sex Transm Dis* 1983; 10:202–204.

43. Centers for Disease Control: Revision of the CDC surveillance case definition of acquired immunodeficiency syndrome. *JAMA* 1987; 258:1143–1154.

44. Sarosi GA, Johnson PC: Disseminated histoplasmosis in HIV infected patients. *Clin Infect Dis,* in press.

45. Wheat LJ, Connolly-Stringfield PA, Baker RL, et al: Disseminated histoplasmosis in the acquired immune deficiency syndrome: Clinical findings, diagnosis and review of the literature. *Medicine (Baltimore)* 1990; 69:361–374.

46. Mandell W, Goldberg DM, Neu HC: Histoplasmosis in patients with the acquired immune deficiency syndrome. *Am J Med* 1986; 81:974–978.

47. Salzman SH, Smith RL, Aranda CP: Histoplasmosis in patients at risk for the acquired immunodeficiency syndrome in a nonendemic setting. *Chest* 1988; 93:916–921.

48. Davies SF, Sarosi GA: Role of serodiagnostic tests and skin tests in the diagnosis of fungal disease. *Clin Chest Med* 1987; 8:135–146.

49. Wheat LJ, Kohler RB, French MLU: Immunoglobulin M and G histoplasmal antibody response in histoplasmosis. *Am Rev Respir Dis* 1983; 128:65–70.

50. Wheat LJ, Kohler RB, Tewari RP: Diagnosis of disseminated histoplasmosis by detection of *Histoplasma capsulatum* antigen in serum and urine specimens. *N Engl J Med* 1986; 314:83–88.

51. Mycosis Study Group: Treatment of blastomycosis and histoplasmosis with ketoconazole. *Ann Intern Med* 1985; 103:861–873.

52. Sarosi GA, Voth DW, Dahl BA, et al: Disseminated histoplasmosis: Results of long-term follow-up. *Ann Intern Med* 1971; 75:511–516.

53. McKinsey DS, Gupta MR, Riddler SA, et al: Long-term amphotericin B therapy for disseminated histoplasmosis in patients with the acquired immunodeficiency syndrome (AIDS). *Ann Intern Med* 1989; 111:655–659.

54. Gilchrist TC: Protozoan dermatitis. *J Cutan Genitourin Dis* 1894; 12:496–499.

55. Gilchrist TC, Stokes WR: A case of *pseudo-lupus vulgaris* caused by a blastomyces. *J Exp Med* 1898; 3:53–78.

56. Martin DS, Smith DT: Blastomycosis I. A review of the literature. *Am Rev Tuberc* 1939; 39:275–304.

57. Schwarz J, Baum GL: Blastomycosis. *Am J Clin Pathol* 1951; 11:999–1029.

58. Sarosi GA, Davies SF: Blastomycosis. State of the art. *Am Rev Respir Dis* 1979; 120:911–938.

59. Smith JR Jr, Harris JS, Conant NF, et al: An epidemic of North American blastomycosis. *JAMA* 1951; 158:641–645.

60. Furcolow ML, Chick EW, Busey JD, et al: Prevalence and incidence studies of human and canine blastomycosis. I. Cases in the U.S., 1895–1968. *Am Rev Respir Dis* 1970; 102:60–67.

61. Kepron MD, Schoemperlen B, Hershfield ES, et al: North American blastomycosis in central Canada. *Can Med Assoc J* 1972; 106:243–246.

62. Tosh FE, Hammerman KJ, Weeks RJ, et al: A common source epidemic of North American blastomycosis. *Am Rev Respir Dis* 1974; 109:525–529.

63. Sarosi GA, Hammerman KJ, Tosh FE, et al: Clinical features of acute pulmonary blastomycosis. *N Engl J Med* 1974; 290:540–543.

64. Denton JD, McDonough ES, Ajello L, et al: Isolation of *Blastomyces dermatitidis* from soil. *Science* 1961; 133:1126–1128.

65. Sarosi GA, Serstock DS: Isolation of *Blastomyces dermatitidis* from pigeon manure. *Am Rev Respir Dis* 1976; 114:1179–1183.

66. Klein BS, Vergeront JM, Weeks RJ, et al: Isolation of *Blastomyces dermatitidis* in soil associated with a large outbreak of blastomycosis in Wisconsin. *N Engl J Med* 1986; 314:529–534.

67. Klein BS, Vergeront JM, DiSalvo AF, et al: Two outbreaks of blastomycosis along rivers in Wisconsin: Isolation of *Blastomyces dermatitidis* from riverbank soil and evidence of its transmission along waterways. *Am Rev Respir Dis* 1987; 136:1333–1338.

68. Sarosi GA, Eckman MR, Davies SF, et al: Canine blastomycosis as a harbinger of human disease. *Ann Intern Med* 1979; 91:733–735.

69. Sanders JS, Sarosi GA, Nollet DJ, et al: Exfoliative cytology in the rapid diagnosis of pulmonary blastomycosis. *Chest* 1977; 72:193–196.

70. Sarosi GA, King RA: Apparent diminution of the blastomycin skin test: Follow-up of an epidemic of blastomycosis. *Am Rev Respir Dis* 1977; 116:785–788.

71. Klein BS, Vergeront JM, Kaufman L, et al: Serological tests for blastomycosis: Assessment during a large point-source outbreak in Wisconsin. *J Infect Dis* 1987; 155:262–268.

72. Bradsher RW: Development of specific immunity in patients with pulmonary or extrapulmonary blastomycosis. *Am Rev Respir Dis* 1984; 129:430–434.

73. Davies SF, Colbert R, Bradsher RW: Concurrent human and canine histoplasmosis from cutting decayed wood. *Ann Intern Med* 1990; 113:252–253.

74. Baum GL, Lerner PI: Primary pulmonary blastomycosis: A laboratory acquired infection. *Ann Intern Med* 1970; 73:263–265.

75. Sarosi GA, Davies SF, Phillips JR: Self-limited blastomycosis: A report of 39 cases. *Semin Respir Infect* 1986; 1:40–44.

76. Bradsher RW, Rice DC, Abernathy RS: Ketoconazole therapy for endemic blastomycosis. *Ann Intern Med* 1985; 103:872–875.

77. Bradsher BW: Blastomycosis: Fungal infections of the lung update: 1989. *Semin Respir Infect* 1990; 5:105–110.

78. Posadas A: Un nuevo caso de micosis fungoides con psorospermias. *Ann Circ Med Argent* 1892; 15:585–597.

79. Wernicke E: Über einen protozoenbefunde bei mycosis fungoides. *Zentralbl Für Bakt* 1892; 12:859–861.

80. Ophüls W: Further observations on a mould formerly described as a protozoan *(Coccidioides immitis, Coccidioides pyogenes)*. *J Exp Med* 1905; 6:445–446.

81. Ophüls W: Coccidioidal granuloma. *JAMA* 1905; 45:1291–1296.

82. Dickson EC: Coccidioides infection. Part I. *Arch Intern Med* 1937; 59:1029–1044.

83. Dickson EC: Coccidioidomycosis. The preliminary acute infection with fungus coccidioides. *JAMA* 1938; 111:1362–1365.

84. Dickson EC, Gifford MA: Coccidioides infection (coccidioidomycosis) II. The primary type of infection. *Ann Intern Med* 1938; 62:853–871.

85. Drutz DJ, Catanzaro A: Coccidioidomycosis. State of the art. Part I. *Am Rev Respir Dis* 1978; 117:559–585.

86. Smith CE, Beard RR, Rosenberger HG, et al: Effect of season and dust control on coccidioidomycosis. *JAMA* 1946; 132:833–839.

87. Goldstein DM, McDonald JB: Primary pulmonary coccidioidomycosis. Follow-up of 75 cases with 10 more cases from a new endemic area. *JAMA* 1944; 124:557–561.

88. Winn WA, Johnson GH: Primary coccidioidomycosis: A roentgenographic study of 40 cases. *Ann Intern Med* 1942; 17:407–422.

89. Werner SB, Pappagianis D, Heindl I, et al: An epidemic of coccidioidomycosis among archeology students in northern California. *N Engl J Med* 1972; 286:507–512.

90. Flynn NM, Hoeprich PD, Kawachi MM, et al: An unusual outbreak of wind-borne coccidioidomycosis. *N Engl J Med* 1979; 301:358–361.

91. Smith CE, Beard RR, Whiting EG, et al: Varieties of coccidioidal infection in relation to the epidemiology and control of the disease. *Am J Public Health* 1946; 36:1394–1402.

92. Huppert M: Racism in coccidioidomycosis (letter). *Am Rev Respir Dis* 1978; 118:797–798.

93. Pappagianis D, Lindsay S, Beall S, et al: Ethnic background and the clinical course of coccidioidomycosis (letter). *Am Rev Respir Dis* 1979; 120:959–961.

94. Drutz DJ, Catanzaro A: Coccidioidomycosis. State of the art. Part II. *Am Rev Respir Dis* 1978; 117:727–771.

95. Bayer AS: Fungal pneumonias, pulmonary coccidioidal syndromes (part I). *Chest* 1981; 79:575–583.

96. Rowland US, Westphal RE, Hinchcliffe WA: Fatal coccidioidomycosis: Analysis of host factors, in Ajello L (ed): Coccidioidomycosis—current clinical and diagnostic status. Miami, Symposia Specialists, 1977, p 91.

97. Sarosi GA, Parker JD, Doto IL, et al: Chronic pulmonary coccidioidomycosis. *N Engl J Med* 1970; 283:325–329.

98. Rivkin LM, Winn DF, Salyer JM: The surgical treatment of pulmonary coccidioidomycosis. *J Thorac Cardiovasc Surg* 1961; 42:402–412.

99. Winn WA: A long term study of 300 patients wtih cavitary abscess lesions of the lung of coccidioidal origin. *Dis Chest* 1968; 54(suppl I):12–16.

100. Hyde L: Coccidioidal pulmonary cavitation. *Dis Chest* 1968; 54(suppl I):17–21.

101. Cunningham RT, Einstein H: Coccidioidal pulmonary cavities with rupture. *J Thorac Cardiovasc Surg* 1982; 84:172–177.

102. Deresinski SC, Stevens DA: Coccidioidomycosis in compromised hosts: Experience at Stanford University Hospital. *Medicine (Baltimore)* 1975; 54:377–395.

103. Cohen IM, Galgiani JN, Potter D, et al: Coccidioidomycosis in renal replacement therapy. *Arch Intern Med* 1982; 142:489–494.

104. Catanzaro A: Pulmonary mycosis in pregnant women. *Chest* 1984; 86(suppl):14S–18S.

105. Standard PG, Kaufman L: Immunological procedure for the rapid and specific identification of *Coccidioides immitis* cultures. *J Clin Microbiol* 1977; 5:149–153.

106. Warlick MA, Quan SF, Sobonya RE: Rapid diagnosis of pulmonary coccidioidomycosis. Cytologic vs. potassium hydroxide preparation. *Arch Intern Med* 1983; 143:723–725.

107. Sarosi GA, Catanzaro A, Daniel TM, et al: Clinical usefulness of skin testing in histoplasmosis, coccidioidomycosis and blastomycosis: Official statement of The American Thoracic Society. *Am Rev Respir Dis* 1988; 138:1081–1082.

108. Smith CE, Saito MT, Beard RR, et al: Serologic tests in the diagnosis and prognosis of coccidioidomycosis. *Am J Hygiene* 1950; 52:1–21.

109. Sarosi GA, Bates JH, Brads her RW, et al: Chemotherapy of the pulmonary mycoses: Official statement of The American Thoracic Society. *Am Rev Respir Dis* 1988; 138:1078–1081.

110. Galgiani JN, Stevens DA, Graybill JR, et al: Ketoconazole therapy of progressive coccidioidomycosis. Comparison of 400 and 800 mg doses and observations at higher doses. *Am J Med* 1988; 84:603–610.

111. Fish DG, Ampel NM, Galgiani JN, et al: Coccidioidomycosis during human immunodeficiency virus infection. A review of 77 patients. *Medicine (Baltimore)* 1990; 69:384–391.

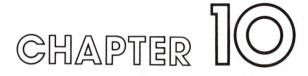

CHAPTER 10

Carbon Monoxide Poisoning

Stephen R. Thom, M.D., Ph.D.

Assistant Professor of Medicine, Chief, Hyperbaric Medicine, Institute for Environmental Medicine, University of Pennsylvania School of Medicine, Philadelphia, Pennsylvania

The pathophysiology of carbon monoxide (CO) poisoning has been investigated for nearly 100 years.[1] Despite this, many questions remain. This review highlights the major pathophysiologic issues associated with CO exposure and discusses clinical aspects of CO poisoning and its treatment.

EPIDEMIOLOGY

Incomplete combustion of any carbon fuel generates CO. Smoke inhalation injury occurs in 80% of the estimated 8,000 annual fire fatalities in the United States; sixty percent of deaths, 3,800 per year,[2] have been attributed to CO. Exposure to automobile exhaust and combustion products from indoor heaters may account for an additional 1,500 accidental deaths and 2,300 suicides each year.[3] Public health officials have demonstrated that, despite generally increased awareness of the CO problem, cursory surveillance of accidental deaths grossly underestimates its significance.[4] The importance of CO among all causes of unintentional poisoning deaths in the United States, therefore, is difficult to establish. Recently, the mortality rate from all gases and vapors-related poisonings is reported to have decreased by 25%.[5] A question remains, however, whether this is due to increased public awareness and fewer poisonings, improved treatment, or underreporting of deaths.

Exposure to CO also results from hepatic metabolism of methylene chloride (dichloromethane), a component of most popular paint strippers.[6] Carboxyhemoglobin (COHb) levels as high as 40% have been recorded after a 6-hour exposure to paint remover.[7] Thus, in addition to the central nervous system depressant effects of this organic solvent, there is also stress due to CO production. Exposure may precipitate myocardial infarction and death in patients with underlying coronary artery disease.[8]

PATHOPHYSIOLOGY

Tissue Oxygen Supply

The exchange of CO between environmental air and the body takes place mainly in the lungs; its dynamics can be described satisfactorily by mathematic models.[9] Inhaled CO diffuses rapidly across the alveolar-capillary membrane and binds to hemoglobin to form COHb, central features of CO toxicology. The relative affinity of CO for hemoglobin is approximately 200-fold greater than that of O_2.[10]

Alveolar ventilation is the most important physiologic variable influencing the rate of COHb formation.[11] CO uptake increases with increased ventilation and decreases with rapid ventilation during resuscitation. However, ventilation has almost no influence on the maximum COHb level achievable, which depends on alveolar CO and O_2 concentrations and atmospheric pressure. There are many estimates of the half-life time for excretion of CO and a decrease in the body COHb burden. Experimental data have demonstrated wide variations between individuals. For example, values for 18 healthy young men breathing air ranged from 128 to 409 minutes, with an average of 320 minutes.[12]

The COHb level reached depends on alveolar CO partial pressure, duration of exposure, metabolic rate, and pulmonary function. The common clinical practice of attempting to predict a patient's "maximum" COHb level at the time of exposure based on an extrapolation from some point after treatment has begun, therefore, may be futile. Moreover, as the blood level has no predictive value for estimating severity of CO poisoning,[13–17] nothing is gained with this practice.

Alveolar O_2 tension (P_{AO_2}) may be normal or decreased depending upon the fraction of O_2 in the inspired air (F_{IO_2}), so arterial O_2 tension (P_{aO_2}) may be normal to low. Oxyhemoglobin saturation, derived in blood gas analysis by calculation, remains in the normal range unless the P_{aO_2} is severely depressed and is independent of oxyhemoglobin and COHb concentrations. Hence, arterial O_2 saturation may be interpreted falsely as being normal when the ratio of oxyhemoglobin to total hemoglobin concentration is low. The oxygen available to tissues may be decreased either by a direct reduction of O_2 content by a low Pa_{O_2}, by the presence of COHb, or by a leftward shift in the oxyhemoglobin dissociation curve caused by the presence of COHb in erythrocytes.

Cellular O_2 utilization also may be impaired by CO. A likely intracellular target for CO is myoglobin, which has a 40-fold greater affinity for CO than for O_2.[18] Coburn has estimated that only 10% to 15% of the CO present in the body is bound to extracellular proteins.[19] CO binds to myoglobin even when CO concentrations are quite low.[20] A one-to-one relationship exists between COHb in blood and carboxymyoglobin level in skeletal or cardiac muscle, even with normal oxygenation.[18, 21, 22] The flux of CO to the extravascular space is augmented greatly during hypoxia. When the Pa_{O_2} drops below 40 mm Hg, 20% to 40% of intravascular CO may shift to myoglobin in the myocytes.[21, 23] However, the significance of CO binding to myoglobin is not entirely clear. Myoglobin is an O_2 carrier protein that may facilitate O_2 diffusion in muscle cells or function as an O_2 store close to mitochondria. Cardiac and striatal muscle dysfunction during acute CO exposure may be due to impaired myoglobin-mediated O_2 transport.[24, 25]

The affinity of mitochondrial cytochrome oxidase for CO is only one-ninth that for O_2, however, some CO binding can occur, especially during hypoxia[26] or when there is a massive CO body burden.[27] Small reductions in cellular respiration due to CO also can be shown in in vitro assays in the presence of O_2, although the physiologic significance of this is uncertain.[28]

Vascular Effects

CO exposure causes vasodilatation that is attributable largely to the associated decrease in arterial O_2 saturation and the leftward shift of the oxyhemoglobin dissociation curve. However, since the increase in tissue perfusion exceeds that necessary to meet O_2 demands, there may be additional mechanisms involved.[29] With this in mind, it is intriguing that endothelium-derived relaxation factor (EDRF), normally taken up and thus "deactivated" by hemoglobin, is not taken up by COHb.[30, 31] This autocoid, putatively identified as nitric oxide, is generated by endothelial cells and causes vascular relaxation by activating smooth muscle guanylate cyclase. The presence of COHb and hence a lower concentration of functional hemoglobin may cause a higher local concentration of EDRF, although this mechanism has not been studied in animal models of CO poisoning. At CO concentrations that probably are greater than usually occur in vivo, CO also will activate guanylate cyclase directly and cause endothelium-independent vascular relaxation.[32]

In addition to its vasomotor influences, CO causes functional and pathologic changes in blood vessel walls. Exposure of humans to 5,000 ppm of CO for short periods to achieve a COHb of 20% to 25% increases vessel permeability, documented by enhanced ^{131}I albumin loss from the intravascular compartment.[33, 34]

Intermittent exposure to CO for 1 day increases the glomerular filtration rate by 50%.[35] Monkeys exposed to CO at 250 ppm for 2 weeks exhibited coronary artery damage consisting of subendothelial edema, fatty streaking, and lipid-loaded cells.[36] A link between CO and atheromatous changes in arterial walls was demonstrated by Astrup and Kjedlsen in rabbits fed high-cholesterol diets, but not in those fed normal diets.[37, 38] An elevated COHb level (>5%) can be used as an index for increased risk for atherosclerosis in humans.[39]

Cardiac

The effects on myocardial function of breathing relatively low concentrations of CO have been studied extensively. In summary, pathologic changes occur in animals after exposures of several weeks to CO sufficient to raise COHb levels to 16% to 20%. Rabbits exhibit myofibrillar necrosis and mitochondrial degeneration after 2 weeks.[40] Coronary artery changes in monkeys have been mentioned already.[36] Dogs exposed for 11 weeks show electrocardiographic and morphologic evidence of damage.[41]

Exposure of animals to high levels of CO (COHb 26% to 75%) for short periods can cause myocardial hemorrhage, multifocal necrosis, leukocyte infiltration, mural thrombi, and degeneration of muscle fibers, as well as lethal dysrhythmias.[41, 42] Ventricular function may be depressed at COHb levels of 20% to 30%.[43] Subendocardial ischemia may occur due to the differential blood flow through regions of the myocardium during a CO stress.[44]

Acute exposure to CO for several hours to achieve COHb levels of 15% to 20% has failed to precipitate spontaneous dysrhythmias in normal or ischemic dog hearts.[45, 46] However, monkeys exposed for 6 hours to only 100 ppm of CO (COHb 9%) exhibited a decreased threshold for induction of ventricular fibrillation.[47] Exposures of humans to 100 to 200 ppm of CO, achieving COHb levels of 4% to 6%, also have failed to cause spontaneous dysrhythmias in normal subjects or patients with coronary artery disease.[48] Interestingly, exposure to 50 to 250 ppm of CO long enough to achieve only 2.5% to 3.5% COHb significantly shortens the time to develop angina and electrocardiographic evidence of myocardial ischemia in exercising patients with coronary artery disease.[49] Thus, the physiologic reserve clearly is compromised by even mild COHb elevations.

Pulmonary

Pulmonary edema in patients with normal heart size and no previous cardiac or pulmonary disease is rather common in serious CO poisoning. Up to 30% of patients may have abnormalities on chest x-ray, with features such as perihilar haze, peribronchial and perivascular cuffing, ground-glass appearance, and intra-alveolar edema.[50] One may see pulmonary changes in patients exposed to automobile exhaust or combustion products from faulty heaters; however, severe pulmonary pathology is associated most often with smoke inhalation by fire victims. Animal studies indicate that brief exposure to smoke, but not to CO only, precipitates pulmonary injury that evolves slowly over 24 to 72 hours.[51, 52] A recent study showed that the pulmonary injury from smoke appears to involve principally the airways and not the alveoli.[53] In this study, lipid peroxidation products were detected in the liver and blood, but not in the lung. Systemic microvascular integrity also was impaired markedly (increased fluid permeability), but pulmonary vascular permeability changed only modestly. Thus, smoke inhalation appeared to cause a systemic oxidative stress that CO alone does not trigger. Studies indicate that the eicosanoid system, or at least sulfidopeptide leukotrienes, are not involved in these effects.[54]

Older studies of lung pathophysiology also failed to identify direct effects of CO on lung morphology or function.[55] It has been speculated that contradictory pulmonary findings following protracted CO exposure[56] were due to systemic compromise, specifically the hypotension and hypoxia, caused by CO. Thus, it now appears that early pulmonary abnormalities cannot be ascribed to direct effects of CO. They may be due to chemical irritants in smoke. It remains unclear, however, whether the systemic stress associated with exposure to CO for more than a few minutes may participate in the evolution of organ compromise. It seems reasonable to consider that the hypoxia and hypotension occurring in some models of both pure CO and smoke-related poisonings, may contribute to organ dysfunction throughout the body.

Cerebral Function and Physiology

Subtle cortical dysfunction occurs in humans with CO levels as low as 5%.[57] Effects detected at such low levels are difficult to reconcile with the minimal compromise in O_2 delivery. Not surprisingly, the detection of abnormalities seems to be related to the sensitivity of the testing method. An exception are studies of visual detection threshold. Early studies suggested that low-level CO caused dysfunction,[58] whereas recent carefully controlled studies have failed to find an effect when COHb levels are less than about 20%.[59]

Animal studies have demonstrated neurophysiologic effects interpreted as direct toxic actions of CO rather than CO compromise of hemoglobin function. An in vivo study of the cat electroretinogram[60] demonstrated abnormalities with only 7.5% COHb. In vitro studies of rat Purkinje cell electrical activity demonstrated impairment with CO levels of 500 to 1,000 ppm.[61] If tissue CO partial pressure is approximately — at most — one half of the inspired partial pressure,[62] this in vitro study would be comparable to breathing 1,000 to 2,000 ppm of CO, sufficient to achieve a COHb level of more than 60%. Ventilation of rats with 5,000 ppm of CO appears to impair cortical cytochrome oxidase activity despite the presence of hemoglobin and O_2.[27] CO-mediated impairment of respiration occurs in isolated, perfused neuronal and muscle cells.[26] As discussed previously, the affinity of the cytochrome system for O_2 is some nine times that of CO. Previously, cytochrome binding by CO had been shown only when there was concurrent hypoxia.[63, 64]

Both central and peripheral nervous system pathology can be caused by CO poisoning. Peripheral problems, although rare, have been reported by several observers.[13, 65] Demyelination and abnormal conduction of peripheral nerves also has been shown in rats.[66] Clinical central nervous system pathology exhibits several patterns.[67] Extensive multifocal cerebral white matter changes are found most often among patients who suffer severe poisoning with prolonged coma (e.g., 24 hours). These patients manifest a monophasic, unremitting neurologic deterioration. White matter changes also may be demyelinative (Grinker's myelinopathy), with relative sparing of axons. This form is seen classically in patients with an initial "pseudo"-recovery who relapse several days to weeks later and present with so-called delayed neurologic deterioration (discussed later), although it may be seen acutely as well. Gray matter changes, most specifically necrosis of the globus pallidus, are considered a pathologic hallmark of CO poisoning, but they also can arise following other hypoxic-ischemic brain insults.[68] As with other insults, now popularly described as postischemic reperfusion injuries, pathologic changes may be seen in the cerebellum, hippocampus, and substantia nigra.[67–69] Computed tomographic and magnetic resonance scanning have demonstrated lesions in the globus pallidus as well as in the white matter among surviving CO poisoning victims.[70–72] Formerly, these changes were documented only at autopsy.

Animal studies have demonstrated central nervous system pathology similar to that seen in humans. The physiologic changes required to cause neuropathology in animals are instructive for clinical evaluations of relative risk; this will be stressed further later in this chapter. Ginsberg et al.,[73] using rhesus monkeys, and Okeda et al.,[74] using cats, found that the magnitude of white matter lesions correlates with the degree of hypotension and systemic acidosis incurred during CO exposure. Okeda found that cats with unilateral carotid artery ligations exhibited both the gray and white matter changes ipsilateral to the ligation; similar lesions occurred in cats after nitrogen hypoxia and systemic hypotension.[74, 75] Importantly, neither hypoxia nor hypotension alone produced pathology. CO seems a relatively unique toxic agent, since it precipitates both hypoxia and hypotension concurrently.

Analogies between CO poisoning and central nervous system postischemic reperfusion pathology have been mentioned already. Postischemic reperfusion injury is a form of oxidative stress that arises following ischemic-hypoxic insults. There are numerous potential mechanisms for the resulting pathology.[76] The idea that CO-mediated injury may be due to a form of postischemic reperfusion injury has come from animal studies and similarities between CO-mediated and hypoxic-ischemic brain pathology. In keeping with this supposition, brain oxidative stress quantified by products of lipid peroxidation has been found after but not during CO poisoning in a rat model.[77] The biochemical changes occurred only after a period of relative hypoxia (mean COHb 40%) that culminated in loss of consciousness and systemic hypotension.

Necrosis of the globus pallidus following CO poisoning has been correlated with variations in local brain blood flow.[78] At a time of systemic hypotension among cats exposed to 3,000 ppm of CO, only those who also showed a marked decrease in local blood flow in the globus pallidus developed pathology. Interestingly, at the same time that pallidal blood flow was low, flows in other regions of the brain—specifically the putamen and claustrum—were above normal. Regional differences in blood flow in response to CO poisoning have been noted in other,[29] but not all,[79] studies. Conjecture about the mechanism of the sensitivity of the globus pallidus of humans and animals has focused on the regional arterial supply. Vascularity is poor relative to other portions of the basal ganglia,[80] and there are few anastomoses among the branches. Neuroanatomists describe vascular branching as often occurring perpendicular to the vascular trunk; these channels then apparently double back opposite to the principal direction of flow. Although these observations are intriguing, they do not necessarily explain the pathology; paradoxic local vasoconstriction of the vessel walls has been suggested also. There may be still other peculiarities involving regions of the basal ganglia, such as high local iron concentrations, which might predispose this area to oxidative stress. That some peculiarity may exist in the local vasculature is supported by a remarkable degree of wall damage noted in this region in pathologic specimens.[67]

In summary, although considerable information on the neuropathology of CO has been obtained, the conclusions we can reach are essentially the same as those stated in 1950 by Lilienthal in his review of the subject[81]

> . . . nervous tissue, particularly central, is especially vulnerable to damage during CO intoxication. There is evidence that the effects stem from combined vascular and specific neuronal damage, but the mechanisms which operate are not defined, and, indeed, some would appear to be common to all agents which lead to anoxia generally in the central nervous system.

Congenital Effects

Fetal exposure to CO occurs by transplacental diffusion and possibly by facilitated diffusion.[82] Although fetal hemoglobin binding of CO proceeds more slowly than in the maternal circulation, at equilibrium, the fetal COHb level will exceed the maternal level due to the greater affinity of fetal hemoglobin for CO. The chief effect of maternal CO exposure is O_2 desaturation, which in turn causes prompt fetal hypoxemia. A decrease in fetal Po_2 occurs in proportion to maternal and fetal COHb levels; the fetus, therefore, is challenged to increase its cardiac output to compensate for even mild reductions in O_2 tension.[82, 83] Fetal cardiomegaly has been shown in an animal model of moderate CO exposure (200 ppm).[84]

Evidence indicates that low-level chronic maternal CO exposure slows development both in utero and postpartum.[85–87] Acute high-level exposures are often catastrophic. Clinical reports cover a spectrum from acute mortality of both mother and fetus to instances where both survive. Poisonings in the first trimester can precipitate somatic and neurologic abnormalities in the fetus, while second- and third-trimester poisonings more typically cause neuropathologic changes consistent with hypoxia. These changes are noted principally in the basal ganglia.[88, 89] Animal studies have established that chronic maternal CO exposures of as little as 30 ppm cause fetal cerebral insults. There is a rough proportionality between the exposure level and the degree of fetal pathology. The lowest levels cause fetal brain edema and low growth rate, while somatic congenital abnormalities and fetal mortality occur at the higher CO levels.[90–92] CO seems to preferentially impair development of the cerebellum, as well as noradrenergic, serotonergic, and aspects of the GABA-ergic neural systems.[93]

As with general clinical aspects of acute CO poisoning, fetal risk is linked closely to signs and symptoms at the time of poisoning and not to a specific COHb level.[94, 95] Animal work corroborates this view. Following brief exposure of pregnant cats to 3,000 ppm of CO, fetal neuropathology was correlated with the degree of maternal acidosis (and presumably cardiovascular decompensation) rather than with blood CO levels.[96]

CLINICAL FINDINGS

In the absence of a clear history of exposure, the diagnosis of CO poisoning can be missed easily. One epidemiologic study suggested that, unless health care workers are extremely vigilant, as many as one third of CO cases may go undiagnosed.[97] This is because most signs and symptoms are nonspecific. Common symptoms include headache, fatigue, malaise, and nausea. The principal concern when patients present with these complaints is preventing continued CO exposure, which may produce life-threatening physiologic compromises. Two historical clues have proven valuable in identifying occult CO poisoning: whether the patient's cohabitants have similar symptoms, and whether gas fuel appliances are used at home.[98]

Signs and Symptoms

Manifestations of serious CO poisoning include cardiopulmonary compromise, ischemic cardiac pain, convulsions, and unconsciousness. While there is a rough correlation between moderate symptoms (such as headache and nausea) and relatively low COHb levels (up to approximately 20%),[12] no correlation exists between the blood level and manifestations of serious poisoning.[13-17] This can be reconciled in part by the experimental evidence discussed earlier. CO-mediated tissue damage may be the result of a cascade of reactions set into motion by the associated hypoxia and ischemia. The inciting agent, the high body burden of CO, may be removed while the secondary reactions continue. Moreover, if physiologic responses to high levels of CO do not occur (e.g., hypotension), the stress of the high CO level alone is insufficient to precipitate pathology. Alternatively, lower CO levels may cause injury if cardiopulmonary compromise occurs. Hence, patients with coronary artery disease and/or a low cardiovascular reserve appear to be at increased risk from CO poisoning.[13-15] Rare clinical reports[99, 100] and one animal study,[101] but not another,[102] indicate that neurologic deficits may arise due to chronic CO exposure that lasts weeks to months. This aspect of CO poisoning is not well described, however, and the pathophysiologic issues are not defined.

Physical signs of CO poisoning are nonspecific. Cutaneous findings on occasion include hemorrhagic bullae, which are likely the result of pressure necrosis when an unconscious victim lies in one position.[103, 104] Rarely, the affected areas are not in a dependent position, but one cannot rule out seizures or some involuntary movement turning the victim prior to rescue. It is exceedingly rare to observe "cherry red" coloration except among those who recently have died. In addition to hypotension or shock, cardiopulmonary effects include dysrhythmias such as atrial fibrillation and atrial or ventricular tachycardia. Findings on electrocardiogram include intraventricular conduction defects and ST segment depression.[48, 10, 10] Pulmonary edema, as discussed earlier, is rather common and may be due to combustion products other than CO or to systemic insults that evolve after acute smoke exposure. Renal dysfunction due to rhabdomyolysis may develop acutely, but more often evolves over the first 24 to 48 hours after CO poisoning. Again, muscle necrosis is thought to be due to ischemic pressure injury, although a direct CO myotoxic effect is thought to occur at times.[104, 107, 108] Acute neurologic findings may include asymmetric reflexes as well as alterations in mental status and convulsions. Rarely, peripheral nerve palsies and transient neurosensory deafness have been reported.[13, 14, 65, 105, 109, 110] Changes in the brain sometimes are observed on computerized tomographic scans taken within 6 hours following poisoning.[70-72] White matter lesions are more predictive of poor prognosis than are gray matter changes.[70] Since magnetic resonance imaging is a sensitive method for assessing white matter changes, it may prove of greater value in the early assessment of CO victims as experience in its use is acquired.[72, 111]

Acute neurologic damage may occur in 14% of patients.[17] In addition to acute neurologic abnormalities, neurologic and psychiatric changes have been described after an apparently successful resuscitation. Delayed neuropsychiatric sequelae occur as a consequence of numerous forms of ischemic-hypoxic cerebral insults.[13-15, 112-115] From 3 to 28 days after CO poisoning, patients may manifest aphasia, apraxia, apathy, disorientation, hallucinations, bradykinesia, cogwheel rigidity, gait disturbances, and fecal and urinary incontinence. Rarely, cortical blindness has occurred. Personality changes reportedly include impulsiveness, so-called affective incontinence, mood changes, violence, and verbal aggressiveness. Approximately 50% to 75% of patients who develop delayed neurologic deterioration slowly will improve spontaneously, but the time taken may be up to 2 years.[13]

The incidence of delayed neurologic sequelae is debated in the literature; there are wide variations in reported rates. This seems to be attributable largely to the manner in which the severity of CO poisoning is estimated. Thus, if all exposures are grouped, delayed neurologic sequelae may occur in only 8% or fewer cases.[13, 14, 115] If, however, one considers only those poisonings severe enough to warrant hospitalization, sequelae occur in approximately 12% of cases. For example, in one Korean report,[13] only 549 of 2,360 patients were admitted, and there were 65 cases of delayed neurologic sequelae. Thus, considering "severe" cases only (e.g., patients admitted), the incidence is 11.8%. Similar observations were made in a follow-up report to this study.[14] Unfortunately, admission criteria were not stated in either report.

Estimating Severity of Poisoning

Reliable objective methods for assessing severity of CO poisoning are not available. The COHb level, when elevated, is a good index for establishing the diagnosis, but is unreliable in determining risk. The blood lactate level may correlate with the duration of exposure, a parameter associated with risk, although the prognostic value of blood lactate levels is uncertain.[116] Serum amylase may be elevated, but it is not helpful for assessing severity of poisoning, since the enzyme is from the salivary gland.[117] Neuroradiologic imaging, as discussed earlier, is helpful, but it has not proven to be sensitive or specific for assessing poisoning severity or prognosis. The electroencephalogram may show slow waves and delta waves[118] as well as diagnose status epilepticus in profoundly injured patients. Despite early indications to the contrary,[119] encephalographic findings have not been found to be of prognostic value.[7, 14, 120] Some clinical tests for assessing neurologic capability have been developed. Myers et al.[121, 122] described an abbreviated cortical function test that they used in clinical decision-making. There also is a very recent atempt to couple SPECT (single positron emission computed tomography) scanning with cortical function testing.[123]

From the array of clinical observations published over the past 40 years, some useful, albeit qualitative, estimations of risk can be made. Coma, hypotension, evidence of cardiac ischemia, and metabolic acidosis are serious clinical findings.[13–16, 124, 125] Regarding neurologic status in particular, any period of unconsciousness seems to be associated with increased risk. Patients with a compromised cardiovascular reserve, for instance those with a history of coronary artery disease and the elderly, seem to be at increased risk.[14, 15] Animal models have shown that the degree and duration of cardiovascular compromise and acidosis are associated with increased neuropathology.[73, 74] One small clinical series reported risk to be proportional to the degree of metabolic acidosis,[126] but larger series have failed to substantiate a reliable correlation.[127-129] Of course, the question of how patients are treated is expected to influence prognosis; this issue will be discussed as follows.

MANAGEMENT

Supporting vital signs and providing supplemental oxygen are the essentials of emergency treatment for CO intoxication. Treating with oxygen, preferably 100% O_2, is recommended because COHb dissociation is hastened by elevated arterial O_2 partial pressures.[130] Unfortunately, assessing the success of aggressive, supportive care is obscured by confusion in estimating the severity of poisoning. Thus, some surveys report only a 1% to 2% mortality rate,[7, 15] while others report a 20% to 30% mortality.[116, 131, 132] A recent paper that detailed the use of 100% O_2 at 1 atm, intensive care using mechanical ventilation, hypothermia, and steroid and diuretic use reported a 30% mortality rate.[17]

Experimental studies of treatment have been hampered by gaps in our understanding of pathophysiology. For example, questions remain about the most appropriate animal model to use. In part, the choice is influenced by whether one is interested in acute mortality or later development of neuropathology. A recent review discussed many of the animal models that have been developed.[133] To our knowledge, the only treatment that has shown benefit in animal trials is the use of pure oxygen at greater than sea level pressure, i.e., hyperbaric oxygen (HBO). In 1972, Pearce et al.[134] demonstrated hypothermia to be of no benefit in improving survival of dogs following CO poisoning, whereas 3 atm absolute (ATA) O_2 without or with hypothermia significantly improved outcome. Recent studies related to the question of CO-mediated delayed neuropathology also suggest therapeutic benefit of HBO. Using lipid peroxidation as an index of delayed oxidative stress following CO poisoning, treatment with O_2 at 3 ATA blocked the chemical change but 2 or 1 ATA did not.[135] Elucidating the mechanism of benefit obviously is hampered by the fact that the mechanism of the CO stress is unknown. Of course, there also is a need to correlate lipid peroxidation with neuropathology. If oxidative stress is driven by impaired mitochondrial function, the HBO benefit may be due to hastening the removal of CO from the cytochrome chain, as was shown recently.[27] The beneficial effect also may be of a more general character and unrelated to the manner in which free radical species are generated and initiate lipid peroxidation. Oxygen at the partial pressures likely to arise when animals or humans are exposed to 2 to 3 ATA O_2 can be shown to antagonize lipid peroxidation in the setting of a neutral or acid pH.[136] The mechanism appears to be based on establishing several lipid free radical termination reactions that do not occur at lower O_2 partial pressures.

Numerous clinical reports related the prompt reversal of CO-induced coma to the administration of HBO.[124, 127, 137–140] More prompt awakening does not necessarily imply lower overall mortality, but several reports from large (e.g., > 100 patients) series suggest that fatalities may number fewer than 4% with HBO.[72, 137, 141] The difficulty in determining severity of poisoning obviously leaves some doubt regarding the significance of the successes in these reports. Using identical criteria for judging the severity of poisoning, Goulon et al.[127] provided comparative data, as well as an index of how prompt treatment must be to be beneficial. Their retrospective study reported a mortality rate of 30.1% among both patients not treated with HBO and those treated with HBO more than 6 hours following poisoning. In contrast, the mortality rate was 13.5% among comparably poisoned patients treated with HBO within 6 hours of discovery.

HBO treatment also appears to diminish morbidity risk. As already mentioned, supportive care results in approximately a 12% incidence of delayed neurologic sequelae in large series.[13, 14] Neurologic sequelae also occurred in 12% (19 of 155) of patients in the Goulon et al. series[127] who either did not receive HBO or were treated more than 6 hours after poisoning. The incidence was 0.7% (1 in 147) when HBO was administered within 6 hours. Myers et al.[121] also reported a 12% incidence of delayed sequelae among patients treated with 100% O_2, but a 0% incidence among those treated with HBO. Further supporting the efficacy of HBO in decreasing the incidence of neurologic sequelae, Norman et al.[142] reported a 1.4% incidence (1 of 70), Norkool et al.[143] reported a 2% incidence (3 of 115 and 1 of 50), and Mathieu et al.[145] reported a 4% incidence (9 of 203). Recently reported was a very ambitious clinical trial designed to assess clinical parameters used to gauge the severity of poisoning as well as to compare the therapeutic effects of several HBO treatments with use of 100% O_2 at 1 atm.[146] Unfortunately, the method used to assess the efficacy of treatment was the incidence of neuropsychiatric sequelae based on a self-assessment questionnaire. Also approximately half of each group began treatment more than 6 hours following poisoning. The authors reported an alarming 35% to 45% incidence of "sequelae" in all groups, which immediately brings into question the reliability and sensitivity of a self-test. The reported conclusions of the study are that, in the absence of loss of consciousness, there is no benefit to administering one hyperbaric treatment (2 ATA O_2 for approximately 2 hours) compared to 100% O_2 at 1 atm, and with loss of consciousness, there is no benefit to using two HBO treatments separated by 12 hours, rather than just one treatment.

Several authors have argued that treatment of CO poisoning should consist only of supportive measures and the administration of 100% O_2 until controlled prospective studies are carried out.[128, 147, 148] To be sure, such trials would solidify perceptions of clinical care. It seems, however, that to embark on such a plan ignores extensive clinical experience. Moreover, the fact that animal trials also demonstrate the efficacy of HBO treatment makes it difficult to insist on clinical trials.

We feel the weight of clinical and experimental information supports the use of HBO for CO poisoning. There is legitimate concern regarding the transfer of critically ill patients with unstable vital signs from an initial receiving hospital to a facility providing hyperbaric therapy. As clinical data suggest that the benefit of HBO treatment diminishes when there is a delay of more than 6 hours,[127] expeditious transport is a very important issue. Fortunately, there have been only rare complications associated with this practice.[149]

The criteria used as indications for HBO therapy are not strictly standardized and vary among treating centers. Our facility has taken the view that treatment should be based solely on clinical findings and not on a particular COHb level. Patients in coma, those with cardiovascular instability, and those with severe acidosis (pH < 7.25) or a history of unconsciousness are treated. Although it is not our practice, many centers also treat patients with COHb levels of 25%,[137] 30%,[142] or 40$^+$%[143, 150] irrespective of symptoms, as well as patients with abnormal scores on a psychometric test.[121, 145]

A special situation requiring additional clinical considerations is CO poisoning of pregnant women. The pathophysiologic aspects of congenital CO poisoning have been discussed earlier. A central question that remains is whether aggressive treatment improves fetal outcome after CO poisoning. Because fetal hemoglobin affinity for CO is higher than that of the mother, there will be a higher steady-state level and longer elimination half-life for CO in the fetus than in the mother. Based on a mathematic model, Hill et al.[151] recommended that a pregnant woman should receive 100% O_2 for up to five times as long as is necessary to reduce the maternal COHb to normal. The next question, of course, is whether hyperbaric oxygen should be used more liberally in these cases. There are several compelling clinical reports that suggest that resolution of fetal distress and improved status at delivery may have occurred because of timely utilization of hyperbaric oxygen.[152, 153] To our knowledge, there is only one relevant pregnant animal study. Following a 20-minute exposure of rats to 5,000 ppm of CO, treatment with 3 ATA O_2 markedly diminished fetal death compared to no treatment.[154] Unfortunately, there was no 100% O_2, 1 ATA treatment group. In this study and in others,[155] the application of HBO under protocols similar to those used clinically have been found to cause no fetal injuries and only transient restriction of the ductus arteriosus.[156]

General protocols for treating patients with HBO vary slightly from center to center and usually include exposure to 2.5 to 3.0 ATA for 46 minutes to 2 hours. The inherent toxicity of O_2 must be addressed, of course, whenever HBO is used therapeutically. To summarize briefly, the human organ systems most susceptible to the toxic effects of O_2 are the lungs, brain, and eyes. Pulmonary O_2 toxicity has been studied extensively; it is known that HBO at 2 to 3 ATA can impair pulmonary mechanics (e.g., elasticity), vital capacity, and gas exchange.[157–160] These changes are observed, however, only when the duration of exposure is much greater than that used clinically. Alterations in pulmonary function in association with the standard clinical use of HBO have not been observed.[161, 162] Central nervous system O_2 toxicity—manifested as a grand mal seizure—occurs in approximately 1 in 10,000 patients with current clinical HBO protocols.[163, 164] Pathologic changes in association with isolated O_2-mediated seizures have not been found in studies with guinea pigs, rabbits, or humans.[165] The toxic effects of O_2 on the eyes are thought of most typically in the context of retrolental fibroplasia. There is no report of retrolental fibroplasia following HBO treatment of young children, which may reflect merely that this practice is uncommon. Intermittent HBO treatments can cause myopia, usually among older patients treated for several weeks. This change is virtually always temporary; reversal occurs within approximately 6 weeks after terminating treatment.[166] Of course, this extended course of therapy is beyond that appropriate for treating CO poisoning.

SUMMARY

CO poisoning causes in excess of 7,000 deaths annually, making it among the leading causes of poisoning deaths in this country. CO compromises oxygenation by impairing hemoglobin function, and possibly the function of other heme-containing proteins. The two organ systems most affected by CO are the cardiovascular and central nervous systems. Acute exposure can disrupt vasomotor tone, increase vessel permeability, and cause cardiac dysrhythmias and infarction. Chronic exposures cause pathologic changes in arteries as well as the myocardium. Neurologic abnormalities may be caused by chronic CO exposure; acute, high-level exposures typically are required to precipitate neuropathology. Acute or delayed neurologic problems may be seen.

Relative risk among patients suffering CO poisoning is difficult to quantify, and any reliance on the COHb level is inappropriate. Clinical findings including hypotension, cardiac ischemia, coma, and loss of consciousness are associated with increased risk. With serious poisoning, the mortality rate may be as high as 30%, the rate of acute neurologic damage 14%, and the rate of delayed neuropsychiatric sequelae 12%. It is notable that these statistics are reported for cases where treatment involved supportive care and 100% O_2 at 1 ATA. The use of HBO, at least within 6 hours of poisoning, appears to decrease mortality to 13% or less and delayed neurologic sequelae to 4% or less. Animal trials support the clinical observations that hyperbaric O_2 provides an extra benefit over ambient pressure O_2, and the effect cannot be ascribed merely to an enhanced removal of COHb. Precisely what the mechanism of the benefit is will require more research. It may relate to improved mitochondrial function, or possibly to newly described biochemical reactions and aspects of the so-called postischemic reperfusion injury.

REFERENCES

1. Haldane J: The action of carbonic oxide on man. *J Physiol* 1895; 18:430–462.
2. Birky MM, Clarke FB: Inhalation of toxic products from fires. *Bull N Y Acad Med* 1981; 57:997–1013.

3. Gregg MB: Carbon Monoxide intoxication a preventable environmental health hazard. *MMWR* 1982; 31:529–531.

4. Baron RC, Backer RC, Sopher IM: Fatal unintended carbon monoxide poisoning in West Virginia from nonvehicular sources. *AJPH* 1989; 79:1656–1658.

5. Goldman RA: Unintentional poisoning mortality - United States, 1980–1986. *MMWR* 1989; 38:529–531.

6. Steward TD, Fisher TN, Hosko MJ, et al: Carboxyhemoglobin elevation after exposure to dichlormethane. *Science* 1972; 176:295–296.

7. Langehennig PL, Seeler RA, Berman E: Paint removers and carboxyhemoglobin. *N Engl J Med* 1981; 295:1137.

8. Stewart RD, Hake CL: Paint remover hazard. *JAMA* 1976; 235:398–401.

9. Coburn RF, Forster RE, Kane PB: Considerations of the physiological variables that determine the blood carboxyhemoglobin concentration in man. *J Clin Invest* 1965; 44:1899–1910.

10. Rodkey FL, O'Neal JD, Collison HA, et al: Relative affinity of hemoglobin S and hemoglobin A for carbon monoxide and oxygen. *Clin Chem* 1974; 20:83–84.

11. Hauck H: Parameters influencing carbon monoxide kinetics. *Exp Pathol* 1989; 37:170–176.

12. Peterson JE, Stewart RD: Absorption and elimination of carbon monoxide by inactive young men. *Arch Environ Health* 1970; 21:165–171.

13. Choi S: Delayed neurologic sequelae in carbon monoxide intoxication. *Arch Neurol* 1983; 40:433–435.

14. Min SK: Brain syndrome associated with delayed neuropsychiatric sequelae following acute carbon monoxide intoxication. *Acta Psychiatr Scand* 1986; 73:80–86.

15. Garland H, Pearce J: Neurological complications of carbon monoxide poisoning. *Q J Med* 1967; 144:445–455.

16. Winter PM, Miller JN: Carbon monoxide poisoning. *JAMA* 1976; 236:1502–1504.

17. Krantz T, Thisted B, Strom J, et al: Acute carbon monoxide poisoning. *Acta Anaesthesiol Scand* 1988; 32:278–282.

18. Coburn RF, Mayers LB: Myoglobin O_2 tension determined from measurements of carboxymyoglobin in skeletal muscle. *Am J Physiol* 1971; 220:66–74.

19. Coburn RF: The carbon monoxide body stores. *Ann N Y Acad Sci* 1970; 174:11–22.

20. Kreuzer F, Hoofd LJC: Facilitated diffusion of CO and oxygen in the presence of hemoglobin or myoglobin. *Adv Exp Med Biol* 1976; 75:207–215.

21. Sokal JA, Majka J, Palus J: The content of carbon monoxide in the tissues of rats intoxicated with carbon monoxide in various conditions of acute exposure. *Arch Toxicol* 1984; 56:106–108.

22. Coburn RF, Ploegmakers F, Gondric P, et al: Myocardial myoglobin oxygen tension. *Am J Physiol* 1979; 236:H307–H313.

23. Luomanmaki K, Coburn RF: Effects of metabolism and distribution of carbon monoxide on blood and body stores. *Am J Physiol* 1969; 217:354–363.

24. Chen KC, McGrath JJ: Response of the isolated heart to carbon monoxide and nitrogen anoxia. *Toxicol Appl Pharmacol* 1985; 81:363–370.

25. King CE: Maximal O_2 uptake limitation in contracting skeletal muscle during carbon monoxide hypoxia. *Adv Exp Biol Med* 1989; 248:705–712.

26. Chance B, Erecinska M, Wagner M: Mitochondrial responses to carbon monoxide toxicity. *Ann N Y Acad Sci* 1970; 174:193–204.

27. Brown SD, Piantadosi CA: In vivo binding of carbon monoxide to cytochrome C oxidase in rat brain. *J Appl Physiol* 1990; 68:604–610.

28. Walum E, Varnbo I, Peterson A: Effects of dissolved carbon monoxide on the respiratory activity of perfused neuronal and muscle cell cultures. *Clin Toxicol* 1985; 23:299–308.

29. Koehler RC, Jones Jr MD, Traystman RJ: Cerebral circulatory response to carbon monoxide and hypoxic hypoxia in the lamb. *Am J Physiol* 1982; 243:H27–H32.

30. Martin W, Villani GM, Jothianandan D, et al: Blockade of endothelium-dependent and glyceryl trinitrate-induced relaxation of rabbit aorta by certain ferrous hemoproteins. *J Pharmacol Exp Ther* 1985; 233:679–685.

31. Ignarro LJ, Byrns RE, Buga GM, et al: Endothelium-derived relaxing factor from pulmonary artery and vein possesses pharmacologic and chemical properties identical to those of nitric oxide radical. *Circ Res* 1987; 61:866–879.

32. Graser T, Vedernikov YP, Li DS: Study on the mechanism of carbon monoxide induced endothelium-independent relaxation in porcine coronary artery and vein. *Biochem Biophys Acta* 1990; 4:293–296.

33. Parving HH, Ohlsson K, Buchardt-Hansen HJ, et al: Effect of carbon monoxide on capillary permeability to albumin and macroglobulin. *Scand J Clin Lab Invest* 1972; 29:381–388.

34. Siggaard-Anderson J, Bonde-Peterson F, Hanson TI, et al: Plasma volume and vascular permeability during hypoxia and carbon monoxide exposure. *Scand J Clin Lab Invest* 1968; 22(suppl 103):39–48.

35. Pauli HG, Truniger B, Larsen JK, et al: Renal function during prolonged exposure to hypoxia and carbon monoxide. *Scand J Clin Lab Invest* 1968; 22(suppl 103):55–60.

36. Thomsen H, Klein J: Carbon monoxide induced atherosclerosis in primates. An electron microscope study on the coronary arteries of macachirus monkeys. *Atherosclerosis* 1974; 20:233–240.

37. Kjedlsen K, Astrup P, Wanstrup J: Ultrastructural intimal changes in rabbit aorta after a moderate carbon monoxide exposure. *Atherosclerosis* 1972; 16:67–82.

38. Hugod C, Hawkins L, Kjeldsen K, et al: Effect of carbon monoxide exposure on aorta and coronary intimal morphology in the rabbit. A revaluation. *Atherosclerosis* 1978; 30:333–342.

39. Wald M, Howard S, Smith PG, et al: Association between atherosclerotic diseases and carboxyhemoglobin levels in tobacco smokers. *BMJ* 1973; 1:761–765.

40. Kjedlsen K, Thomson HK, Astrup P: The effects of carbon monoxide on myocardium. Ultra structural changes in rabbits after a moderate chronic exposure. *Circ Res* 1974; 34:339–348.

41. Ehrich WE, Bellet S, Lewey FH: Cardiac changes from CO poisoning. *Am J Med Sci* 1944; 208:511–523.

42. Ginsberg MD, Myers RE, McDonagh BF: Experimental carbon monoxide encephalopathy in the primate. II. Clinical aspects, neuropathology, and physiologic correlation. *Arch Neurol* 1974; 30:209–216.

43. Cramlet SH, Erickson HH, Gorman HA: Ventricular function following acute carbon monoxide exposure. *J Appl Physiol* 1975; 39:482–486.

44. Einzig S, Nicoloff DM, Lucas RV: Myocardial perfusion abnormalities in carbon monoxide poisoned dogs. *Can J Physiol Pharmacol* 1980; 58:396–405.

45. Verrier RL, Mills AK, Skornik WA: *Acute Effects of Carbon Monoxide on Cardiac Electrical Stability*. Cambridge, Mass, Health Effects Institute, 1990.

46. Vanoli E, DeFerrari GM, Stramba-Badiale M, et al: Carbon monoxide and lethal arrhythmias in conscious dogs with a healed myocardial infarction. *Am Heart J* 1989; 117:348–357.

47. DeBias DA, Banerjee CM, Birkhead NC, et al: Effects of carbon monoxide inhalation on ventricular fibrillation. *Arch Environ Health* 1976; 31:38–42.

48. Anderson EW, Andelman RJ, Strauch JM, et al: Effects of low-level carbon monoxide exposure on onset and duration of angina pectoris. *Ann Intern Med* 1973; 79:46–50.

49. Allred FN, Bleecker ER, Chaitman BR, et al: Short-term effects of carbon monoxide exposure on the exercise performance of subjects with coronary artery disease. *N Engl J Med* 1989; 321:1426–1432.

50. Stone S, Higashihana T, Kotake T, et al: Pulmonary manifestations in acute carbon monoxide poisoning. *AJR Am J Roentgenol* 1974; 120:865–871.

51. Sugi K, Theissen JL, Traber LD, et al: Impact of carbon monoxide on cardiopulmonary dysfunction after smoke inhalation injury. *Circ Res* 1990; 66:68–75.

52. Shimazu T, Ikeuch H, Hubbard GB, et al: Smoke inhalation injury and the effect of carbon monoxide in the sheep model. *J Traum* 1990; 30:170–175.

53. Demling RH, LaLonde C: Moderate smoke inhalation produces decreased oxygen delivery, increased oxygen demands, and systemic but not lung parenchymal lipid peroxidation. *Surgery* 1990; 108:544–552.

54. Quinn DA, Robinson D, Jung W, et al: Role of sulfidopeptide leukotrienes in synthetic smoke inhalation injury in sheep. *J Appl Physiol* 1990; 68:1962–1969.

55. Fisher AB, Hyde RW, Baue AE, et al: Effect of carbon monoxide on function and structure of the lung. *J Appl Physiol* 1969; 26:4–12.

56. Fein A, Grossman RF, Jones JG, et al: Carbon monoxide effect on alveolar epithelial permeability. *Chest* 1980; 78:726–731.

57. Schultze JH: Effects of mild carbon monoxide intoxication. *Arch Environ Health* 1963; 7:524–530.

58. McFarland RA: The effects of exposure to small quantities of carbon monoxide on vision. *Ann NY Acad Sci* 1970; 174:301–312.

59. Hudnell HK, Benignus VA: Carbon monoxide exposure and human visual detection thresholds. *Neurotoxicol Teratol* 1989; 11:363–371.

60. Ingenito AJ, Durlacher L: Effects of carbon monoxide on the b-wave of the cat electroretinogram: Comparisons with nitrogen hypoxia, epinephrine, vasodilator drugs and changes in respiratory tidal volume. *J Pharmacol Exp Ther* 1979; 211:638–646.

61. Raybourn MS, Cork C, Schimmerling W, et al: An in vitro electrophysiological assessment of the direct cellular toxicity of carbon monoxide. *Toxicol Appl Pharmacol* 1978; 46:769–779.

62. Gothert M, Lutz F, Malorny G: Carbon monoxide partial pressure in tissue of different animals. *Environ Res* 1970; 3:303–309.

63. Keilin D, Hartree EF: Cytochrome and cytochrome oxidase. *Proc R Soc Lond [Biol]* 1939; 127:167–191.

64. Wald G, Allen DW: The equilibrium between cytochrome oxidase and carbon monoxide. *J Gen Physiol* 1957; 40:593–608.

65. Snyder RD: Carbon monoxide intoxication with peripheral neuropathy. *Neurology* 1970; 20:177–180.

66. Grunnet ML, Petajan JH: Carbon monoxide-induced neuropathy in the rat. *Arch Neurol* 1976; 33:158–163.

67. Lapresle J, Fardeau M: The central nervous system and carbon monoxide poisoning, in Bour H, Ledingham IM (eds): *Carbon Monoxide Poisoning*. Amsterdam, Elsevier Publishing, 1967, pp 31–74.

68. Ginsberg MD: Carbon monoxide intoxication: Clinical features, neuropathology and mechanisms of injury. *Clin Toxicol* 1985; 23:281–288.

69. Brierley JB: Cerebral hypoxia, in Blackwood W, Corsellis JAN (eds): *Greenfield's Neuropathology*. Chicago, Year Book Medical Publishers, 1976, pp 43–60.

70. Miura T, Mitomo M, Kawai R, et al: CT of the brain in acute carbon monoxide intoxication: Characteristic features and prognosis. *AJNR* 1985; 6:739–742.

71. Nardizzi LR: Computerized tomographic correlate of carbon monoxide poisoning. *Arch Neurol* 1979; 36:38–39.

72. Vieregge P, Klostermann W, Blumm RG, et al: Carbon monoxide poisoning: Clinical, neuro-physiological, and brain imaging observations in acute disease and follow-up. *J Neurol* 1989; 236:478–481.

73. Ginsberg MD, Myers RE: Experimental carbon monoxide encephalopathy in the primate. I. Physiologic and metabolic aspects. *Arch Neurol* 1974; 30:202–208.

74. Okeda R, Funata N, Takano T, et al: The pathogenesis of carbon monoxide encephalopathy in the acute phase physiological morphological correlation. *Acta Neuropathol (Berl)* 1981; 54:1–10.

75. Okeda R, Matsuo T, Kuroiwa T, et al: Experimental study on pathogenesis of the fetal brain damage by acute carbon monoxide intoxication of the pregnant mother. *Acta Neuropathol (Berl)* 1986; 69:244–252.

76. Hallenbeck JM, Dutka AJ: Background review and current concepts of reperfusion injury. *Arch Neurol* 1990; 47:1245–1254.

77. Thom SR: Carbon monoxide-mediated brain lipid peroxidation in the rat. *J Appl Physiol* 1990; 68:997–1003.

78. Song SY, Okeda R, Funata N, et al: An experimental study of the pathogenesis of the selective lesion of the globus pallidus in acute carbon monoxide poisoning in cats. *Acta Neuropathol (Berl)* 1983; 61:232–238.

79. MacMillan V: Regional cerebral blood flow of the rat in acute carbon monoxide intoxication. *Can J Physiol Pharmacol* 1975; 53:644–650.

80. Alexander L: The vascular supply of the striopallidum. *A Research Nerv Ment Dis Proc* 1942; 21:77–132.

81. Lilienthal JL: Carbon monoxide. *Pharmacol Rev* 1950; 2:324–354.

82. Longo LD: The biological effects of carbon monoxide on the pregnant woman, fetus, and new-born infant. *Am J Obstet Gynecol* 1977; 129:69–103.

83. Longo LD: Carbon monoxide: Effects on oxygenation of the fetus in utero. *Science* 1976; 194:523–524.

84. Clubb FJ, Penney DG, Baylerian MS, et al: Cardiomegaly due to myocyte hyperplasia in perinatal rats exposed to 200 ppm carbon monoxide. *J Mol Cell Cardiol* 1986; 18:477–486.

85. Tachi N, Aoyama M: Postnatal growth in rats prenatally exposed to cigarette smoke or carbon monoxide. *Bull Environ Contam Toxicol* 1990; 45:641–648.

86. Miller HE, Hassanein K, Hensleigh PA: Fetal growth retardation in relation to maternal smoking and weight gain in pregnancy. *Am J Obstet Gynecol* 1976; 125:55–60.

87. Fechter LC, Mactutus CF, Storm JE: Carbon monoxide and brain development. *Neurotoxicology* 1986; 7:463–474.

88. Ginsberg MD, Myers RE: Fetal brain injury after maternal carbon monoxide intoxication. *Neurology* 1976; 26:15–23.

89. Longo LD: Carbon monoxide in the pregnant mother and fetus and its exchange across the placenta. *Ann N Y Acad Sci* 1970; 141:313–341.

90. Fechter LD, Annua Z: Toxicity of mild prenatal carbon monoxide exposure. *Science* 1977; 1977:680–682.

91. Astrup P, Olsen HM, Trolle D, et al: Effect of moderate carbon monoxide exposure on fetal development. *Lancet* 1972; 2:1220–1222.

92. Williams IR, Smith E: Blood picture, reproduction and general condition during daily exposure to illuminating gas. *Am J Physiol* 1935; 110:611–615.

93. Storm JE, Fechter LD: Prenatal carbon monoxide exposure differentially affects postnatal weight and monoamine concentration of rat brain regions. *Toxicol Appl Pharmacol* 1985; 81:139–146.

94. Copel JA, Bowen F, Bolognese RJ: Carbon monoxide intoxication in early pregnancy. *Obstet Gynecol* 1982; 59:265–285.

95. Caravati EM, Adams CJ, Joyce SM, et al: Fetal toxicity associated with maternal carbon monoxide poisoning. *Ann Emerg Med* 1988; 17:714–717.

96. Okeda R, Matsuo T, Kuroiwa T, et al: Experimental study on pathogenesis of the fetal brain damage by acute carbon monoxide intoxication of the pregnant mother. *Acta Neuropathol (Berl)* 1986; 69:244–252.

97. Barret L, Danel V, Faure J: Carbon monoxide poisoning, a diagnosis frequently overlooked. *Clin Toxicol* 1985; 23:309–313.

98. Heckerling PS, Leikin JB, Maturen A: Occult carbon monoxide poisoning: Validation of a prediction model. *Am J Med* 1988; 84:251–256.

99. Beck HG: The clinical manifestations of chronic carbon monoxide poisoning. *Ann Clin Med* 1926; 5:1088–1096.

100. Beck HG: Slow carbon monoxide asphyxiation. *JAMA* 1936; 107:1025–1029.

101. Lewey FH, Drabkin DL: Experimental chronic carbon monoxide poisoning of dogs. *Am J Med Sci* 1944; 208:502–511.

102. Stupfel M, Bouley G: Physiological and biochemical effects on rats and mice exposed to small concentrations of carbon monoxide for long periods. *Ann N Y Acad Sci* 1970; 174:342–368.

103. Myers RAM, Snyder SK, Majerus TC: Cutaneous blisters and carbon monoxide poisoning. *Ann Emerg Med* 1985; 14:603–606.

104. Nagy R, Greer KE, Hatman LE: Cutaneous manifestations of acute carbon monoxide poisoning. *Cutis* 1979; 24:381–383.

105. Thompson N, Henry JA: Carbon monoxide poisoning: Poisons unit experience over five years. *Human Toxicol* 1983; 2:335–338.

106. Carnevali R, Omboni E, Rossan M, et al: Electrocardiographic changes in acute carbon monoxide poisoning. *Minerva Med* 1987; 78:175–178.

107. Slevin J: Carbon monoxide induced muscle necrosis. *Arch Neurol* 1979; 36:523–524.

108. Bessoudo R, Gray J: Carbon monoxide poisoning and non-oliguric acute renal failure. *Can Med Assoc J* 1978; 119:41–44.

109. Burney RE, Wu SC, Nemiroff MJ: Mass carbon monoxide poisoning: Clinical effects and results of treatment in 184 victims. *Ann Emerg Med* 1982; 11:394–399.

110. Baker SR, Lilly DJ: Hearing loss from acute carbon monoxide intoxication. *Ann Otol Rhinol Laryngol* 1977; 86:323–328.

111. Horowitz AL, Kaplan R, Sarpel G: Carbon monoxide toxicity: MR imaging in the brain. *Radiology* 1987; 162:787–788.

112. Plum F, Posner JB, Hain RF: Delayed neurological deterioration after anoxia. *Arch Intern Med* 1962; 110:56–63.

113. Smith JS, Brandon S: Morbidity from acute carbon monoxide poisoning at three-year follow-up. *BMJ* 1973; 1:318–321.

114. Meigs JW, Hughes JPW: Acute carbon monoxide poisoning. *Arch Indust Hyg Occupant Med* 1952; 6:344–356.

115. Shillito FH, Drinker CK, Shaughnessy TJ: The problem of nervous and mental sequelae in carbon monoxide poisoning. *JAMA* 1936; 106:669–674.

116. Sokal JA, Kralkowska E: The relationship between exposure duration, carboxyhemoglobin, blood glucose, pyruvate and lactate and the severity of intoxication in 39 cases of acute carbon monoxide poisoning in man. *Arch Toxicol* 1985; 57:196–199.

117. Takahashi M, Maemura K, Sawada Y, et al: Hyperamylasemia in acute carbon monoxide poisoning. *J Trauma* 1982; 22:311–314.

118. Ginsburg R, Romano J: Carbon monoxide encephalopathy: Need for appropriate treatment. *Am J Psychiatry* 1976; 133:317–320.

119. Tatetsu S, Toya G, Wash KD: The EEG and prognosis in carbon monoxide poisoning. *Brain Nerve* 1967; 19:210–217.

120. Neufeld MY, Swanson JW, Klass DW: Localized EEG abnormalities in acute carbon monoxide poisoning. *Arch Neurol* 1981; 38:524–527.

121. Myers RAM, Snyder SK, Emhoff TA: Subacute sequelae of carbon monoxide poisoning. *Ann Emerg Med* 1985; 14:1163–1167.

122. Myers RAM, Messier LD, Jones DW, et al: New directions in the research and treatment of carbon monoxide exposure. *Am J Emerg Med* 1983; 2:226–230.

123. Augustine EA, Littman EB, Stern LW, et al: Neuropsychological and SPECT scan correlates of acute carbon monoxide toxicity. *J Clin Exp Neuropsychol* 1990; 12:69.

124. Smith G, Sharp GR: Treatment of carbon-monoxide poisoning with oxygen under pressure. *Lancet* 1960; 1:905–906.

125. Ginsberg MD: Carbon monoxide intoxication: Clinical features, neuropathology and mechanisms of injury. *Clin Toxicol* 1985; 23:281–288.

126. Larkin JM, Brahos GJ, Moylan JA: Treatment of carbon monoxide poisoning: Prognostic factors. *J Trauma* 1976; 16:111–114.

127. Goulon M, Barois A, Rapin M, et al: Carbon monoxide poisoning and acute anoxia due to breathing coal gas and hydrocarbons. *Ann Med Interne (Paris)* 1969; 120:335–349.

128. Strohl KP, Feldman NT, Saunders NA, et al: Carbon monoxide poisoning in fire victims: A reappraisal of prognosis. *J Trauma* 1980; 20:78–80.

129. Myers RAM, Britten JS: Are arterial blood gases of value in treatment decisions for carbon monoxide poisoning? *Crit Care Med* 1989; 17:139–142.

130. Roughton FJW, Darling RD: The effect of carbon monoxide on the oxyhemoglobin dissociation curve. *Am J Physiol* 1944; 141:17–31.

131. Richardson JC, Chambers RA, Heywood PM: Encephalopathies of anoxia and hypoglycemia. *Arch Neurol* 1959; 1:178–182.

132. Simpson CA: Carbon monoxide poisoning in New Castle-upon-Tyne. *New Castle Med J* 1963; 28:67–70.

133. Penney DG: Acute carbon monoxide poisoning: Animal models: A review. *Toxicology* 1990; 62:123–160.

134. Pearce EC, Zacharias A, Alday Jr JM, et al: Carbon monoxide poisoning: Experimental hypothermic and hyperbaric studies. *Surgery* 1972; 72:229–237.

135. Thom SR: Antagonism of carbon monoxide-mediated brain lipid peroxidation by hyperbaric oxygen. *Toxicol Appl Pharmacol* 1990; 105:340–344.

136. Thom SR, Elbuken ME: Oxygen-dependent antagonism of lipid peroxidation. *Free Radic Biol Med* 1991; 413–426.

137. Kindwall EP: Carbon monoxide poisoning treated with hyperbaric oxygen. *Resp Ther* 1975; pp 29–33.

138. Myers RAM, Snyder SK, Linberg S, et al: Value of hyperbaric oxygen in suspected carbon monoxide poisoning. *JAMA* 1981; 246:2478–2480.

139. Ziser A, Shupak A, Halpern P, et al: Delayed hyperbaric oxygen treatment for acute carbon monoxide poisoning. *BMJ* 1984; 289:960.

140. Yee LM, Brandon GK: Successful reversal of presumed carbon monoxide-induced semicoma. *Aviat Space Environ Med* 1983; 54:641–643.

141. Norman JN, Ledingham IM: Carbon monoxide poisoning: Investigations and treatment. *Prog Brain Res* 1967; 24:101–122.

142. Norman JN, MacIntyre J, Shearer JR, et al: Use of a one-man mobile pressure chamber in the treatment of carbon monoxide poisoning. *BJM* 1970; 2:333–335.

143. Norkool DM, Kirkpatrick JN: Treatment of acute carbon monoxide poisoning with hyperbaric oxygen: A review of 115 cases. *Ann Emerg Med* 1985; 14:1168–1171.

144. Lamy M, Hauguet M: Fifty patients with carbon monoxide intoxication treated with hyperbaric oxygen therapy. *Acta Anaesthesiol Belg* 1969; 1:49–53.

145. Mathieu D, Nolf M, Durocher A, et al: Acute carbon monoxide poisoning risk of late sequelae and treatment by hyperbaric oxygen. *Clin Toxicol* 1985; 23:315–324.

146. Raphael JC, Elkharrat D, Guincestre MCJ, et al: Trial of normobaric and hyperbaric oxygen for acute carbon monoxide intoxication. *Lancet* 1989; 2:414–419.

147. Olson KR: Carbon monoxide poisoning: Mechanisms, presentation, and controversies in management. *J Emerg Med* 1984; 1:233–243.

148. Grube BJ, Marvin JA, Heimbach DM: Therapeutic hyperbaric oxygen: Help or hindrance in burn patients with carbon monoxide poisoning? *J Burn Care Rehabil* 1988; 9:249–252.

149. Sloan EP, Murphy DG, Hart R, et al: Complications and protocol considerations in carbon monoxide-poisoned patients who require hyperbaric oxygen therapy: Report from a ten-year experience. *Ann Emerg Med* 1989; 18:629–634.

150. Broome JR, Pearson RR: Hyperbaric oxygen for carbon monoxide poisoning. *BMJ* 1987; 295:225.

151. Hill EP, Hill JR, Power GG, et al: Carbon monoxide exchanges between the human fetus and mother: A mathematical model. *Am J Physiol* 1977; 232:H311–H323.

152. VanHoesen KB, Camporesi EM, Moon RE, et al: Should hyperbaric oxygen be used to treat the pregnant patient for acute carbon monoxide poisoning? *JAMA* 1989; 261:1039–1043.

153. Hollander DI, Nagery DA, Welch R, et al: Hyperbaric oxygen therapy for the treatment of acute carbon monoxide poisoning in pregnancy. *J Reprod Med* 1987; 32:615–617.

154. Cho SH, Yun DR: The experimental study on the effect of the hyperbaric oxygenation on the pregnancy wastage of the rats in acute carbon monoxide poisoning. *Seoul J Med* 1982; 23:67–75.

155. Gilman SC, Bradley ME, Greene KM, et al: Fetal development: Effects of decompression sickness and treatment. *Aviat Space Environ Med* 1983; 54:1040–1042.

156. Assali NS, Kirschbaum THL, Dilts DV: Effects of hyperbaric oxygen on uteroplacental and fetal circulation. *Circ Res* 1968; 22:573–588.

157. Fisher AB, Hyde RW, Puy RJM, et al: Effect of oxygen at 2 atmospheres on the pulmonary mechanics of normal man. *J Appl Physiol* 1968; 24:529–536.

158. Clark JM, Lambertsen CJ: Alveolar-arterial O_2 differences in man at 0.2, 1.0, 2.0, and 3.5 ata inspired Po_2. *J Appl Physiol* 1971; 30:753–763.

159. Puy RJM, Hyde RW, Fisher AB, et al: Alterations in the pulmonary capillary bed during early O_2 toxicity in man. *J Appl Physiol* 1968; 24:537–543.

160. Caldwell PRB, Lee WL, Schildkraut HS, et al: Changes in lung volume, diffusion capacity, and blood gases in men breathing oxygen. *J Appl Physiol* 1966; 21:1477–1483.

161. Clark JM, Lambertsen CJ: Pulmonary oxygen toxicity: A review. *Pharmacol Rev* 1971; 23:37–133.

162. Hart GB, Strauss MB, Riker J: Vital capacity of quadriplegic patients treated with hyperbaric oxygen. *J Am Paraplegia Soc* 1984; 7:113–114.

163. Davis JC: Hyperbaric medicine: Patient selection, treatment procedures, and side effects, in Davis JC, Hunt TK (eds): *Problem Wounds.* New York, Elsevier, 1988, pp 225–235.

164. Hart GB, Strauss MB: Central nervous system oxygen toxicity in a clinical setting, in Bove AA, Bachrack AJ, Greenbaum LJ (eds): *Undersea and Hyperbaric Physiology IX.* Bethesda, Undersea and Hyperbaric Medicine Society, 1987, pp 695–699.

165. Clark JM: Oxygen toxicity, in Bennett PB, Elliott DH (eds): *The Physiology and Medicine of Diving and Compressed Air Work.* London, Balliere, 1983, pp 200–238.

166. Lyne AJ: Ocular effects of hyperbaric oxygen. *Trans Ophthalmol Soc UK* 1978; 98:66–68.

CHAPTER 11

Drug-Induced Pulmonary Disease

Richard J. Pisani, M.D.

Assistant Professor of Thoracic Disease and Critical Care Medicine, Mayo Medical School, Mayo Clinic, Rochester, Minnesota

Edward C. Rosenow, III, M.D.

Arthur M. and Gladys D. Gray Professor of Medicine, Thoracic Disease and Internal Medicine, Mayo Medical School, Mayo Clinic, Rochester, Minnesota

Accompanying the explosion in the number of medications used to treat disease is a simultaneous increase in untoward side effects. In light of the fact that they encounter the entire cardiac output, it is not surprising that the lungs frequently would be involved in toxicity caused by chemicals that make it into the systemic circulation. Over the last 30 years, the number of drugs known to affect the lungs adversely has increased from just a few to almost 100 and the clinicopathologic manifestations of drug-induced pulmonary disease (DIPD) have diversified.

Medical knowledge in this area is growing rapidly, and tends to develop in a systematic fashion. Initially, an association is made between an adverse pulmonary reaction and a particular medication. The first articles usually are case reports and, if the toxicity is commonplace, series of patients may be presented. Once it appears that the association is more than casual, epidemiologic studies may appear trying to identify the patient population at greatest risk. In addition, attempts are made to establish animal models. These serve several purposes. First, they more strongly suggest that the relationship between the drug and the toxicity is a causal one. Second, they permit hypothesis testing regarding the mechanism underlying such a relation. Finally, they may increase our understanding of pulmonary disease that, although not caused by medication, has similar clinical features (e.g., pulmonary fibrosis). More recent research has applied newer diagnostic techniques such as bronchoalveolar lavage (BAL) and computerized tomography to study patients with DIPD.

In this chapter, we will review the current state of knowledge regarding DIPD. We will not discuss ionizing radiation or oxygen administration beyond their contributions to the damage caused by medications. Excellent reviews of toxicity due to these treatment modalities have appeared recently.[1, 2]

In addition, we will not discuss the pulmonary consequences caused by certain drugs indirectly inasmuch as they cause a patient to become immunocompromised. This area also has been reviewed recently.[3] The chapter is divided into five sections. The first section addresses the physiologic and histopathologic changes that can be produced by DIPD. Section two will review current understanding of the possible mechanisms by which drugs cause such changes. The last three sections are more clinically oriented and attempt to approach this area from the perspective of the practicing physician interested in using this text as a resource. Section three presents the clinical features of eight commonly encountered forms of DIPD in detail. Section four summarizes the drugs known to cause each of five different clinical presentations. Finally, a physician may encounter a patient who has developed pulmonary symptoms while taking a newly released medication and ask, "what information is necessary to establish the drug as the causative factor?" Section five establishes some guidelines for the diagnosis of DIPD, even in patients taking a drug not known to cause DIPD.

PATTERNS OF LUNG INJURY BY DRUGS

Illness due to DIPD most often presents in association with some type of alteration in the structural integrity of the lung manifested by a limited array of histopathologic findings despite being caused by a large number of drugs. If the clinician postpones obtaining biopsy specimens so as to observe a patient's progress once a possible source of DIPD has been discontinued, the roentgenographic features may provide the only clue as to what type of injury has occurred. This is particularly true in cases that reverse quickly. Nonetheless, published information regarding the lung's histopathologic response to DIPD has been well summarized.[4] The basic histopathologic patterns encountered are listed in Table 1.

Interstitial pneumonitis (also called diffuse alveolar damage by some) is a nonspecific pathologic entity characterized by varying degrees of interstitial/alveolar edema, leukocyte margination, thickening of alveolar ducts, alveolar collapse, and denudation of type I cells.[5] When examined under the electron microscope, the epithelium shows evidence of damage. There usually is some cellular infiltrate to

TABLE 1.
Histopathologic Patterns in Drug-Induced
Pulmonary Disease

Common
Interstitial pneumonitis/diffuse alveolar damage
Pulmonary fibrosis
Type II pneumocyte proliferation/atypia
Eosinophilia
Uncommon
Granuloma formation
Bronchiolitis obliterans
Alveolar hemorrhage
Lipoid pneumonia
Thrombotic angiopathy
Pulmonary veno-occlusive disease
Alveolar proteinosis

be found in the alveolar air spaces and/or the interstitium. The lesion may be labeled desquamative interstitial pneumonia (DIP) or lymphocytic interstitial pneumonia (LIP) if the pathologist notes a prominence of either macrophages or lymphocytes, respectively.[6, 7] In some cases, the identification of LIP might be predicted by the combination of a diffuse interstitial infiltrate on chest roentgenogram and a lymphocytosis on BAL.[8]

Presumably, the natural history of ongoing diffuse alveolar damage is the ultimate development of pulmonary fibrosis. This conclusion is based in part on studies of the histopathologic progression consequent to bleomycin-induced lung injury in mice.[9] In this model, early inflammatory changes characterized by perivascular and interstitial edema, epithelial proliferation, and cellular infiltration evolve into dense fibrosis and volume loss within 4 to 8 weeks. During this transition, the interstitium may be distorted by dense rounded collections of immature fibroblasts and connective tissue matrix called Masson's nodules. In humans, bleomycin induces diffuse fibrosis usually involving the lower lung regions preferentially, as would be expected in usual interstitial pneumonia (UIP). However, other patterns of involvement have been described, including nodular fibrosis, which might be mistaken for metastatic malignancy based on the x-ray appearance.[10]

Type II pneumocyte proliferation, typically associated with type II cellular atypia, is a characteristic pathologic feature of lung injury caused by antineoplastic agents ("cytotoxic" injury). This type II hyperplasia is part of a reparative response to damage that primarily affects type I cells. These are more susceptible to damage at the alveolar level due to their greater surface area and paucity of biosynthetic organelles that might permit self-repair. Since they are terminally differentiated, type I pneumocytes depend upon maturation of type II cells to replace them if damaged. Early repair is characterized by the appearance of cuboidal cells lining the alveolar space, causing the alveolus to resemble an acinar space. These cuboidal cells are proliferating type II pneumocytes. The presence of chemotherapeutic agents known to interfere with DNA synthesis during type II cell differentiation leads to cellular atypia characterized by large hyperchromatic nuclei, bizarre nuclear chromatin appearance, enlarged nucleoli, and increased cellular size. Unfortunately, such changes are not specific for cytotoxic DIPD, having been seen also with damage caused by oxygen[11] and viral disease.[4]

Eosinophilia in a lung biopsy specimen should raise the possibility of DIPD along with other disorders such as chronic eosinophilic pneumonia, vasculitis, allergic bronchopulmonary aspergillosis, and parasitic infection. Peripheral eosinophilia may or may not be present when pulmonary eosinophilic infiltration is caused by DIPD. Three different histopathologic patterns have been described. One is characterized by eosinophilic accumulation in air spaces with or without similar involvement in the interstitial compartment. Vasculitis typically is not seen and eosinophilic abscesses are rare. Clinically, this pattern is associated with multiple drugs and tends to resolve within 1 month of drug cessation.[12] The second pattern includes hypersensitivity pneumonitis, vasculitis, and tissue eosinophilia and had been seen almost exclusively in association with acute DIPD secondary to nitrofurantoin[13] until a similar histopathology was described recently in association with L-tryptophan ingestion.[14] The third pattern demonstrates extensive fibrosis and interstitial eosinophilia without an eosinophilic airspace exudate. Peripheral eosinophilia usually is not associated. The histopathology closely resembles that of UIP and, if reversibility occurs upon drug discontinuation, it is likely to regress slowly without the addition of corticosteroids, which are variably effective. Its appearance has been limited primarily to DIPD associated with chronic nitrofurantoin[15] or gold[16] ingestion. Clinically, the first two patterns of eosinophilia have been labeled as "hypersensitivity pneumonitis," but this term probably should not be used to describe the histopathologic changes. Lymphocyte-predominant interstitial pneumonia and granulomatous reactions also have been called hypersensitivity pneumonitis, particularly when the BAL shows a lymphocytosis with a decreased helper/suppressor ratio.

Histopathologic changes that occur less commonly with DIPD are shown on the bottom of Table 1. Each reaction usually is associated with a small number of drugs. Granuloma formation is identified readily by the pathologist, but is atypical for most DIPD, with the exception of its unique relation to intravenous drug abuse.[17] In such cases, talc (magnesium silicate) contained in medications intended for oral use is injected intravenously by addicts. Granulomas tend to appear first in the pulmonary arterioles, but with chronic addiction may be seen predominantly in the interstitium. Bronchiolitis obliterans is characterized by obstructive lung disease due to blockage of small airways with proliferating granulation tissue. Its association with penicillamine[18] and gold[19] remains questionable because of its known association with rheumatoid arthritis, for which these drugs are used. A more convincing association is its link to sulfasalazine, based on a recent case report in which reversal and recurrence were related to discontinuation and rechallenge with the drug.[20] Alveolar hemorrhage is characterized by airspace filling with red blood cells and hemosiderin-laden macrophages. After publishing a case report regarding the association of alveolar hemorrhage to cocaine smoking,[21]

Murray et al. later reported that 35% of individuals who died of acute cocaine intoxication had significant numbers of hemosiderin-laden macrophages in their lungs.[22] Lipoid pneumonia, thrombotic angiopathy, and pulmonary veno-occlusive disease are some of the other less frequently encountered histopathologic findings attributed to DIPD.

Amiodarone produces its own unique collection of histopathologic changes, which has been described as a phospholipidosis.[23] Multiple cell types in the lung as well as nonpulmonary cells accumulate a variety of phospholipids. In the lung, this effect is seen most readily in alveolar macrophages, which develop a foamy appearance. This appearance is due to the presence of lamellar bodies, which can be identified readily by light microscopy after staining with toluidine blue. These changes are characteristic of amiodarone exposure. A recent study has demonstrated that they are not specific for DIPD related to amiodarone.[24] Autopsy specimens from five patients who had been taking amiodarone but were without pulmonary symptoms were examined; three of the five had foamy alveolar macrophages.

DIPD also can manifest itself by altering lung function without causing major structural changes. Table 2 lists physiologic changes associated with DIPD. Noncardiogenic pulmonary edema and bronchospasm frequently are initiated by exposure to certain medications. Neuromuscular respiratory failure, pulmonary hypertension, pleural effusion, and pneumomediastinum are less commonly drug-related. Diagnosis of DIPD in these situations is often difficult for many reasons. First, these disorders often can present acutely and may be life-threatening. This leaves little time for extensive history-taking regarding drug ingestion in cases where attention must be focused on immediate therapeutic support. Second, there rarely will be any histopathologic data to suggest a particular group of causative agents. Third, physician familiarity with these reactions probably is not as great as with those that cause structural damage. β-Blocker-induced bronchospasm is an exception to this rule because of its high incidence. Most of these entities, however, occur infrequently and medical information about them often is limited to a small number of case reports. Section four of this chapter should provide a resource to increase familiarity with this type of DIPD.

TABLE 2.
Physiologic Changes Seen in Drug-Induced
Pulmonary Disease

Common
Bronchospasm
Neurogenic pulmonary edema
Uncommon
Neuromuscular respiratory failure
Pulmonary hypertension
Pleural effusion
Pneumomediastinum/pneumothorax

MECHANISMS OF LUNG INJURY

Despite the sizeable number of drugs causing DIPD, only a few have been studied in animal models of pulmonary toxicity. The possible mechanisms of DIPD caused by bleomycin,[25] cyclophosphamide,[26] and amiodarone[27] have been reviewed recently. BAL cells from humans have been studied in patients with DIPD due to methotrexate or gold, and other less common drug hypersensitivity reactions. Despite the considerable amount of research that has been done, however, our understanding of the mechanisms of DIPD remains limited and speculative.

Before even speculation can begin, normal mechanisms of lung defense, inflammation, and repair should be reviewed. To this end, we have constructed Figures 1 and 2, which depict such mechanisms schematically. In this model, antigenic stimulation (e.g., bacteria) elicits one or more immunologic responses as a first step. If antigen is engulfed by alveolar or interstitial macrophages, it then can be presented to T lymphocytes. If there are memory T cells present (second expo-

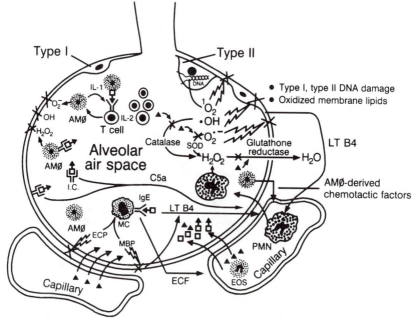

FIG 1.
Possible mechanisms of lung injury. See text. IL-1 = interleukin-1; IL-2 = interleukin-2; AMØ = alveolar macrophage; I.C. = immune complex; MC = mast cell; MBP = major basic protein; ECP = eosinophil cationic protein; ECF = eosinophil chemotactic factor; LT B4 = leukotriene B$_4$; EOS = eosinophil; PMN = polymorphonuclear cell; SOD = superoxide dismutase. The *closed triangles* indicate the drug or drug metabolite (hapten); the *open squares* indicate the conjugate; the two signs connected indicate the antigen; and the *crossed lines* indicate injury to alveolar capillary membrane; type I cells.

Repair

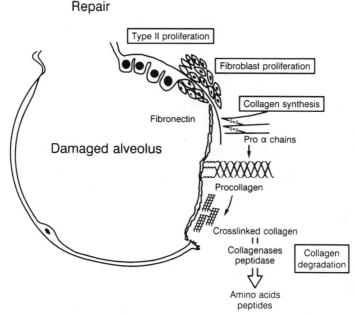

FIG 2.
Schematic representation of pulmonary repair process.

sure to antigen), this interaction can produce T cell proliferation and lymphokine secretion, the latter enhancing neutrophil chemotaxis, macrophage phagocytosis, and both B and T cell proliferation and differentiation. This sequence likely would result in histopathologic changes of either lymphocyte-predominant interstitial pneumonia or granuloma formation. If antigen encounters sensitized plasma cells, specific antibody production could lead to immune complex formation and subsequent activation of the complement cascade. C5a would be a powerful chemoattractant for polymorphonuclear cells, yet also would be capable of activating macrophages. In this scenario, a neutrophilic alveolitis would be the dominant histopathologic finding. Finally, if antigen was engaged by IgE bearing mast cells, the resultant release of eosinophil chemotactic factor (ECF) and leukotriene B_4 (LTB_4) would recruit eosinophils to the lung.

Although each of the different effector cells has a unique composition of cytotoxic substances that can be used in the process of destroying foreign material, all rely on the production of reactive oxygen species such as hydrogen peroxide (H_2O_2), hydroxyl radical (OH·), superoxide anion (O_2^-), and singlet oxygen ($^1O_2$). While much of the damage caused by these species is contained within the cells in which they are generated, inevitably some oxidant material escapes the intracellular milieu and, if left unchecked, causes damage to host tissue.[28] One of the most well-established clinical examples of oxidant tissue damage is oxygen-induced lung injury. Supranormal levels of oxygen have been shown to inhibit protein synthesis, damage DNA, alter membrane lipids, and reduce surfactant synthesis.[2] Peroxidation of membrane lipids may lead to production of lipoxygenase pathway metabolites of arachidonic acid such as LTB_4 and thus amplify the potential for damage by recruiting polymorphonuclear leukocytes to the area.[29] In order to prevent this, an elaborate antioxidant defense system is in place.

Superoxide dismutase (SOD) catabolizes O_2 by converting it to H_2O_2. Catalase and glutathione peroxidase convert H_2O_2 into water. The latter enzyme requires sufficient amounts of reduced glutatione (GSH), which is regenerated by another enzyme, glutathione reductase. Although glutathione is the principal nonenzymatic intracellular antioxidant, others such as α-tocopherol (vitamin E), ascorbate, and β-carotene play a role. Despite the presence of these antioxidants in a normal host, some damage is likely to occur to host tissue, as exemplified by the persistence of a radiographic infiltrate long after the acute infection of bacterial pneumonia has resolved.

Repair after lung injury (see Fig 2) is a complex and poorly understood process, but one capable of regenerating lung tissue that has normal architectural appearance and gas exchange function. Among the phenomena required to produce healthy repair are (1) normal lung cell regeneration and differentiation, (2) adequate fibroblast proliferation and matrix deposition, and (3) appropriate resorption and remodeling of matrix proteins. The histopathologic correlate to malfunction in cellular regeneration would be type II atypia, whereas uncontrolled collagen synthesis and deposition would culminate in fibrosis. It would be oversimplifying to say that fibrosis is prevented by an adequate balance between connective tissue deposition and resorption. The complexity of this process is illustrated by some provocative observations regarding the possible role suppressor T cells play in regulating this process.[30] Experimentally induced fibrosis (by bleomycin) was shown to be produced by depletion of suppressor T cells using cyclophosphamide, and to be prevented, despite cyclophosphamide treatment, by resupplying these cells. Future research is likely to uncover other cell-matrix interactions. Clearly, Figure 2 is an oversimplification; nonetheless, it provides a framework upon which the experimental findings regarding the mechanisms of lung injury can be reviewed coherently.

Within this framework, there are many places at which drugs could interfere with lung homeostasis. A comprehensive review of these mechanistic possibilities has been published[31, 32] that details the methodology and results of experimental inquiry into this area, including a presentation of studies with directly conflicting results. Rather than recapitulate this body of diverse experimental findings, we will present only data that clearly demonstrate a potential means by which drugs could interact with processes outlined in Figure 1 so as possibly to produce DIPD. These are summarized in Table 3 for quick reference. It is important to emphasize that the majority of these data represent possible mechanisms. In other words, demonstration that bleomycin administration can lead to the production of toxic oxygen intermediates[33] does not prove that this action is critical to the mechanism of bleomycin-induced DIPD. Doxorubicin (Adriamycin), a drug not known to produce DIPD, is clearly capable of generating oxygen radicals.[60] We think that, in order for a study to claim that a particular drug activity is mechanistically critical,

TABLE 3.

Summary of Experimental Data Showing How Drugs Might Alter Normal Inflammatory Response and Repair Mechanisms*

Specific Mechanism Studied/Experimental Design and Findings	Drug(s) Studied and Reference
Sequence of histopathologic changes	
Cellular damage and infiltrate precedes fibrosis (hamster)	Bleomycin[34]
Type I pneumocyte followed by fibrosis (mice)	Cyclophosphamide[35]
Oxidant generation/antioxidant depletion	
Generation of reactive oxygen intermediates (in vitro)	Bleomycin[33]
Protection from injury by hypoxia (rat)	Bleomycin[36]
Toxicity is augmented by hyperoxia (mice)	Bleomycin, cyclophosphamide[37]
Inhibition of glutathione reductase (rats, mice)	BCNU[38-41]
Increased levels of glutathione disulfide (rats)	BCNU[38]
Metabolic abnormality in lung	
Decreased lung levels of bleomycin hydroxylase (mice, rabbits)	Bleomycin[41]†
Increased concentration of bleomycin in lung (mouse/human)	Bleomycin[42]
Arachidonic acid metabolism/lipid peroxidation	
Pretreatment with lipoxygenase inhibitor led to chemotactic inhibition of fibrosis (mice)	Bleomycin[43]
Pretreatment with cyclooxygenase inhibitor reduces collagen accumulation (hamsters)	Bleomycin[44]
Increased lipid peroxidation (rats)	Cyclophosphamide[45]
Matrix deposition and repair	
Increased lung fibroblast proliferation (hamsters)	Bleomycin[46]
Increased lung prolyl hydroxylase activity (rats)	Bleomycin[47]
Increased messenger RNA for matrix proteins (mice)	Bleomycin[48]† Cyclophosphamide[49]†
Genetic predisposition to injury	
Susceptible animals do not metabolize toxic drug (mice)	Bleomycin[50]†
Susceptible animals have diminished DNA repair (mice)	Bleomycin[48]†
Immunologic mechanisms	
Supernatant of DIPD lung/BAL is chemotactic and activates neutrophils (rat lung explant)	Bleomycin[51]
T suppressor cells downregulate fibrosis (mice)	Bleomycin/cyclophosphamide[31]
Autoantibody production (rats)	Bleomycin[52]
Lymphocytic alveolitis in DIPD patients but not other patients on medication (human BAL)	Methotrexate[53]†
Immune complex formation (human)	Captopril[54]
Leukocyte migration inhibition in DIPD but not other patients on medication (human)	Propranolol,[55]† amiodarone[56]†
Lymphocyte transformation studies suggest hypersensitivity to drug causing DIPD (human)	Gold/naproxen,[57] gold,[58] nitrofurantoin[59]

*BCNU = carmustine; DIPD = drug-induced pulmonary disease; BAL = bronchoalveolar lavage.
†Studies that have begun to unravel the mechanistic puzzle of DIPD.

at least one of two criteria must be met: (1) the results must prove not only that a drug known to produce DIPD has a particular effect on lung homeostasis, but that such activity must be absent or attenuated in drugs known not to cause DIPD; or (2) the results must suggest why, at the same dosage of medication, the lung tissue of one person develops DIPD while that of another is spared. Some experimental observations, particularly in recent years, have met one or both of these criteria and have begun to unravel the mechanistic puzzle presented by DIPD. These studies are indicated on Table 3 by a dagger.

Upon reviewing Table 3, it is clear that there are numerous ways in which drugs could disturb normal lung homeostasis. The frequency of disturbances caused by bleomycin most likely is due to the fact that it is the most-studied of the drugs that cause DIPD. With time, other drugs will be shown to be capable of similar effects. In any case, the purpose of the list is not to indict a particular agent as most toxic, but rather to summarize how the mechanism of DIPD is being studied. Not included in Figure 1 or Table 3 is information regarding underlying mechanisms behind noncardiogenic pulmonary edema, bronchospasm, or other less frequently seen presentations of DIPD.

Aspirin has been the best-studied of drugs known to cause pulmonary edema. Studies in sheep treated with aspirin demonstrated increased pulmonary lymph flow despite relatively unchanged pulmonary arterial pressures.[61] This observation, coupled with the finding that human pulmonary edema due to aspirin is isosmotic with plasma,[62] demonstrated that aspirin produces a capillary leak. The fact that aspirin-related edema is seen in aspirin overdose has led some to speculate that the pulmonary edema is related to central nervous system alterations. Others have suggested that alterations in arachidonic acid metabolism caused by aspirin's blockade of the cyclooxygenase pathway are important. Hypotheses about the mechanism of pulmonary edema caused by other drugs are similarly speculative.

A review of the mechanisms of bronchospasm is beyond the scope of this chapter. However, the phenomenon of angiotensin-converting enzyme (ACE) inhibitor–induced cough is raising some interesting questions about the relationship of bronchospasm and cough. ACE inhibitors increase the sensitivity of the cough reflex to capsaicin,[63] apparently by blocking the breakdown of substance P and bradykinin.[64] Recently, it has been noted that the majority of patients with ACE-induced cough had occult bronchial hyperreactivity,[65] which was not seen in other patients taking ACE inhibitors without cough. It is possible that substance P or bradykinin plays a role in triggering clinically relevant bronchospasm in individuals with occult bronchial hyperreactivity.

DRUG-INDUCED PULMONARY DISEASE: CLINICAL FEATURES DUE TO WELL-DESCRIBED ETIOLOGIC AGENTS

In this section, we will describe the clinical features of DIPD caused by agents that are now well-established pulmonotoxic agents. Since most clinicians are aware that these drugs do cause DIPD, the question at issue is not, "could this drug be causing my patient's symptoms?" but rather, "do my patient's findings match those of DIPD caused by this drug?" Cytotoxic chemotherapeutic agents will be presented first, followed by noncytotoxic agents.

Cytotoxic lung injury is a difficult problem clinically for several reasons: (1) it can be fatal; (2) it is readily confused with pulmonary infection, which also commonly complicates cancer chemotherapy; and (3) decisions to discontinue a drug, even if DIPD is proven, may be hard if the drug is fighting cancer successfully. A large number of cytotoxic agents have been shown to cause DIPD. They are shown in Table 4. Those drugs in bold print are more frequent offenders and have generated a larger number of case reports and experimental studies. We will focus our attention on those and refer the reader to three recent reviews of cytotoxic lung injury[66-68] for a discussion of the other drugs, all of which will be presented from a different perspective in the next section.

Certain clinical features are common to most of the cytotoxic agents. Presenting symptoms usually include dyspnea, fever, and nonproductive cough. Onset can be acute, but is more typically subacute or chronic; weight loss is common. The chest x-ray characteristically shows a diffuse interstitial pattern, and may be relatively normal when symptoms first appear. Hilar adenopathy could be a clue to a methotrexate DIPD, but is otherwise uncommon. Pulmonary function tests typically show a reduction in diffusion capacity for carbon monoxide (DLCO) and lung volumes without a decrease in flows. Decreases in DLCO often precede obvious loss

TABLE 4.
Chemotherapeutic Drugs Known to Cause
Drug-Induced Pulmonary Disease

Alkylating
  Busulfan
  Cyclophosphamide
  Chlorambucil
  Melphalan
Antibiotic
  Bleomycin
  Mitomycin C
Antimetabolite
  Methotrexate
  Mercaptopurine
  Azathioprine
  Cytosine arabinoside
Nitrosamines
  BCNU (carmustine)
  CCNU (lomustine)
  Methyl CCNU (semustine)
Other
  Procarbazine
  Zinostatin
  VP-16

of volume and may be a harbinger of incipient DIPD. Cellular atypia may be seen in sputum[69] or BAL[70] specimens, but this finding has not been proven to be a predictor of DIPD. Increased uptake on gallium-67 scan has been seen in patients with DIPD, and may be seen even in patients with normal chest x-rays. Whether it is an early indicator of incipient lung damage or a nonspecific drug effect remains unknown.

Bleomycin

Bleomycin is an antitumor antibiotic used to treat a number of squamous cell cancers as well as germ cell tumors and lymphomas. It can be given by subcutaneous, intramuscular, and intravenous routes. Most of the drug is excreted by the kidneys in its biologically active form, and drug accumulation at standard doses should not occur unless the creatinine clearance has fallen to 30 mL/min.[71] Because of its bone marrow–sparing effect, it often is added to multidrug regimens. Besides its pulmonary toxicity, it also causes toxicity in the skin and mucous membranes.

Treatment protocols employing bleomycin, by regularly evaluating pulmonary function, have shown that up to 20% of patients will develop pulmonary disease and that approximately 1% of such reactions will be fatal. Incidence estimates are quite variable, however, from as low as 2%[72] to as high as 40%.[73] The variability stems from differences in diagnostic criteria and intensity of pulmonary follow-up across studies. Incidence also may be greater when bleomycin is used with other modalities, including radiation, as compared to when it is used alone.

Risk factors for bleomycin DIPD include: total dose >450 units, radiotherapy involving the chest, supplemental oxygen, and renal insufficiency. Age does not appear to influence risk until it exceeds 70 years, at which point it jumps from 5% to 15%.[74] The evidence that renal failure is a risk factor for bleomycin lung toxicity is fairly convincing now.[75] In particular, special precautions should be used when combining bleomycin and cis-platinum in the same regimen. Concern over high inspired oxygen concentrations after treatment with bleomycin was heightened following a report describing the deaths of five patients being treated for testicular cancer after exposure to supplemental oxygen at concentrations of between 35% and 42%.[76] Others have observed the same phenomenon and recommend pretreatment with corticosteroids if supplemental oxygen use is anticipated.[77] Formerly, many authors advocated regular monitoring of the DLCO as a screening test for development of DIPD while on bleomycin, some recommending drug discontinuation on the basis of a fall in DLCO. More recently, the following observations have been made regarding the DLCO: (1) it does not change with low-dose bleomycin (<300 units)[78]; (2) it tends to fall in smokers on bleomycin, regardless of whether they have or develop DIPD[79]; and (3) it is ineffective in predicting clinically detectable DIPD.[80] Based on these observations, clinical decision-making based on reductions of DLCO should be done cautiously, if at all.

Patients with bleomycin-induced pneumonitis/fibrosis present with the symptoms described above, and a lesser number may complain of pleuritic or substernal chest pain. Fine rales may appear before chest x-ray changes or symptoms. The chest x-ray appearance typically is one of diffuse interstitial infiltrates; however, in its earliest stages, an alveolar pattern may be seen. Also seen early in many cases is a small area of infiltrate in the costophrenic angles. Loss of lung volume is quite common and the hemidiaphragms will be elevated to some degree in the majority of patients with diffuse involvement.[81] Care must be taken not to presume that nodular densities on the chest x-ray indicate metastatic disease, since several case reports have shown that bleomycin DIPD may present as nodular lesions[10] that, in some cases, may even cavitate.[82] While computed tomographic scanning may be more sensitive than chest x-ray at detecting early parenchymal changes, it also can be misleading. When used to follow patients treated with bleomycin for germ cell tumors, computed tomography detected nodular densities in one fourth of patients that, when biopsied, revealed nonspecific pneumonitis.[83]

Pulmonary function tests in patients receiving, or about to receive, bleomycin are problematic for several reasons. The DLCO may be decreased artificially secondary to anemia. Measurements may be confounded by the presence of lung metastases, analgesic effect, or patient weakness. Last, initial pretreatment values may be decreased falsely if they are obtained postoperatively (e.g., staging laparotomy). Once interstitial DIPD has developed, however, one can expect to see evidence of restrictive disease of variable severity. Gallium scans show increased uptake in patients with bleomycin-induced toxicity, but also can be diffusely positive before symptoms or chest x-ray abnormalities develop. The clinical significance of such a finding is uncertain.

In terms of eventual outcome, patients with mild respiratory impairment often have complete reversal of pulmonary abnormalities upon drug discontinuation. Even those with severe acute impairment usually return to normal if they can survive the acute phase of their illness.[84] Radiographic resolution may take 6 to 12 months. One study documented improvement in pulmonary function with steroid treatment and relapse upon tapering in some patients.[85] Unfortunately, no randomized trials have documented the efficacy of steroids with any certainty.

Over 90% of patients with bleomycin-related DIPD have fibrosis/pneumonitis; however, two other clinical syndromes have been described. A small number of patients develop an eosinophilic pneumonitis with or without peripheral eosinophilia, which usually reverses rapidly. All of the patients have pulmonary infiltrates (typically alveolar), but only half have symptoms.[86] Finally, a small number of patients (estimated at 3%) will develop acute chest pain during continuous intravenous infusion of bleomycin.[87] The pain may mimic myocardial ischemia and sometimes will abate upon reducing the flow rate of the infusion. Awareness of this phenomenon, therefore, may save some patients unnecessary cardiologic evaluation.

Busulfan

Busulfan is an alkyl sulfonate used almost exclusively in the treatment of chronic granulocytic leukemia. The average time from initial use to the development of symptoms is about 4 years, but there is great variability and some can develop symptoms in less than 2 months. The incidence of DIPD complicating busulfan use is 4%, and both children and adults may be affected. Duration of therapy appears to be a risk factor and, although there is not a clear dose-toxicity relationship, patients receiving a total dose of less than 500 mg usually are not afflicted.[88] Busulfan use does not appear to cause significant alterations in pulmonary functions. Chest x-ray may show an alveolar pattern more frequently than in other cytotoxic lung injury because of some of the unique histopathologic findings, such as desquamation of dysplastic type II pneumocytes into the alveolar space and alveolar proteinosis. Mortality of busulfan lung is estimated at 50%, but this figure may be misleading because (1) many of the case reports come from the premechanical ventilation era and (2) many patients have coincident infections or leukemic infiltrates. Clinical response to corticosteroids varies. Busulfan has been used more recently in the conditioning regimens used for bone marrow transplantation. The role it plays in contributing to the interstitial pneumonitis many patients develop posttransplant is unknown.

BCNU (Carmustine)

BCNU is a nitrosourea that is lipophilic and therefore able to cross the blood-brain barrier. It often is used simultaneously with corticosteroids. It has been found to cause DIPD in between 1% and 30% of patients treated. It is more likely to cause toxicity when the cumulative dose exceeds 1,500 mg/m²,[89] but there have been numerous reports of DIPD occurring at lower total doses, and one case of irreversible respiratory compromise after a single dose.[90] Such cases apparently are rare, and a more recent study reported no DIPD in 182 patients with cumulative doses of less than 900 mg/m².[91] Besides the dose, patient age, pretreatment lung disease, and a low platelet count with the first cycle of treatment all appear to be risk factors for DIPD.[92] Onset of symptoms is variable in pace and time of appearance in relation to treatment. Many patients do not develop symptoms until after BCNU has been discontinued. Unlike other cytotoxic drugs, BCNU rarely is associated with fever when lung toxicity develops. Chest x-ray findings vary and upper lobe predominance may be seen. A recent report showed that, in children who survived treatment for gliomas and were reevaluated 13 to 17 years after therapy, six of eight had abnormal chest x-rays with upper-zone fibrotic changes.[93] Pulmonary function tests usually show restriction, which oftentimes will not reverse despite drug cessation. Histopathologic findings are notable for the high incidence of bland fibrosis. Surprisingly, granulomatous changes have been observed in a few patients. The mortality appears to be higher than with almost any other drug; one series has reported a 70% mortality.[94] It appears that this is a form of DIPD that tends not to reverse with drug discontinuation. The benefit of corticosteroids is questionable, since many patients develop symptoms while taking them for their brain tumor. Anecdotal reports of clinical improvement of DIPD with resumption or increased doses of corticosteroids raise hope that they may be beneficial.

Methotrexate

Methotrexate is an antimetabolite frequently used in combination chemotherapy regimens to treat acute leukemia, sarcomas, and breast cancer, primarily. In recent years, it also has been used at lower doses to treat nonmalignant conditions such as psoriasis, rheumatoid arthritis, and asthma. The incidence of lung toxicity is estimated to be 7%. Methotrexate DIPD has a number of unique features that distinguish it from other drugs that cause cytotoxic lung injury.

First, the majority of patients present with a syndrome that resembles hypersensitivity pneumonitis. Systemic complaints of malaise, headache, myalgias, fever, and chills may overshadow pulmonary symptoms. A rash is common, seen in roughly 20% of patients. Onset usually is acute or subacute, with most patients developing symptoms within 6 weeks of starting treatment. Eosinophilia may be seen in 40% of patients.[95] The basis for comparison to hypersensitivity pneumonits stems not only from the clinical similarities, but also from BAL findings, which, in one report, showed a T suppressor–dominant alveolitis like that seen in hypersensitivity pneumonitis.[96] More recent data confirmed a BAL lymphocytic alveolitis, but found T helper predominance.[53] Despite this discrepancy, histopathologic review typically shows an abundant mononuclear cell infiltrate without the cytologic atypia so often encountered with other cytotoxic agents. Clearly, the mechanism of this process is not identical to that of hypersensitivity pneumonitis, since some patients who have developed DIPD and recovered have been able to resume methotrexate without sequelae. Nonetheless, as would be expected with this type of presentation, recovery usually is prompt upon withdrawal of methotrexate. Mortality is low, estimated at about 1%.

Second, the radiographic manifestations are unusual in that a significant number of patients (10% to 15%) develop hilar adenopathy or pleural effusions. The latter may be the only radiologic finding in some patients, whose only symptom related to methotrexate DIPD is acute pleuritis.[97] Third, unlike many other cytotoxic agents, age, irradiation, cumulative dose, and underlying lung disease do not appear to be risk factors for methotrexate pneumonitis. It has been suggested, however, that the incidence may decrease if patients are given the drug less frequently (every 2 to 4 weeks rather than every week).

Fourth, methotrexate does not appear to have an adverse affect on pulmonary function tests. When 38 adolescents with osteogenic sarcoma were tested serially while receiving methotrexate at doses up to 250 g/m^2, only 1 patient was noted to have an abnormality, mild restriction related to pleuritis.[98] Finally, a small number of patients taking methotrexate have developed acute respiratory failure secondary presumably to noncardiogenic pulmonary edema. Although this has been described most often in patients receiving methotrexate intrathecally, one case involved oral administration after a prior history of intrathecal treatment.[99]

In light of the fact that cumulative dose does not appear to alter DIPD risk, it is not surprising that recently there have been reports of series of patients developing methotrexate pneumonitis while receiving low-dose therapy for nonmalignant disorders, usually rheumatoid arthritis.[100, 101] In one of these reports,[101] many of the patients also had been taking nitrofurantoin chronically. Overall, pneumonitis affects between 5% and 10% of these patients. Despite its usually benign course, methotrexate pneumonitis, if not detected and treated, can progress to a fibrotic process with a poorer outcome.

Pulmonary disease related to noncytotoxic drug ingestion is problematic for several reasons. First, only a few drugs have established a track record of causing DIPD on a regular basis (to be discussed in this section). Most often, knowledge regarding DIPD will be limited to one or more case reports. As a result, most nonpulmonary and even some pulmonary physicians will be unaware that a particular drug could cause DIPD. Second, unlike cytotoxic agents, whose administration is controlled by the physician, noncytotoxic drug use usually is controlled by the patient, who oftentimes fails to give a complete drug history. Diuretics, analgesics, vitamins/amino acids (e.g., L-tryptophan), ophthalmologic preparations, and even antibiotics (nitrofurantoin) are atop the list of drugs most often forgotten. It is a rare patient who volunteers their use of illicit drugs such as cocaine or heroin. Third, DIPD related to these compounds often is acute in onset and sometimes is life-threatening. Knowledge of the connection between illness and medication may not be of immediate importance, but once patients are stabilized, they should be questioned about their medications to prevent the possibility of similar responses in the future.

Nitrofurantoin

Pulmonary reactions to nitrofurantoin represent one of the most frequent forms of DIPD. The Swedish Adverse Drug Reaction Committee reported 921 adverse reactions to nitrofurantoin, of which 43% were due to acute pneumonitis, and 5% were due to chronic pneumonitis.[102] Over 170 of the patients previously had used nitrofurantoin and half had experienced an untoward reaction at that time. Despite the large number of cases reported, the incidence is low (.02% to 1%), as is the case with most noncytotoxic DIPD.

Acute nitrofurantoin DIPD is typified by the acute onset of dyspnea and fever; nonproductive cough is seen in two thirds of cases. A smaller number of patients present with pleuritic chest pain, which may be mistaken for myocardial ischemia or pulmonary embolism. Most patients are female and are taking nitrofurantoin for urinary tract infection. Onset is rapid and usually starts within hours to days of treatment initiation.[103] The time to the onset of symptoms is related inversely to the number of previous drug exposures.[13] Dosage does not appear to be a risk factor. Physical examination reveals rales in most patients. Leukocytosis and eosinophilia are seen in one third of patients. The chest x-ray may show diffuse or unilateral involvement, with an alveolar or interstitial process that tends to involve the bases. It may be normal in the small number of patients who present with acute bronchospasm. Pleural effusions, usually unilateral, are seen in one third of patients. These findings obviously are nonspecific, and there is no test that assures the diagnosis. Knowledge of this reaction and appropriate inquiry could prevent unnecessary hospitalization and antibiotic therapy for suspected pneumonia. Hospitalization for acute nitrofurantoin DIPD is an unusual occurrence, with only three instances reported from a recent review of over 16,000 first courses of treatment.[104] Mortality from this acute presentation is approximately 1%.

The chronic form of nitrofurantoin DIPD presents as insidious onset of dyspnea on exertion and cough. The lung histology and radiographic changes mimic usual interstitial pneumonitis. The acute form does not predispose a patient to this reaction. Although the literature is controversial as to the benefit of corticosteroids in this subset, our experience suggests that they often will be necessary to see clinical improvement. One approach is to observe the patient for several months after drug discontinuation, and to initiate a steroid trial if he has failed to improve during that time.

Amiodarone

Amiodarone is an iodinated benzofuran that has been used extensively in recent years for the treatment of malignant cardiac dysrhythmias. Unfortunately, it frequently causes side effects involving thyroid, bone marrow, peripheral nerve, liver, coagulation, and lung function. The DIPD caused by amiodarone is one of the most serious side effects. Estimates of incidence vary from 0% to 61%,[105] but a recent study's estimate of 6% is probably accurate.[106] Patients are most likely to develop lung toxicity during the first year of use. Toxicity appears to be be much less in patients taking lower dosages, as evidenced by a recent study in which only 1 of 43 patients taking amiodarone developed DIPD while taking an average dose of 205 mg/day for 3 years.[107] Blood levels of amiodarone of more than 1 μg/mL are important for arrhythmia control, but have not been shown to correlate with DIPD development.

Patients with DIPD present in one of two ways. Most commonly, they complain of dyspnea, nonproductive cough, weight loss, and fever of insidious onset. Chest x-ray shows a slowly evolving diffuse interstitial process. One third of patients present with an acute syndrome characterized by fever and rapidly developing alveolar infiltrates on chest x-ray. Pleuritic pain is seen often. These features prompt consideration of congestive heart failure, pneumonia, or pulmonary embolism—not uncommon entities in this subset of severely ill patients. Physical examination may reveal rales or a pleural rub, the latter heard more often in those complaining of pleurisy. Laboratory findings are nonspecific, but an elevated sedimentation rate is seen in the majority of patients with DIPD, a finding less likely to be noted in congestive heart failure or embolism.

Pulmonary function changes associated with DIPD include a reduction in lung volume and DLCO. It was hoped that serial pulmonary function tests in patients taking amiodarone might be able to predict DIPD by a fall in DLCO, but a recent prospective study showed that such an approach was ineffective.[108] Of 91 patients (mean dose 367 mg/day) studied, 4 developed DIPD and all had a more than 20% reduction in DLCO. Unfortunately, 15 other patients without clinical evidence of lung disease also had a more than 20% drop. These patients remained asymptomatic for a year while still taking amiodarone. The positive predictive value of the drop in DLCO, therefore, was 21%. In light of the fact that as many as 45% of patients on amiodarone will die within a short period of discontinuation (mostly from cardiac disease),[109] it seems inappropriate to base such a decision on a reduction in DLCO without other findings.

Although the acute and chronic forms of amiodarone lung tend to present with alveolar and interstitial x-ray patterns, respectively, various other x-ray patterns have been reported, including (1) mass lesions,[110] (2) necrotizing pneumonitis,[111] (3) multiple nodules,[112] and (4) pleural effusion.[113] Hilar adenopathy does not occur. Although computed tomographic scanning may show high-density pulmonary infiltrates unique to amiodarone due to its iodine content, the sensitivity and specificity of these findings remains uncertain. In contrast, a recent study of gallium-67 scanning in patients taking amiodarone suggested that positive uptake is likely to be seen in DIPD but not in other non–amiodarone-related pulmonary conditions.[114] Unfortunately, clearly documented cases of DIPD occasionally have been associated with a negative scan. The expense, high radiation dose, and delay in obtaining results (48 to 72 hours) raise questions about the clinical utility of the test.

BAL can show two abnormalities in patients with amiodarone lung toxicity: (1) characteristic foamy alveolar macrophages and (2) lymphocytic alveolitis with a T suppressor predominance in most cases. The former is a sign of amiodarone use, but is not specific for toxicity.[115] The latter tends to recede as symptoms abate and has some specificity, since such an alveolitis would be unlikely in congestive heart failure and pulmonary embolism. The observation that BAL lymphocytes from patients with amiodarone DIPD but not from asymptomatic amiodarone users produce leukocyte migration inhibition upon reincubation with amiodarone is exciting.[56] This sort of approach could lead to a relatively noninvasive diagnostic test for certain types of DIPD.

The unique histopathologic findings associated with amiodarone ingestion, but not specifically for amiodarone DIPD, were discussed in detail in the first section of this chapter. What was not mentioned was the clinical significance of the lack of such findings; they are a necessary although not sufficient finding in making the diagnosis with certainty. Accompanying the lamellar inclusions and foamy alveolar macrophages, one also should see interstitial pneumonitis or, less commonly, alveolar hemorrhage if DIPD is present.

It is clear from the aforementioned that there is no diagnostic test that is highly specific for amiodarone DIPD. Management of patients in whom the diagnosis is suspected based on compatible symptoms and chest x-ray, therefore, should be guided by doing what is best for the patient rather than by a need to confirm DIPD. For example, if there is strong clinical suspicion of DIPD, and another potentially antiarrhythmic agent is available, a reasonable course would be to discontinue the drug before pursuing more invasive tests such as BAL. On the other hand, if amiodarone is the only available antiarrhythmic, a more aggressive evaluation to find supportive histopathologic changes and exclude other diagnostic possibilities is in order. Two notes of caution are called for, however. First, in patients in whom pulmonary embolism is suspected, it has been reported that pulmonary angiography has precipitated fatal adult respiratory distress syndrome.[116] Appropriate caution should be exercised, therefore, before pursuing angiography in these patients. Second, even a certain diagnosis of DIPD should not automatically mandate drug discontinuation. Even in these patients, the greatest threat to life is cardiac disease, not DIPD.[117] Corticosteroids have been used effectively in such circumstances with or without an accompanying reduction in amiodarone dose.

Penicillamine

Although primarily used in the treatment of rheumatoid arthritis, penicillamine is used also in Wilson's disease and macroglobulinemia. It has seen use more recently in scleroderma lung disease and primary biliary cirrhosis. The overall incidence of associated DIPD is small and probably inestimable, yet it merits discussion in this section since the manifestations of penicillamine DIPD are many. It can cause (1) a Goodpasture's-like syndrome, (2) pneumonitis/fibrosis, (3) hypersensitivity pneumonitis, (4) drug-induced lupus, and possibly (5) bronchiolitis obliterans.[118]

Although more than ten case reports of penicillamine-related Goodpasture's syndrome have appeared in print, the incidence of this presentation is probably less than 1%, based on the fact that no cases were detected in a prospective study of over 200 patients under treatment.[119] Onset is acute and appears with a variable latency after first exposure. Patients present with dyspnea, cough, hemoptysis, and hematuria. Hypoxemia or hemoptysis may be profound enough to require intubation and mechanical ventilation. Chest x-ray shows diffuse alveolar infiltrates.

Laboratory abnormalities include increased creatinine, urinary red blood cell casts, and, surprisingly, a negative antiglomerular basement membrane antibody. Renal biopsies tend to show an acute necrotizing glomerulonephritis without the linear immunofluorescence pattern typical of Goodpasture's syndrome. Lung biopsies show alveolar hemorrhage but no vasculitis or linear immunofluorescence. Treatment includes drug discontinuation, mechanical ventilatory and dialysis support as needed, and some form of immunotherapy. Current recommendations include cyclophosphamide, corticosteroids, and plasmapheresis.

Pneumonitis/fibrosis and hypersensitivity reaction are also rare, with under ten cases reported. Clinically, presentation is similar to that with other drugs that cause these syndromes: subacute onset of dyspnea and cough, diffuse interstitial infiltrates, and restrictive pulmonary function tests. Typically, symptoms reverse upon drug discontinuation, although steroids have been used successfully in some cases. Some of these patients may have drug-induced systemic lupus erythematosus.

Over ten cases of bronchiolitis obliterans related to penicillamine have been reported. The typical presentation is subacute and includes dyspnea and cough, but rarely fever. Physical examination may reveal an "inspiratory squeak" on auscultation. Chest x-ray may show an alveolar or interstitial infiltrate, but more often is normal or hyperinflated. Pulmonary function is unique in that it shows reduction in flows, which is atypical for most other forms of parenchymal DIPD. Histopathologic changes were discussed earlier; however, some feel that the bronchiolitis associated with penicillamine can be distinguished by the absence of polypoid inflammatory masses that cause bronchial lumen obstruction in non-DIPD cases.

Unfortunately, whether this syndrome really is caused by penicillamine is open to debate, since it clearly can occur spontaneously in patients with rheumatoid arthritis. Although one case has been described during treatment for eosinophilic fasciitis,[18] it remains possible that bronchiolitis may be due to the underlying disease in this case as well. Whatever the cause, bronchiolitis occurring in patients who have taken penicillamine has an ominous prognosis; 5 of 13 patients have died despite aggressive treatment. Two cases have shown clinical improvement with azathioprine and cyclophosphamide, but overall therapeutic experience is too limited to make any final recommendations.

Cocaine

Cocaine is an alkaloid derived from the leaves of the *Erythroxylon cocapla* plant and used primarily by inhalation of the hydrochloride salt. This salt decomposes upon heating and, therefore, cannot be smoked. When intended for inhalation, it usually is prepared as a powder and typically is diluted by a variety of fillers. Free-base cocaine ("crack") is prepared by alkalinizing the hydrochloride salt with ammonia or baking soda. It has a lower melting point than the powder form and can be smoked by cigarette or glass water pipe. It is absorbed readily by the lungs and, unlike the powder, usually achieves rapid elevations in plasma drug levels. In some studies of frequent users, the intravenous route of administration is most common. Taken in either form, by any route, it is extremely addictive. In the late 1980s, it was estimated that 30 million Americans had tried cocaine and that 5 million were regular users. In addition to acute effects of drug intoxication such as seizures, blurred vision, and dysphoria, there are organ-specific toxicities that may occur at lower doses and even by the nasal route. These include life-threatening dysrhythmia, myocardial infarction, cardiomyopathy, endocarditis, aortic dissection, stroke, and DIPD. Typically, afflicted individuals are young and healthy; some are experimenting with the drug for the first time.

Cocaine-related DIPD has not been a typical entry in most discussions of this subject, although it has been the subject of two recent reviews.[120, 121] It certainly fits well in this section, since (1) internists and pulmonologists are very likely to encounter cocaine users, and (2) cocaine is associated with a greater variety of lung problems than any other drug. This becomes evident upon review of Table 5, which lists the forms of cocaine DIPD described to date.

The incidence of DIPD in cocaine abusers appears to be higher than that seen with any other drug; 25% to 60% of free-base users complain of respiratory symptoms such as cough, chest pain, dyspnea, and bloody or black sputum production.[122] In one study conducted at a chemical dependency center, abnormalities in DLCO were seen in 10 of 19 consecutive free-base users studied.[123] Among a population in which the most common route of administration was intravenous, chest pain was the most frequent respiratory complaint.[124] Among free-basers, dyspnea is the most prominent symptom.

TABLE 5.
Pulmonary Complications of Cocaine Abuse*

Common
Pneumothorax/pneumomediastinum (FB)
"Filler" granulomatosis (IV, N)
Obstructive changes (FB)
Dyspnea, reduced DLCO (FB)
Pulmonary edema (FB, IV, N)
Pulmonary hypertension (IV, N)
Uncommon
Interstitial pneumonitis (FB)
Pulmonary artery coarctation (N)
Bronchospasm (FB)
Tracheal injury/stenosis (FB)
Pulmonary needle embolism (IV)
Bronchiolitis obliterans (FB)

*N = intranasal; IV = intravenous; FB = free-base or inhaled smoke.

Pulmonary edema, similar to that seen with narcotic abuse, has been reported with each route of cocaine administration, including "body packers," individuals smuggling cocaine intestinally who are unfortunate enough to have a bag rupture.[125-128] Individuals present with acute onset of dyspnea and are noted to have diffuse alveolar infiltrates on chest x-ray, without cardiomegaly. They are afebrile and auscultation may reveal rales of bronchial breath sounds. Atrial blood gases show hypoxemia and a widened alveolar-arterial gradient. Complete reversal of these abnormalities is noted within 48 hours. The mechanism is unknown, but it has been postulated to be secondary to transient left ventricular failure arising from the increased afterload associated with cocaine's vasoconstrictive effect. In an animal model of intravenous cocaine-induced pulmonary edema in mice, administration of propranolol before or after cocaine resulted in a profound reduction in mortality (from 100% to 18%), which in part supports this theory.[129] Although β-blockade usually would be considered to exacerbate congestive failure, if the mechanism was due to vasoconstrictive afterload and tachycardic diastolic dysfunction, then β-blockade might improve hemodynamics.

Barotrauma also is a frequent problem and justifies performing a chest x-ray in any cocaine user who complains of chest pain. In one series of chest x-rays taken in 71 consecutive patients complaining of chest pain after smoking crack, 2 had pneumothorax, 1 had pneumomediastinum, and 1 had hemopneumothorax.[130] The majority will have subcutaneous emphysema and half will have Hamman's sign.[131] The mechanism is uncertain.

Alveolar hemorrhage is seen also.[21] As mentioned earlier, an autopsy series of chronic abusers frequently showed hemosiderin-laden macrophages.[22] The acute presentation mimics that described for pulmonary edema. A decreased hemoglobin without other sources of blood loss should suggest the possibility of chronic alveolar hemorrhage. Occasionally, this subset will present with massive hemoptysis.

Talc granulomatosis from intravenous injection has been mentioned already earlier in this chapter.[17] The clinician should be aware that this phenomenon can occur also subsequent to inhalational cocaine exposure as well.[132] Patients present with the subacute onset of dyspnea with or without an interstitial infiltrate on chest x-ray. The diagnosis has been made by transbronchial biopsy, which reveals numerous nonnecrotizing granulomas in the interstitium and bronchial wall. Giant cells may contain needle-shaped crystals. It may be suggested by a decrease in the DLCO, which may continue to drop even if cocaine is discontinued. In addition to talc, cellulose granulomas have been described with inhalations as well.[133]

Pulmonary eosinophilia has been described in two contexts. First, one patient has been reported who has had three separate episodes of fever, transient pulmonary infiltrates, and bronchospasm after inhalation. The illness was associated with pruritus, peripheral eosinophilia, and an elevated IgE level.[134] Two other patients have been described who presented with fever, hemoptysis, and hypoxemic respiratory failure. Histopathology in these patients revealed interstitial pneumonia with a prominent eosinophilic infiltrate and alveolar hemorrhage. Clinical improvement with corticosteroids was rapid.[120]

Other less frequently reported syndromes include thermal injury to the upper airway with consequent tracheal stricture,[135] pulmonary needle embolism,[136] and pulmonary hypertension due to multiple coarctations of the pulmonary artery.[137] There is a limited amount of data associating free-base cocaine smoking with asthma,[138] but it appears that many chronic users have decreased expiratory flow rates.[139]

Initially, it was suggested that free-base inhalation caused a decrease in DLCO in cocaine users.[140] Recently, however, when larger numbers of patients were studied and the effect of marijuana or tobacco use was considered, cocaine did not appear to cause a drop in the mean DLCO.[139] In light of the fact that autopsy studies have demonstrated histopathologic evidence of medial hypertrophy in 20% of individuals dying of cocaine intoxication,[22] it seems reasonable to suspect that a subset of chronic users has pulmonary vascular disease. Future studies should clarify whetner a decrease in DLCO identifies these patients. In the meantime, cocaine abuse should be placed in the differential of pulmonary hypertension.

It is clear from the foregoing information that cocaine can cause both chronic and acute life-threatening pulmonary disease with an alarming frequency. In light of the fact that many of these patients will not volunteer a history of cocaine abuse, it is incumbent upon their physicians to raise the question of cocaine when any of these presentations are encountered.

DRUG-INDUCED PULMONARY DISEASE: DIFFERENTIAL DIAGNOSIS OF COMMON CLINICAL PRESENTATIONS

This section is intended to serve as a reference for the clinician who has entertained the possibility that their patient's pulmonary problems may be due to a medication. We have divided the clinical manifestations into five major categories: (1) pneumonitis/fibrosis (Table 6), (2) pulmonary edema (Table 7), (3) pulmonary infiltrates and peripheral eosinophilia (Table 8), (4) pleural effusion (Table 9), and (5) bronchospasm (Table 10). Each category contains a list of potentially causative agents. For each drug, one reference is provided to serve as a starting point for more detailed study. Space does not permit a detailed discussion of this many drugs, but a few comments about each of the categories are in order.

Pneumonitis/fibrosis is used in this section as a clinical, rather than a histologic, descriptive term. The prototype for this entity is the typical DIPD associated with bleomycin, presented in detail earlier. Also included in this category are patients who have a hypersensitivity pneumonitis picture without a peripheral eosinophilia. Typical presenting symptoms include cough, dyspnea, and fever. Chest x-ray usually shows diffuse interstitial involvement with varying degrees of acinar opacification or honeycomb changes. Pulmonary function tests typically show restrictive changes and reduced DLCO, while flow rates remain stable. Prognosis is variable, but can be life-threatening in some patients.

TABLE 6.
Drug-Induced Pulmonary Disease Associated With
Pneumonitis/Fibrosis

Acyclovir[142]
Azathioprine[143]
Bacille Calmette-Gúerin[144]
Bleomycin[81]
Bromocriptine[145]
Busulfan[90]
Captopril[54]
Carbamazepine[146]
Cocaine[132]
Cyclophosphamide[147]
Dantrolene[148]
Desipramine[149]
Diclofenac[150]
Gold salts[151]
Ibuprofen[150]
Imipramine[152]
Isoniazid[153]
Ifosfamide[154]
Lomustine[155]
Melphalan[156]
Mercaptopurine[157]
Methotrexate[95]
Mineral oil/oily nose drops[158]
Mitomycin[159]
Naproxen[160]
Nilutamide[161]
Oxyphenbutazone[162]
Phenylbutazone[163]
Phenytoin[164]
Piroxicam[150]
Procarbazine[165]
Propranolol[55]
Semustine[166]
Sulfasalazine[167]
Sulindac[168]
Tocainide[169]
Trimethoprim/sulfamethoxazole[170]
Tryptophan[171]
Zinostatin[172]

Pulmonary edema secondary to drugs typically presents acutely. Patients may have life-threatening hypoxemia due to the dense alveolar infiltrates readily seen on chest x-ray. Mechanical ventilatory support may be required, but symptoms usually resolve over 48 to 72 hours. Many of the drugs associated with this reaction are illegal and information regarding their use may not be offered readily. Although familiarity with these agents might not alter the immediate supportive care measures taken, it could prevent unnecessary diagnostic procedures for less likely causes of pulmonary edema.

TABLE 7.
Drugs Associated With Pulmonary Edema

Bupivcaine[173]
Cocaine[126]
Cytosine arabinoside[174]
Dextran[175]
Chlordiazepoxide[176]
Diltiazem[177]
Ethchlorvynol[178]
Haloperidol[179]
Heroin[180]
Hydrochlorothiazide[181]
Interleukin-2[182]
Lidocaine[183]
Methadone[180]
Methotrexate[184]
Morphine[180]
Naloxone[185]
Propoxyphene[180]
Protamine[186]
Ritodrine[187]
Salicylates[188]
Terbutaline[187]

Pulmonary infiltrates associated with peripheral eosinophilia also have been called hypersensitivity pneumonitis. We have avoided that term, since some apparent hypersensitivity reactions usually do not have a peripheral eosinophilia. Patients who do have elevations in their peripheral eosinophil count share certain clinical features. They can present acutely or subacutely with cough, dyspnea, and fever. Other organ systems frequently are involved and, in some patients, rash, myalgia, hepatitis, or even lymphadenopathy may overshadow pulmonary complaints. The chest x-ray may show diffuse or focal infiltrates, which usually are more alveolar than interstitial. Outcome commonly is excellent, with rapid clinical improvement upon drug cessation in most cases. When required, corticosteroids usually are effective. The route of drug administration may be unusual, as in the case of benzalkonium nose drops or sulfur-containing vaginal creams. Therefore, the clinician must make a point of inquiring about any drugs that might be taken by such routes if peripheral eosinophilia is discovered.

Drugs known to cause pleural effusions often are associated with pulmonary infiltrates as well (e.g., nitrofurantoin), but this is not always the case. Other drugs, such as methysergide, may cause effusions alone. Subacute development of a pleural effusion also may be due to the development of drug-induced lupus erythematosus, most often related to hydralazine or procainamide. The antinuclear antibody assay is positive in all such patients, but the test for double-stranded DNA is negative.

TABLE 8.
Drugs Associated With Pulmonary Infiltrates and
Peripheral Eosinophilia

Benzalkonium[189]
Bleomycin[86]
Captopril[54]
Carbamazepine[190]
Chlorpropamide[191]
Cromolyn sodium[192]
Dantrolene[148]
Dapsone[193]
Desipramine[194]
Imipramine[152]
Methotrexate[95]
Nitrofurantoin[13]
Naproxen[195]
Para-aminosalicylic acid[196]
Penicillamine[197]
Penicillin[198]
Phenytoin[199]
Pyramethamine[193]
Sulfasalazine[200]
Sulfonamides[201]
Tryptophan[202]

Finally, drug-induced bronchospasm can be caused by agents other than β-blockers and salicylates. β-blockers are not equal in their tendency to precipitate bronchospasm. Metoprolol, atenolol, and labetalol are all less likely to cause bronchospasm than are propranolol, nadolol, or timolol. Timolol is unusual, since it has been associated with fatal bronchospasm in patients taking the ophthalmologic preparation for glaucoma, reemphasizing the need for careful questioning about substances being taken by *all* routes. The patient or family should be asked

TABLE 9.
Drugs Associated With Pleural Effusions

Amiodarone[113]
Bromocriptine[145]
Dantrolene[148]
Ethchlorvynol[178]
Hydralazine[203]
Isoniazid[204]
Methotrexate[96]
Methysergide[205]
Nitrofurantoin[13]
Practolol[206]
Procainamide[207]
Tryptophan[167]

TABLE 10.

Drugs Associated With Bronchospasm or Cough

Angiotensin converting enzyme inhibitors[208]
Beclomethasone[209*]
β-Agonists[210]
β-Blockers[211]
Cocaine[138*]
Contrast media[212]
Dipyridamole[213]
Lidocaine[214*]
Methotrexate[215]
Nonsteroidal anti-inflammatory drugs
    (NSAIDS)[211]
Pentamidine[216*]
Polymyxin[217*]
Propaphenone[218]
Salicylates[211]

*Inhalational exposure.

to bring with them all drug containers, including those for over-the-counter preparations, which have been used in the last 6 months. A call to the pharmacist may be useful on occasion, since many pharmacists have a computer record of all prescriptions filled. The incidence of cough in patients taking ACE inhibitors is between 1% and 25%, depending on the manner of questioning. These drugs probably cause cough by a mechanism unrelated to the adrenergic nervous system, but they are capable of increasing bronchial reactivity.

DRUG-INDUCED PULMONARY DISEASE: SOME RECOMMENDATIONS REGARDING DIAGNOSIS AND MANAGEMENT

Unfortunately, when patients develop DIPD, there is not a diagnostic test that can establish the diagnosis. As can be seen above, even open lung biopsy is either nonspecific or, as in the case of amiodarone-related changes, specific for drug effect, but not for drug toxicity. Pulmonary function, laboratory, and chest x-ray findings all are similarly nonspecific. This does not imply that they are without value. There are three main reasons for conducting a full evaluation including these diagnostic measures. First, they may help to rule out or diminish the likelihood of DIPD. As an example, a normal gallium scan makes amiodarone toxicity highly unlikely. Second, tests may exclude competing diagnoses. In the case of amiodarone again, an abnormal sedimentation rate argues against pulmonary embolism or congestive heart failure. Finally, pulmonary function and chest x-ray can serve as excellent objective markers of improvement upon discontinuation of a drug suspected to be causing DIPD. We definitely do not recommend rechallenging a patient with a suspected drug as a means of establishing a diagnosis. Ultimately, therefore, the degree of certainty with which the diagnosis of DIPD can be made depends upon (1) the extent to which competing diagnoses have been ruled out, and (2) the observation of clinical improvement over time after drug cessation. In situations where DIPD has been known to progress despite discontinuation (e.g., BCNU), a certain degree of uncertainty will persist and clinical judgment will be required for management decisions. Hopefully, the information provided above will help in some such circumstances.

Most of the references in section IV are illustrative case reports of DIPD related to a particular drug. In some cases, they are the only such report for a particular drug. Many of these have appeared only recently and, since a review almost 20 years ago,[141] the number of drugs associated with DIPD has grown exponentially. These observations make it clear that *any* drug, even one for which no pulmonary toxicity has been described, should be suspected of causing DIPD. That being the case, it might be helpful to the clinician to have some criteria that might serve as guidelines in establishing a probable case of DIPD that has not been reported previously. These are shown in Table 11. Of note is the fact that histopathology is not required. However, it may be beneficial for two reasons. First, it may eliminate more strongly other diagnostic possibilities. Second, it may start to establish a foundation for future knowledge and descriptions of the particular drug reaction under investigation.

The value of BAL in identifying DIPD is just beginning to be recognized. Hopefully, over the next few years, tests will become standardized and sensitivity/specificity will be determined. In the meantime, the diagnostic utility of BAL depends largely on the completeness of the controls used in any particular experiment. To strengthen the diagnostic significance, two controls should be present. First, BAL from asymptomatic patients taking the medication under suspicion should not show any activity. Second, in vitro assays showing increased activity in the presence of the suspected drug should show attenuated activity when exposed under similar conditions to one or more drugs the patient is not taking.

TABLE 11.
Drug-Induced Pulmonary Disease: Criteria for Diagnosis

1. Patient is taking medication at the time symptoms develop, or within a few weeks, rarely months
2. Latency of symptom onset after initiation of drug is weeks to months; however, acute reactions such as pulmonary edema or bronchospasm can occur soon after only one dose
3. Symptoms abate/improve within 1 month of drug discontinuation, sooner in acute reactions
4. Objective data such as diffusing capacity (DLCO), vital capacity, Pao_2 also show improvement after the drug has been stopped
5. Other likely diagnostic possibilities have been eliminated
6. If performed, bronchoalveolar lavage studies examining leukocyte migration inhibition or lymphocyte proliferation upon exposure to the suspected drug should be positive
7. Findings recur with rechallenge; not recommended, but occasionally occurs because diagnosis is not entertained during first exposure or patient inadvertently resumes medication

SUMMARY

In summary, the clinician must be constantly alert to the possibility that the drug(s) a patient is taking or has taken recently may be contributing to his pulmonary symptoms and chest roentgenographic findings. One of the biggest problems in diagnosing DIPD is the incomplete history of medication use given by many patients. It is important, therefore, for the physician to probe beyond routine questions and ask directly about drugs taken (1) by nonoral routes, (2) intermittently without medical guidance, and (3) illegally. This is compounded by the fact that, with rare exceptions, there are no tests diagnostic of DIPD. Hopefully, technical advances will bring new tools to aid in the diagnosis of DIPD. Animal research is critical to such progress. Nonetheless, DIPD should be suspected if, after being observed on multiple occasions, a patient's symptoms and clinical features resolve upon drug discontinuation. Careful documentation of such an association should permit clinicians to report possible cases of DIPD related to drugs that previously had not been known to cause pulmonary disease.

REFERENCES

1. Rosiello RA, Merrill WW: Radiation-induced lung injury. *Clin Chest Med* 1990; 11:65–71.

2. Jackson RM: Molecular, pharmacologic, and clinical aspects of oxygen-induced lung injury. *Clin Chest Med* 1990; 11:73–86.

3. Rosenow EC III: Diffuse pulmonary infiltrates in the immunocompromised host. *Clin Chest Med* 1990; 11:55–64.

4. Smith GJ: The histopathology of pulmonary reactions to drugs. *Clin Chest Med* 1990; 11:95–115.

5. Katzenstein AL, Bloor CM, Liebow AA: Diffuse alveolar damage. The role of oxygen, shock, and related factors. *Am J Pathol* 1976; 85:210–288.

6. Liebow AA, Steer A, Billingsley JG: Desquamative interstitial pneumonia. *Am J Med* 1965; 36:369–404.

7. Liebow AA, Carrington CB: Diffuse pulmonary lymphoreticular infiltrations associated with dysproteinemia. *Med Clin North Am* 1973; 57:809–843.

8. Munn NJ, Baughman RP, Ploysongsang Y, et al: Bronchoalveolar lavage in acute drug-hypersensitivity pneumonitis probably caused by phenytoin. *South Med J* 1984; 77:1594–1596.

9. Adamson IY, Bowden DH: The pathogenesis of bleomycin-induced pulmonary fibrosis in mice. *Am J Pathol* 1974; 77:185–198.

10. Dineen MK, Englander LS, Huben RP: Bleomycin-induced nodular pulmonary fibrosis masquerading as metastatic testicular cancer. *J Urol* 1986; 136:473–475.

11. Deneke SM, Fanburg BL: Normobaric oxygen toxicity of the lung. *N Engl J Med* 1980; 303:76–86.

12. Liebow AA, Carrington CB: The eosinophilic pneumonias. *Medicine (Baltimore)* 1969; 48:251–285.

13. Hailey FJ, Glascock HW Jr, Hewitt WF: Pleuropneumonic reactions to nitrofurantoin. *N Engl J Med* 1969; 281:1087–1090.

14. Travis WD, Kalafer ME, Robin HS, et al: Hypersensitivity pneumonitis and pulmonary vasculitis with eosinophilia in a patient taking an L-tryptophan preparation. *Ann Intern Med* 1990; 112:301–303.

15. Rosenow EC III, DeRemee RA, Dines DE: Chronic nitrofurantoin pulmonary reaction. *N Engl J Med* 1968; 279:1258–1262.

16. Winterbauer RH, Wilske KR, Wheelis RF: Diffuse pulmonary injury associated with gold treatment. *N Engl J Med* 1976; 294:919–921.

17. Waller BF, Brownlee WJ, Roberts WC: Self-induced pulmonary granulomatosis. A consequence of intravenous injection of drugs intended for oral use. *Chest* 1980; 78:90–94.

18. Epler GR, Snider GL, Gaensler EA, et al: Bronchiolitis and bronchitis in connective tissue disease. A possible relationship to the use of penicillamine. *JAMA* 1979; 242:528–532.

19. Fort JG, Scovern H, Abruzzo JL: Intravenous cyclophosphamide and methylprednisolone for the treatment of bronchiolitis obliterans and interstitial fibrosis associated with cryotherapy. *J Rheumatol* 1988; 15:850–854.

20. Sullivan SN: Sulfasalazine lung. Desensitization to sulfasalazine and treatment with acrylic coated 5-ASA and azodisalicylate. *J Clin Gastroenterol* 1987; 9:461–463.

21. Murray RJ, Albin RJ, Mergner W, et al: Diffuse alveolar hemorrhage temporally related to cocaine smoking. *Chest* 1988; 93:427–429.

22. Murray RJ, Smialek JE, Golle M, et al: Pulmonary artery medical hypertrophy in cocaine users without foreign particle microembolization. *Chest* 1989; 96:1050–1053.

23. Lullmann HL, Lullmann-Rauch R, Wasserman O: Drug-induced phospholipidoses. *Crit Rev Toxicol* 1975; 4:185–218.

24. Myers JL, Kennedy JI, Plumb VJ: Amiodarone lung: Pathologic findings in clinically toxic patients. *Hum Pathol* 1987; 18:349–354.

25. Chandler DB: Possible mechanisms of bleomycin-induced fibrosis. *Clin Chest Med* 1990; 11:21–30.

26. Patel JM: Metabolism and pulmonary toxicity of cyclophosphamide. *Pharmacol Ther* 1990; 47:137–146.

27. Martin WJ II: Mechanisms of amiodarone pulmonary toxicity. *Clin Chest Med* 1990; 11:131–138.

28. Babior BM: Oxidants from phagocytes: Agents of defense and destruction. *Blood* 1984; 64:959–966.

29. Martin TR, Altman LC, Albert RK, et al: Leukotriene B4 production by the human alveolar macrophage: A potential mechanism amplifying inflammation in the lung. *Am Rev Respir Dis* 1984; 129:106–111.

30. Schrier DJ, Phan SH: Modulation of bleomycin-induced pulmonary fibrosis in the BALB/C mouse by cyclophosphamide-sensitive T cells. *Am J Pathol* 1984; 116:270–278.

31. Cooper JA Jr, White DA, Matthay RA: Drug-induced pulmonary disease. Part 1: Cytotoxic drugs. *Am Rev Respir Dis* 1986; 133:321–340.

32. Cooper JA, White DA, Matthay RA: Drug-induced pulmonary disease. Part 2: Noncytotoxic drugs. *Am Rev Respir Dis* 1986; 133:488–505.

33. Oberley LW, Buettner GR: The production of hydroxyl radicals by bleomycin and iron (II). *FEBS Let* 1979; 97:47–49.

34. Snider GL, Celli BR, Goldstein RH, et al: Chronic interstitial pulmonary fibrosis produced in hamsters by endotracheal bleomycin. *Am Rev Respir Dis* 1978; 117:289–297.

35. Kumar RK, Truscott JY, Rhodes GC, et al: Type 2 pneumocyte response to cyclophosphamide-induced pulmonary injury: Functional and morphological correlation. *British Journal of Experimental Pathology* 1988; 69:69–80.

36. Berend N: Protective effect of hypoxia on bleomycin lung toxicity in the rat. *Am Rev Respir Dis* 1984; 130:307–308.

37. Hakkinen PJ, Whiteley JW, Witschi HR: Hyperoxia, but not thoracic X-irradiation, potentiates bleomycin- and cyclophosphamide-induced lung damage in mice. *Am Rev Respir Dis* 1982; 126:281–285.

38. Kehrer JP: The effect of BCNU (carmustine) on tissue glutathione reductase activity. *Toxicol Lett* 1983; 17:63–68.

39. Smith AC, Boyd MR: Preferential effects of BCNU on pulmonary glutathione reductase and glutathione/glutathione disulfide ratios: Possible implications for lung toxicity. *J Pharmacol Exp Ther* 1984; 229:658–663.

40. Hardwick SJ, Adam A, Smith LL, et al: A novel lung slice system with compromised antioxidant defenses. *Environ Health Perspect* 1990; 85:129–133.

41. Lazo JS, Humphreys CJ: Lack of metabolism as the biochemical basis of bleomycin-induced pulmonary toxicity. *Proc Natl Acad Sci U S A* 1983; 80:3064–3068.

42. Ohnuma T, Holland JF, Masuda H, et al: Microbiological assay of bleomycin: Inactivation, tissue distribution, and clearance. *Cancer* 1974; 33:1230–1238.

43. Phan SH, Kunkel SL: Inhibition of bleomycin-induced pulmonary fibrosis by nordihydroguiaretic acid. *Am J Pathol* 1986; 124:343–352.

44. Chandler DB, Young K: The effect of diclofenac acid (Voltaren) on bleomycin-induced pulmonary fibrosis in hamsters. *Prostaglandins Leukot Essent Fatty Acids* 1989; 38:9–14.

45. Patel JM: Stimulation of cyclophosphamide-induced pulmonary lipid peroxidation by oxygen. *Toxicology* 1987; 45:79–91.

46. Chandler DB, Hyde DM, Giri SN: Morphometric estimates of cellular changes during the development of bleomycin-induced pulmonary fibrosis in hamsters. *Am J Pathol* 1983; 112:170–177.

47. Kelley J, Newman RA, Evans JN: Bleomycin-induced pulmonary fibrosis in the rat. *J Lab Clin Med* 1980; 96:954–964.

48. Harrison JH Jr, Hoyt DG, Lazo JS: Acute pulmonary toxicity of bleomycin: DNA scission and matrix protein mRNA levels in bleomycin-sensitive and -resistant strains of mice. *Mol Pharmacol* 1989; 36:231–238.

49. Hoyt DG, Lazo JS: Early increases in pulmonary mRNA encoding procollagens and transforming growth factor-beta in mice sensitive to cyclophosphamide-induced pulmonary fibrosis. *J Pharmacol Exp Ther* 1989; 249:38–43.

50. Filderman AE, Genovese LA, Lazo JS: Alterations in pulmonary protective enzymes following systemic bleomycin treatment in mice. *Biochem Pharmacol* 1988; 37:1111–1116.

51. Moseley PL, Shasby DM, Brady M, et al: Lung parenchymal injury induced by bleomycin. *Am Rev Respir Dis* 1984; 130:1082–1086.

52. Schrier DJ, Phan SH, Ward PA: Cellular sensitivity to collagen in bleomycin-treated rats. *J Immunol* 1982; 129:614–617.

53. White DA, Rankin JA, Stover DE, et al: Methotrexate pneumonitis. Bronchoalveolar lavage findings suggest an immunologic disorder. *Am Rev Respir Dis* 1989; 139:18–21.

54. Schatz PL, Mesologites D, Hyun J, et al: Captopril-induced hypersensitivity lung disease. *Chest* 1989; 95:685–687.

55. Gauthier-Rahman S, Akoun GM, Milleron BJ, et al: Leukocyte migration inhibition in propranolol-induced pneumonitis. *Chest* 1990; 97:238–241.

56. Akoun GM, Gauthier-Rahman S, Liote HA, et al: Leukocyte migration inhibition in amiodarone-associated pneumonitis. *Chest* 1988; 94:1050–1053.

57. McFadden RG, Fraher LJ, Thompson JM: Gold-naproxen pneumonitis—a toxic drug interaction? *Chest* 1989; 96:216–218.

58. Geddes DM, Brostoff J: Pulmonary fibrosis associated with hypersensitivity to gold salts. *BMJ* 1976; 1:1444.

59. Back O, Liden S, Ahlstedt S: Adverse reactions to nitrofurantoin in relation to cellular and humoral immune mechanisms. *Clin Exp Immunol* 1977; 28:400–406.

60. Muindi JR, Sinha BK, Gianni L, et al: Hydroxyl radical production and DNA damage induced by anthracycline-iron complex. *FEBS Lett* 1984; 172:226–230.

61. Bowers RE, Brigham KL, Owen PJ: Salicylate pulmonary edema: The mechanism in sheep and review of the clinical literature. *Am Rev Respir Dis* 1977; 115:261–268.

62. Hormaechea E, Carlson RW, Rogove H, et al: Hypovolemia, pulmonary edema and protein changes in severe salicylate poisoning. *Am J Med* 1979; 66:1046–1050.

63. Morice AH, Brown MJ, Higgenbottam T: Cough associated with angiotensin converting enzyme inhibition. *J Cardiovasc Pharmacol* 1989; 13(suppl 3):S59–62.

64. Just PM: The positive association of cough with angiotensin-converting enzyme inhibitors. *Pharmacotherapy* 1989; 9:82–87.

65. Kaufman J, Casanova JE, Riendl P, et al: Bronchial hyperreactivity and cough due to angiotensin-converting enzyme inhibitors. *Chest* 1989; 95:544–548.

66. Snyder LS, Hertz MI: Cytotoxic drug-induced lung injury. *Semin Respir Infect* 1988; 3:217–228.

67. Twohig KJ, Matthay RA: Pulmonary effects of cytotoxic agents other than bleomycin. *Clin Chest Med* 1990; 11:31–54.

68. Lehne G, Lote K: Pulmonary toxicity of cytotoxic and immunosuppressive agents—a review. *Acta Oncol* 1990; 29:113–124.

69. Bedrossian CW, Corey BJ: Abnormal sputum cytopathology during chemotherapy with bleomycin. *Acta Cytol* 1978; 22:202–207.

70. Huang MS, Colby TV, Goellner JR, et al: Utility of bronchoalveolar lavage in the diagnosis of drug-induced pulmonary toxicity. *Acta Cytol* 1989; 33:533–538.

71. Crooke ST, Comis RL, Einhorn LH, et al: Effects of variations in renal failure on the clinical pharmacology of bleomycin administered as an IV bolus. *Cancer Treatment Reports* 1977; 61:1631–1636.

72. Einhorn LH, Donohue J: Cis-diamminedichloroplatinum, vinblastine, and bleomycin combination chemotherapy in disseminated testicular cancer. *Ann Intern Med* 1977; 87:293–298.

73. De Lena M, Guzzon A, Monfardini S, et al: Clinical radiologic and histopathologic studies on pulmonary toxicity induced by treatment with bleomycin. *Cancer Chemotherapy Reports* 1972; 56:343–356.

74. Blum RH, Carter SK, Agre K: A clinical review of bleomycin—a new antineoplastic agent. *Cancer* 1973; 31:903–914.

75. Rabinowits M, Souhami L, Gil RA, et al: Increased pulmonary toxicity with bleomycin and cis-platin chemotherapy combinations. *Am J Clin Oncol* 1990; 13:132–138.

76. Goldiner PL, Carlon GC, Cvitkovic E, et al: Factors influencing postoperative morbidity and mortality in patients treated with bleomycin. *BMJ* 1978; 1:1664–1667.

77. Ingrassia TS III, Ryu JH, Trastek VF, et al: Oxygen-exacerbated bleomycin pulmonary toxicity. *Mayo Clin Proc* 1991; 66:173–178.

78. Lampert B, Eichler F, Meunier J, et al: Pulmonary function assessment during bleomycin therapy. *Biomed Pharmacother* 1985; 39:87–93.

79. Hansen SW, Groth S, Sorensen PG, et al: Enhanced pulmonary toxicity in smokers with germ-cell cancer treated with cis-platinum, vinblastine and bleomycin: A long-term follow-up. *Eur J Cancer* 1989; 29:733–736.

80. McKeage MJ, Evans BD, Atkinson C, et al: Carbon monoxide diffusing capacity is a poor predictor of clinically significant bleomycin lung. *J Clin Oncol* 1990; 8:779–783.

81. Balikian JP, Jochelson MS, Bauer KA, et al: Pulmonary complications of chemotherapy regimens containing bleomycin. *Am J Roentgenol* 1982; 139:455–496.

82. Talcott JA, Garnick MB, Stomper PC, et al: Cavitary lung nodules associated with combination chemotherapy containing bleomycin. *J Urol* 1987; 138:619–620.

83. Trump DL, Bartel E, Pozniak M: Nodular pneumonitis after chemotherapy for germ cell tumors. *Ann Intern Med* 1988; 98:431–432.

84. Van Barneveld PW, Sleijfer DT, Van Der Mark TW, et al: Natural course of bleomycin-induced pneumonitis. *Am Rev Respir Dis* 1987; 135:48–51.

85. White DA, Stover DE: Severe bleomycin-induced pneumonitis. Clinical features and response to corticosteroids. *Chest* 1984; 86:723–728.

86. Holoye PY, Luna MA, Mackay B, et al: Bleomycin hypersensitivity pneumonitis. *Ann Intern Med* 1978; 88:47–49.

87. White DA, Schwartzberg LS, Kris MG, et al: Acute chest pain syndrome during bleomycin infusions. *Cancer* 1987; 59:1582–1585.

88. Ginsberg SJ, Comis RL: The pulmonary toxicity of antineoplastic agents. *Semin Oncol* 1982; 9:34–51.

89. Selker RG, Jacobs SA, Moore PB, et al: BCNU-induced pulmonary fibrosis. *Neurosurgery* 1980; 7:560–565.

90. Lieberman A, Ruoff M, Estey E, et al: Irreversible pulmonary toxicity after single course of BCNU. *Am J Med Sci* 1980; 279:53–56.

91. Weinstein AS, Diener-West M, Nelson DF, et al: Pulmonary toxicity of carmustine in patients treated for malignant glioma. *Cancer Treatment Reports* 1986; 70:943–946.

92. Aronin PA, Mahaley MS Jr, Rudnick SA, et al: Prediction of BCNU pulmonary toxicity in patients with malignant gliomas: An assessment of risk factors. *N Engl J Med* 1980; 303:183–188.

93. ODriscoll BR, Hasleton PS, Taylor PM, et al: Active lung fibrosis up to 17 years after chemotherapy with carmustine (BCNU) in childhood. *N Engl J Med* 1990; 323:378–382.

94. Durant JR, Norgard MJ, Murad TM, et al: Pulmonary toxicity associated with bischloroethylnitrosurea (BCNU). *Ann Intern Med* 1979; 90:191–194.

95. Sostman HD, Matthay RA, Putman CE, et al: Methotrexate-induced pneumonitis. *Medicine (Baltimore)* 1976; 55:371–388.

96. Akoun GM, Mayaud CM, Touboul JL, et al: Methotrexate-induced pneumonitis. Diagnostic value of bronchoalveolar lavage cell data (letter). *Arch Intern Med* 1986; 146:804–805.

97. Urban C, Nirenberg A, Caparros B, et al: Chemical pleuritis as the cause of acute chest pain following high-dose methotrexate treatment. *Cancer* 1983; 51:34–37.

98. Wall MA, Wohl ME, Jaffe N, et al: Lung function in adolescents receiving high-dose methotrexate. *Pediatrics* 1979; 63:741–746.

99. Lascari AD, Strano AJ, Johnson WW, et al: Methotrexate-induced sudden fatal pulmonary reaction. *Cancer* 1977; 40:1393–1397.

100. St Clair EW, Rice JR, Snyderman R: Pneumonitis complicating low-dose methotrexate therapy in rheumatoid arthritis. *Arch Intern Med* 1985; 145:2035–2038.

101. Searles G, McKendry RJ: Methotrexate pneumonitis in rheumatoid arthritis: Potential risk factors. Four case reports and a review of the literature. *J Rheumatol* 1987; 14:1164–1171.

102. Holmberg L, Boman G, Bottinger LE, et al: Adverse reactions to nitrofurantoin. Analysis of 921 reports. *Am J Med* 1980; 69:733–738.

103. Prakash UBS: Pulmonary reaction to nitrofurantoin. *Semin Respir Dis* 1980; 2:71–75.

104. Jick SS, Jick H, Walker AM, et al: Hospitalizations for pulmonary reactions following nitrofurantoin use. *Chest* 1989; 96:512–515.

105. Martin WJ II, Rosenow EC III: Amiodarone pulmonary toxicity—recognition and pathogenesis (part I). *Chest* 1988; 93:1067–1075.

106. Dusman RE, Stanton MS, Miles WM, et al: Clinical features of amiodarone-induced pulmonary toxicity. *Circulation* 1990; 82:51–59.

107. Foresti V, Carini L, Lovagnini-Scher CA, et al: Amiodarone lung toxicity: Role of pulmonary function tests. *Int J Clin Pharmacol Res* 1987; 7:373–380.

108. Gleadhill IC, Wise RA, Schonfeld SA, et al: Serial lung function testing in patients treated with amiodarone: A prospective study. *Am J Med* 1989; 86:4–10.

109. Dean PJ, Groshart KD, Porterfield JG, et al: Amiodarone-associated pulmonary toxicity. A clinical and pathological study of 11 patients. *Am J Clin Pathol* 1987; 87:7–13.

110. Arnon R, Raz I, Chajek-Shaul T, et al: Amiodarone pulmonary toxicity presenting as a mass. *Chest* 1988; 93:425–427.

111. Pollak PT, Sami M: Acute necrotizing pneumonitis and hyperglycemia after amiodarone therapy. Case report and review of amiodarone-associated pulmonary disease. *Am J Med* 1984; 76:935–939.

112. Patel P, Honeybourne D, Watson RD: Amiodarone-induced pulmonary toxicity mimicking metastatic lung disease. *Postgrad Med J* 1987; 63:393–394.

113. Gonzales-Rothi RJ, Hannan SE, Hood CI, et al: Amiodarone pulmonary toxicity presenting as bilateral exudative pleural effusions. *Chest* 1987; 92:179–182.

114. Zhu YY, Botvinick E, Dae M, et al: Gallium lung scintigraphy in amiodarone pulmonary toxicity. *Chest* 1988; 93:1126–1131.

115. Israel-Biet D, Venet A, Caubarrere I, et al: Bronchoalveolar lavage in amiodarone pneumonitis. Cellular abnormalities and their relevance to pathogenesis. *Chest* 1987; 91:214–221.

116. Wood DL, Osborn MJ, Rooke J, et al: Amiodarone pulmonary toxicity: Report of two cases associated with rapidly progressive fatal adult respiratory distress syndrome after pulmonary angiography. *Mayo Clin Proc* 1985; 60:601–603.

117. Kennedy JI, Myers JL, Plumb VJ, et al: Aminodarone pulmonary toxicity: Clinical, radiologic, and pathologic correlations. *Arch Intern Med* 1987; 147:50–55.

118. Zitnik RJ, Cooper JA Jr: Pulmonary disease due to antirheumatic agents. *Clin Chest Med* 1990; 11:139–149.

119. Stein HB, Patterson AC, Offer RC, et al: Adverse effects of d-penicillamine in rheumatoid arthritis. *Ann Intern Med* 1980; 92:24–49.

120. Forrester JM, Steele AW, Waldron JA, et al: Crack lung: An acute pulmonary syndrome with a spectrum of clinical and histopathologic findings. *Am Rev Respir Dis* 1990; 142:462–467.

121. Heffner JE, Harley RA, Schabel SI: Pulmonary reactions from illicit substance abuse. *Clin Chest Med* 1990; 11:151–162.

122. Zerkin E, Novey J: Cocaine free base abuse: A new smoking disorder. *J Psychoactive Drugs* 1982; 14:321–349.

123. Itkonen J, Schnoll S, Glassroth J: Pulmonary dysfunction in "freebase"-cocaine users. *Arch Intern Med* 1984; 144:2195–2197.

124. Brody SL, Slovis CM, Wrenn KD: Cocaine-related problems: Consecutive series of 233 patients. *Am J Med* 1990; 88:325–331.

125. Hoffman CK, Goodman PC: Pulmonary edema in cocaine smokers. *Radiology* 1989; 172:463–465.

126. Kline JN, Hirasuna JD: Pulmonary edema after freebase cocaine smoking—not due to an adulterant. *Chest* 1990; 97:1009.

127. Wetli CV, Fishbain DA: Cocaine induced psychosis and sudden death in recreational cocaine use. *J Forensic Sci* 1985; 30:873–880.

128. Wetli CV, Mittlemann RE: The "body packer syndrome"—toxicity following ingestion of illicit drugs packaged for transportation. *J Forensic Sci* 1981; 26:492–500.

129. Robin ED, Wong RJ, Ptashne KA: Increased lung water and ascites after massive cocaine overdosage in mice and improved survival related to beta-adrenergic blockage. *Ann Intern med* 1989; 110:202–207.

130. Eurman DW, Potash HI, Eyler WR, et al: Chest pain and dyspnea related to "crack" cocaine smoking: Value of chest radiology. *Radiology* 1989; 172:459–462.

131. Seaman ME: Barotrauma related to inhalational drug abuse. *J Emerg Med* 1990; 8:141–149.

132. Oubeid M, Bickel JT, Ingram EA, et al: Pulmonary talc granulomatosis in a cocaine sniffer. *Chest* 1990; 98:237–239.

133. Cooper CB, Bai TR, Heyderman E, et al: Cellulose granuloma in the lungs of a cocaine sniffer. *BMJ* 1983; 286:2021–2022.

134. Kissner DG, Lawrence WD, Selis JE, et al: Crack lung: Pulmonary disease caused by cocaine abuse. *Am Rev Respir Dis* 1987; 136:1250–1252.

135. Taylor RF, Bernard GR: Airway complications from freebasing cocaine. *Chest* 1989; 95:476–477.

136. Hart BL, Newell JD II, Davis M: Pulmonary needle embolism from intravenous drug abuse. *Can Assoc Radiol J* 1989; 40:326–327.

137. Agrons GA, Maslack MM, Parry CE, et al: Multiple coarctations of the pulmonary artery: Scintigraphic appearance. *Clin Nucl Med* 1990; 15:19–21.

138. Rebhun J: Association of asthma and freebase smoking. *Ann Allergy* 1988; 60:339–342.

139. Tashkin DP, Simmons MS, Coulson AH, et al: Respiratory effects of cocaine "freebasing" among habitual users of marijuana with or without tobacco. *Chest* 1987; 92:638–644.

140. Weiss RD, Goldenheim PD, Mirin SM, et al: Pulmonary dysfunction in cocaine smokers. *Am J Psychiatry* 1981; 138:1110–1112.

141. Rosenow EC III: The spectrum of drug-induced pulmonary disease. *Ann Intern Med* 1972; 77:977–991.

142. Pusateri DW III, Muder RR: Fever, pulmonary infiltrates, pleural effusion following acyclovir therapy for herpes zoster ophthalmicus. *Chest* 1990; 98:754–756.

143. Bedrossian CW, Sussman J, Conklin RH, et al: Azathioprine-associated interstitial pneumonitis. *Am J Clin Pathol* 1984; 83:148–154.

144. Kesten S, Title L, Mullen B, et al: Pulmonary disease following intravesical BCG treatment. *Thorax* 1990; 45:709–710.

145. McElvaney NG, Wilcox PG, Churg A, et al: Pleuropulmonary disease during bromocriptine treatment of Parkinson's disease. *Arch Intern Med* 1988; 148:2231–2236.

146. De-Swert LF, Ceuppens JL, Teuwen D, et al: Acute interstitial pneumonitis and carbamazepine therapy. *Acta Paediatr Scand* 1984; 73:285–288.

147. Spector JI, Zimbler H, Ross JS: Early-onset cyclophosphamide induced interstitial pneumonitis. *JAMA* 1979; 242:2842–2853.

148. Miller DH, Haas LF: Pneumonitis, pleural effusions, and pericarditis following treatment with dantrolene. *J Neurol Neurosurg Psychiatry* 1984; 47:553–554.

149. Mutnick A, Schneiweiss F: Desipramine-induced pulmonary interstitial eosinophilia. *Drug Intelligence and Clinical Pharmacy* 1982; 16:966–967.

150. Weber JC, Essingman WK: Pulmonary alveolitis and NSAID—fact or fiction? *Br J Rheumatol* 1986; 25:5–6.

151. Evans RB, Ettensohn DB, Fawaz-Estrup F, et al: Gold lung: Recent developments in pathogenesis, diagnosis, and therapy. *Semin Arthritis Rheum* 1987; 16:196–205.

152. Carlson DH, Healy J: Pulmonary hypersensitivity to imipramine (letter). *South Med J* 1982; 75:514.

153. Miyai M, Tsubota T, Asano K: Isoniazid-induced interstitial pneumonia. *Respir Med* 1989; 83:517–519.

154. Baker WJ, Fistel SJ, Jones RV, et al: Interstitial pneumonitis associated with ifosamide therapy. *Cancer* 1990; 65:2217–2221.

155. Cordonnier C, Vernant JP, Mital P, et al: Pulmonary fibrosis subsequent to high doses of CCNU for chronic leukemia. *Cancer* 1983; 51:1814–1818.

156. Goucher G, Rowland V, Hawkins J: Melphalan-induced pulmonary interstitial fibrosis. *Chest* 1980; 77:805–806.

157. Sostman HD, Matthay RA, Putman CE: Cytotoxic drug-induced lung disease. *Am J Med* 1977; 62:608–615.

158. Lipinski JK, Weisbrod GL, Sanders DE: Exogenous lipoid pneumonitis. *J Can Assoc Radiol* 1980; 31:92–98.

159. Orwoll ES, Kiessling PJ, Patterson JR: Interstitial pneumonia from mitomycin. *Ann Intern Med* 1978; 89:352–355.

160. Buscaglia AJ, Cowden FF, Brill H: Pulmonary infiltrates associated with naproxen. *JAMA* 1984; 251:65–66.

161. Akoun G, Liote H, Liote F, et al: Provocation test coupled with bronchoalveolar lavage in diagnosis of drug (nilutamide)-induced hypersensitivity pneumonitis. *Chest* 1990; 97:495–498.

162. Cameron DC: Diffuse pulmonary disorder caused by oxyphenbutazone (letter). *BMJ* 1975; 2:500.

163. Thurston JG, Marks P, Trapnell D: Lung changes associated with phenylbutazone treatment (letter). *BMJ* 1976; 2:1422–1423.

164. Michael JR, Rudin ML: Acute pulmonary disease caused by phenytoin. *Ann Intern Med* 1981; 95:452–454.

165. Jones SE, Moore M, Blank N, et al: Hypersensitivity to procarbazine (Matulane) manifested by fever and pleuropulmonary reaction. *Cancer* 1972; 29:498–500.

166. Lee W, Moore RP, Wampler GL: Interstitial pulmonary fibrosis as a complication of prolonged methyl-CCNU therapy. *Cancer Treatment Reports* 1978; 62:1355–1358.

167. Moseley RH, Barwick KW, Dobuler K, et al: Sulfasalazine-induced pulmonary disease. *Dig Dis Sci* 1985; 30:901–904.

168. Takimoto CH, Lynch D, Stulbarg MS: Pulmonary infiltrates associated with sulindac therapy. *Chest* 1990; 97:230–232.

169. Perlow GM, Jain BP, Pauker SG, et al: Tocainide-associated interstitial pneumonitis. *Ann Intern Med* 1981; 94:489–490.

170. Ulstad DR, Ampel NM, Shon BY, et al: Reaction after re-exposure to trimethoprim-sulfamethoxazole. *Chest* 1989; 95:937–938.

171. Trazelaar HD, Myers JL, Drage CW, et al: Pulmonary disease associated with l-tryptophan-induced eosinophilia-myalgia syndrome. *Chest* 1990; 97:1032–1036.

172. Seltzer SE, Griffin T, D'Orsi C, et al: Pulmonary reaction associated with neocarzinostatin therapy. *Cancer Treatment Reports* 1978; 6:1271–1272.

173. Wright RS, Feuerman T, Brown J: Neurogenic pulmonary edema after trigeminal nerve blockade. *Chest* 1989; 96:436–438.

174. Haupt HM, Hutchins GM, Moore GW: Ara-C lung: Noncardiogenic pulmonary edema complicating cytosine arabinoside therapy of leukemia. *Am J Med* 1981; 70:256–261.

175. Jedeikin R, Olsfanger D, Kessler I: Disseminated intravascular coagulopathy and adult respiratory distress syndrome: Life-threatening complications of hysteroscopy. *Am J Obstet Gynecol* 1990; 162:44–45.

176. Richman S, Harris RD: Acute pulmonary edema associated with Librium abuse. *Radiology* 1972; 103:57–58.

177. Humbert VH Jr, Munn NJ, Hawkins RF: Noncardiogenic pulmonary edema complicating massive diltiazem overdose. *Chest* 1991; 99:258–260.

178. Miller KS, Sahn SA: Bilateral exudative pleural effusions following intravenous ethchlorvynol administration. *Chest* 1989; 95:464–465.

179. Mahutte CK, Nakasato SK, Light RW: Haloperidol and sudden death due to pulmonary edema. *Arch Intern Med* 1982; 142:1951–1952.

180. Brashear RE: Effects of heroin, morphine, methadone, and propoxyphene on the lung. *Semin Respir Med* 1980; 2:59–69.

181. Kavaru MS, Ahmad M, Amirthalingam KN: Hydrochlorothiazide-induced acute pulmonary edema. *Cleve Clin J Med* 1990; 57:181–184.

182. Mann H, Ward JJ, Samlowski WE: Vascular leak syndrome associated with interleukin-2: Chest radiographic manifestations. *Radiology* 1990; 176:191–194.

183. Elk JR, Wood J, Holladay JT: Pulmonary edema following retrobulbar block. *J Cataract Refract Surg* 1988; 14:216–217.

184. Bernstein ML, Sobel DB, Wimmer RS: Noncardiogenic pulmonary edema following injection of methotrexate into the cerebrospinal fluid. *Cancer* 1982; 50:866–868.

185. Taff RH: Pulmonary edema following naloxone administration in a patient without heart disease. *Anesthesiology* 1983; 59:576–577.

186. Just-Viera JO, Fischer CR, Gago O, et al: Acute reaction to protamine. Its importance to surgeons. *Am Surg* 1984; 50:52–60.

187. Pisani RJ, Rosenow EC III: Pulmonary edema associated with tocolytic therapy. *Ann Intern Med* 1989; 110:714–718.

188. Heffner JE, Sahn SA: Salicylate-induced pulmonary edema: Clinical features and prognosis. *Ann Intern Med* 1981; 95:405–409.

189. Cohen HP, Israel RH: Loeffler's syndrome secondary to "NTZ" nose drops: A self-limited illness. *Respiration* 1979; 38:168–170.

190. Tolmie J, Steer CR, Edmunds AT: Pulmonary eosinophilia associated with carbamazepine. *Arch Dis Child* 1983; 58:833–834.

191. Diffee JJ, Hayes JM, Montesi SA, et al: Chlorpropamide-induced pulmonary infiltration and eosinophilia with multisystem toxicity. *J Tenn Med Assoc* 1986; 79:82–84.

192. Repo UK, Nieiminen P: Pulmonary infiltrates with eosinophilia and urinary symptoms during disodium cromoglycate treatment. A case report. *Scandinavian Journal of Respiratory Diseases* 1976; 57:1–4.

193. Davidson AC, Bateman C, Shovlin C, et al: Pulmonary toxicity of malaria prophylaxis. *BMJ* 1988; 297:1240–1241.

194. Panuska JR, King TR, Korenblat PE, et al: Hypersensitivity reaction to desipramine. *J Allergy Clin Immunol* 1987; 80:18–23.

195. Nader DA, Schillaci RF: Pulmonary infiltrates with eosinophilia due to naproxen. *Chest* 1983; 83:280–282.

196. Wold DE, Zahn DW: Allergic (Loeffler's) pneumonitis occurring during antituberculous chemotherapy. Report of three cases. *American Review of Tuberculosis* 1965; 74:445–453.

197. Davies D, Jones JK: Pulmonary eosinophilia caused by penicillamine. *Thorax* 1980; 35:957–958.

198. Reichlin S, Loveless MH, Kane EG: Loeffler's syndrome following penicillin therapy. *Ann Intern Med* 1953; 38:113–120.

199. Mahatma M, Haponik EF, Nelson S, et al: Phenytoin-induced acute respiratory failure with pulmonary eosinophilia. *Am J Med* 1989; 87:93–94.

200. Wang KK, Bowyer BA, Fleming CR, et al: Pulmonary infiltrates and eosinophilia associated with sulfasalazine. *Mayo Clin Proc* 1984; 59:343–346.

201. Feinmann L: Drug-induced lung disease: Pulmonary eosinophilia and sulfonamides. *Proc R Soc Med* 1975; 68:440–441.

202. Strumpf IJ, Drucker RD, Anders KH, et al: Acute eosinophilic pulmonary disease associated with the ingestion of l-tryptophan-containing products. *Chest* 1991; 99:8–13.

203. Ripe E, Nilsson BS: Pulmonary infiltrations during dihydralazine treatment in a slow isoniazid-inactivator. *Scandinavian Journal of Respiratory Diseases* 1972; 53:56–63.

204. Harmon CE, Portanova JP: Drug-induced lupus: Clinical and serological studies. *Clinics in Rheumatic Diseases* 1982; 8:121–135.

205. Dunn JM, Sloan H: Pleural effusion and fibrosis secondary to Sansert administration. *Ann Thorac Surg* 1973; 15:295–298.

206. MacKay AD, Axford AT: Pleural effusions after practolol (letter). *Lancet* 1976; 1:89.

207. Kaplan AI, Zakher F, Sabin S: Drug-induced lupus erythematosus with in vivo lupus erythematosus cells in pleural fluid. *Chest* 1978; 73:875–876.

208. Bucknall CE, Neilly JB, Carter R, et al: Bronchial hyperreactivity in patients who cough after receiving angiotensin converting enzyme inhibitors. *BMJ* 1988; 296:86–88.

209. Shim CS, Williams MH Jr: Cough and wheezing from beclamethasone dipropionate aerosol are absent after triamcinalone acetonide. *Ann Intern Med* 1987; 106:700–703.

210. Nicklas RA: Paradoxical bronchospasm associated with the use of inhaled beta agonists. *J Allergy Clin Immunol* 1990; 85:959–964.

211. Mecker DP, Wiedemann HP: Drug-induced bronchospasm. *Clin Chest Med* 1990; 11:163–175.

212. Dawson P, Pitfield J, Britlon J: Contrast media and bronchospasm: A study with iopamidol. *Clin Radiol* 1983; 34:227–230.

213. Lette J, Cerino M, Laverdiere M, et al: Severe bronchospasm followed by respiratory arrest during thallium-dipyridamole imaging. *Chest* 1989; 95:1345–1347.

214. McAlpine LG, Thomson NC: Lidocaine-induced bronchoconstriction in asthmatic patients: Relation to histamine airway responsiveness and effect of preservative. *Chest* 1989; 96:1012–1015.

215. Jones G, Mierins E, Karsh J: Methtrexate-induced asthma. *Am Rev Respir Dis* 1991; 143:179–181.

216. Conte JE Jr, Hollander H, Golden JA: Inhaled or reduced-dose intravenous pentamidine for *pneumocystis carinii* pneumonia. *Ann Intern Med* 1987; 107:495–498.

217. Wilson FE: Acute respiratory failure secondary to polymyxin-B inhalation. *Chest* 1981; 79:237–239.

218. Hill MR, Gotz VP, Harman E, et al: Evaluation of the asthmogenicity of propafenone: A new antiarrhythmic drug. *Chest* 1986; 90:689–672.

Index

A

Abdomen: content displacement ventilators in
  ventilatory pump disorders, 72–73
Abuse of cocaine: lung complications due to,
  331
Adenocarcinoma: lymphatic lung, 207
Adenoviruses, 125–126
α-Adrenergic function: increase in airway
  hyperresponsiveness, 172–173
β-Adrenergic dilation: decrease in airway
  hyperresponsiveness, 159–160
Aerosol deposition: increase in airway
  hyperresponsiveness, 150–151
Airflow
  obstruction, 46–54
    pathophysiology, 46–48
    ventilatory strategies for, 48–54
  pressure(s)
    in inverse ratio ventilation, 60
    during pressure-controlled ventilation, 59
    during volume-cycled positive-pressure
      breath, 47
  rates, effect on peak pressure, 52
Airway(s)
  artificial, risks of, 45
  diseases, occupational, 238–242
    assessment techniques, 242
    causes, specific, 240–241
    diagnosis, 242
    management, 242
    mechanisms, 242
    in rural environment, 243
  geometry alterations in airway
    hyperresponsiveness, 154–157
  hyperresponsiveness (see Hyperresponsiveness
    of airway)
  Management System, BiPAP S, 74
  pressure(s)
    continuous positive, in ventilator
      dependence, 78–79
    endotracheal tube resistance on, 80

inspiratory plateau, 52
in inverse ratio ventilation, 60
during pressure-controlled ventilation, 59
-release ventilation in ARDS, 62–63
during volume-cycled positive-pressure
  breath, 47
responsiveness, nonspecific, definition,
  144–147
Allergic alveolitis (see Alveolitis, extrinsic
  allergic)
Allergy: relation to smoking, 242
Alpha-adrenergic function: increase in airway
  hyperresponsiveness, 172–173
Aluminum: and occupational lung disease,
  227–228
Alveolar pressure(s)
  in inverse ratio ventilation, 60
  during pressure-controlled ventilation, 59
  during volume-cycled positive-pressure breath,
    47
Alveolitis, extrinsic allergic
  acute phase, 204
  CT of, high resolution, 201–205
  subacute phase, 204
Amiodarone: causing lung disease, 327–329
Animal confinement-related diseases, 244–245
Antimicrobials in pneumonia (see Pneumonia,
  nosocomial, antimicrobials in)
ARDS, 54–56
  airway pressure-release ventilation in, 62–63
  extended inspiratory time ventilation for,
    60–62
  gas exchange in, extrapulmonary, 63–66
  inverse ratio ventilation for, 60–62
  pathophysiology, 54–55
  pressure-controlled ventilation in, 58–60
  ventilator guidelines for, 57
  ventilatory strategies in, 55–66
  volume-cycled ventilation with PEEP in, 57–58
Asbestos
  -exposure, 208
    atelectasis after, 211

349

Asbestos (cont.)
 general population and, 233–234
 mesothelioma and, 232–233
 mineralogic types, 228–229
 pleural disorders and, benign, 230–231
 -related disorders, 228–234
  cellular features, 229
  molecular features, 229
Asbestosis, 232
 CT of, high-resolution, 206–212
 mild, 209
Asthma
 occupational, 239–240
 ventilatory strategies in, 50–53
Atelectasis: after asbestos exposure, 211
Authority: source of, and ethical
  decision-making, 34
Autonomy: as ethical principle, 31
AutoPEEP: impact on inspiratory effort to
  trigger assisted breath, 48

B

Bacterial species: in lung by different sampling
  techniques, 7
Barotrauma: with mechanical ventilation, 44–45
BCNU: causing lung disease, 324–325
Beneficence: as ethical principle, 30–31
Beryllium: and occupational lung disease, 227
Beta-adrenergic dilation: decrease in airway
  hyperresponsiveness, 159–160
BiPAP S Airway Management System, 74
Blastomycosis, 269–274
 diagnosis, 272–273
 serologic tests, expected sensitivity of, 273
 treatment, 273–274
  recommended, 274
Bleomycin: causing lung disease, 322–323
Brain death: and organ transplant, 35–36
Breath: positive-pressure, volume-cycled, 47
Breathing: intermittent spontaneous, in ventilator
  dependence, 78
Bronchiolitis obliterans: organizing pneumonia,
  CT of, high-resolution, 198–200
Bronchitis: industrial, 238–239
Bronchospasm: associated with drugs, 337
Busulfan: causing lung disease, 324
Byssinosis: occupational, 245

C

Cadmium: in occupational lung disease, 227
Cancer, lung (see Lung cancer)

Cannulation: of extracorporeal carbon dioxide
  removal, 64
Carbon dioxide: removal, extracorporeal,
  cannulation and perfusion circuit of, 64
Carbon monoxide poisoning, 289–309
 cardiac effects, 292
 cerebral function and physiology in, 293–295
 clinical findings, 296–299
 congenital effects, 295–296
 epidemiology, 289–290
 management, 299–302
 oxygen supply in, tissue, 290–291
 pathophysiology, 290–296
 pulmonary effects, 292–293
 severity of, estimation of, 298–299
 signs and symptoms, 296–298
 vascular effects, 291–292
Carcinomatosis: pulmonary lymphatic, CT of,
  high-resolution, 205–206
Cardiopulmonary medicine: ethics in, 29–41
Cardiovascular compromise: and mechanical
  ventilation, 66–69
Carmustine: causing lung disease, 324–325
Catheter: IVOX, 65
Cell: features of asbestos-related disorders, 229
Cerebral function and physiology: in carbon
  monoxide poisoning, 293–295
Chemical gases: occupational, 245
Chemotherapeutic drugs: causing lung disease,
  321
Cocaine
 abuse, lung complications of, 331
 lung disease due to, 330–333
Coccidioidomycosis, 274–282
 diagnosis, 279–281
 disseminated, 279
 pulmonary, persistent, 277–278
 residual pulmonary lesions, 278
 serologic tests, expected sensitivity, 280
 treatment, 281–282
  recommended, 281
Computed tomography, 193–220
 conventional techniques, 195
 high-resolution
  alveolitis, extrinsic allergic, 201–205
  asbestosis, 206–212
  carcinomatosis, pulmonary lymphatic,
   205–206
  diagnostic accuracy of, 213–214
  lung diseases, chronic infiltrative, 196–214
  lung diseases, granulomatous, 200–205
  lung diseases, occupational, 206–214
  lung fibrosis, idiopathic, 196–198

pneumonia, bronchiolitis obliterans
organizing, 198–200
of pneumonia, chronic interstitial, 196–200
sarcoidosis, 200–201
techniques, 195
of lung disease, chronic infiltrative, 193–220
of silicosis, 212–213
Congenital effects: of carbon monoxide
poisoning, 295–296
Consultations: about ethics, 39
Continuous positive airway pressure: in
ventilator dependence, 78–79
Coronaviruses, 128
CO$_2$ removal: extracorporeal, cannulation and
perfusion circuit of, 64
Cough: associated with drugs, 337
Critical illness
malnutrition in, consequences of, 93–95
nutritional support in (*see under* Nutrition)
Cytomegalovirus, 130

D

Decision-making in ethics (*see* Ethics,
decision-making in)
Diaphragm: electrophrenic pacing in ventilatory
pump disorders, 73
Diets: enteral, 103
Drug(s)
associated with
bronchospasm, 337
cough, 337
eosinophilia, peripheral, 336
pleural effusions, 336
pulmonary edema, 335
pulmonary infiltrates, 336
chemotherapeutic, causing lung disease, 321
-induced lung disease (*see* Lung disease,
drug-induced)
lung inflammatory response altered by, 319
lung injury due to, patterns of, 312–316
lung repair mechanisms altered by, 319
Dust: organic dust toxic syndrome in rural
environment, 244

E

Economic issues: and ethics, 31–32
Edema, pulmonary: drugs associated with, 335
Electrolytes
daily requirements, 99
in nutritional support in critical illness,
97–98

Electrophrenic pacing: of diaphragm in
ventilatory pump disorders, 73
Endotracheal tube: resistance on airway and
tracheal pressures, 80
Enteral
diets, 103
nutrition, complications of, 107–108
Eosinophilia: peripheral, associated with drugs,
336
Epithelium
-dependent dilation decrease in airway
hyperresponsiveness, 158–159
permeability increase in airway
hyperresponsiveness, 151–152
Ethic(s), 29–41
brain death and organ transplant, 35–36
in cardiopulmonary medicine, 29–41
consultations, 39
decision-making in, 34–35
effective communication with patients and
family, 34–35
establishing source of authority, 34
economic issues and, 31–32
family, effective communication with,
34–35
government legislation and, advance
directives, 32–33
health care rationing and, 32
intensive care unit and technologic imperative,
29–30
legal precedents and, 33–34
life support (*see* Life support)
patients
effective communication with, 34–35
rights of, recognition of, 35
wishes of, determine early and frequently
review, 35
principles, 30–31
autonomy, 31
beneficence, 30–31
justice, 31
nonmaleficence, 31
theologic issues, 30–31

F

Family: effective communication with, 34–35
Fever: humidifier, in rural environment, 244
Fibrosis: associated with drug-induced lung
disease, 334
Flow (*see* Airflow)
Fungal diseases, 257–287
Future: in life support, 38–39

G

Gas(es)
chemical and toxic, occupational, 245
exchange: extrapulmonary, in ARDS, 63–66
Government legislation: and ethics, 32–33
Granulomatous lung diseases: CT of,
high-resolution, 200–205

H

Health care rationing: and ethics, 32
Heart
compromise and mechanical ventilation, 66–69
effects of carbon monoxide poisoning on, 292
Hemodynamic
consequences of mechanical ventilation, 45
disorders, ventilatory strategies for, 67–69
Herpes simplex viruses: types 1 and 2, 129
Histoplasmosis, 258–268
diagnosis, 266–267
serologic tests, approximate sensitivity of, 267
treatment, 267–268
recommended, 268
Humidifier fever: in rural environment, 244
Hyperresponsiveness of airway, 143–192
mechanisms, 147–173
mechanisms, potential, taxonomy of, 150
mechanisms, response-enhancing, 152–166
airway geometry alterations, 154–157
dilation, beta-adrenergic decrease, 159–160
dilation, epithelium-dependent decrease,
158–159
dilation, nonadrenergic noncholinergic
decrease, 160–161
mediator receptor function alteration,
165–166
neuropeptides, sensory, action increase,
161–164
parasympathetic function alteration, 164–165
smooth muscle alterations, 152–154
mechanisms, stimulus-enhancing, 150–152
aerosol deposition increase, 150–151
epithelial permeability increase, 151–152
mechanisms, stimulus- and response-
enhancing, 167–173
alpha-adrenergic function increase, 172–173
mediators, 167–171
mucociliary clearance alteration, 171–172
secretion alteration in, 171–172
models of, correspondence between, 148–150
nonspecific, 143–192
consequences of, 145–147
sources of, 145–147

responsiveness, nonspecific, definition,
144–147
Hypersensitivity pneumonitis: in rural
environment, 243–244

I

Immunocompromised hosts: unusual pathogens
for nosocomial pneumonia in, 13
Industrial bronchitis, 238–239
Infections
occupational, 245
respiratory, lower, most frequently isolated
pathogens, 11
Influenza viruses, 119–123
Intensive care unit: and technologic imperative,
29–30
IVOX catheter, 65

J

Justice, 31

L

Legal precedents: and ethics, 33–34
Legislation: governmental, and ethics, 32–33
Life support
advanced
withdrawing, 36–38
withholding, 36–37
basic, withholding and withdrawing, 36
future in, 38–39
Lung
(See also Pulmonary)
adenocarcinoma, lymphangitic, 207
cancer
asbestos and, 232
relation to silica, 234–237
carcinomatosis, lymphatic, CT of,
high-resolution, 205–206
coccidioidomycosis, persistent, 277–278
complications of cocaine abuse, 331
disease(s)
chronic infiltrative, listing of, 194
computed tomography of (see under
Computed tomography)
disease, COPD, ventilatory strategies for,
53–54
disease, drug-induced, 311–348
amiodarone, 327–329
associated with fibrosis, 334
associated with pneumonitis, 334
BCNU, 324–325

bleomycin, 322–323
busulfan, 324
chemotherapeutic drugs, 321
cocaine, 330–333
diagnosis, criteria, 338
diagnosis, differential, of common clinical
    presentations, 333–337
diagnosis, recommendations, 337–338
by etiologic agents, well-described, clinical
    features due to, 320–333
histopathologic patterns, 313
management, recommendations, 337–338
methotrexate, 325–326
nitrofurantoin, 326–327
penicillamine, 329–330
physiologic changes in, 315
disease, occupational (*see* Occupational lung
    disease)
effects of carbon monoxide poisoning on,
    292–293
fibrosis, idiopathic, CT of, high-resolution,
    196–198
function test in occupational lung disease,
    222–224
infiltrates associated with drugs, 336
inflammatory response, drugs that might alter,
    319
injury
    by drugs, patterns of, 312–316
    mechanisms of, 316–320
    mechanisms of, possible, 316
    metals and, 225–228
    parenchymal bands, CT of, high-resolution,
        210
    repair mechanisms, drugs that might alter,
        319
    repair process. F schematic representation,
        317
    volume at end-inspiration, 52
Lymphangitic pulmonary adenocarcinoma, 207
Lymphatic carcinomatosis: pulmonary, CT of,
    high-resolution, 205–206

M

Malnutrition: in critical illness, consequences of,
    93–95
Measles virus, 130
Mesothelioma: and asbestos, 232–233
Metal(s)
    hard metal diseases, 226
    and the lung, 225–228
Methotrexate: causing lung disease, 325–326

Micronutrients: in nutritional support in critical
    illness, 98–100
Miner groups and silica (*see* Silica, miner
    groups)
Mineral: daily requirements, 99
Model: of airway hyperresponsiveness,
    correspondence between, 148–150
Monitoring: nutritional support in critical illness,
    106–107
Mortality: in pneumonia, nosocomial, trials, 20
Mouth: positive-pressure ventilation via, in
    ventilatory pump disorders, 73–75
Mucociliary clearance: alteration in airway
    hyperresponsiveness, 171–172
Muscle: smooth, alterations in airway
    hyperresponsiveness, 152–154

N

Neuromuscular disease: mechanical ventilation
    in, 69–75
Neuropeptides: sensory, action increase in
    airway hyperresponsiveness, 161–164
Nitrofurantoin: causing lung disease, 326–327
Nonmaleficence: as ethical principle, 31
Nose: positive-pressure ventilation via, in
    ventilatory pump disorders, 73–75
Nosocomial pneumonia (*see* Pneumonia,
    nosocomial)
Nutrition
    enteral
        complications, 107–108
        diets, 103
    parenteral, 104–106
        complications, 108–111
    support in critical illness, 91–118
        assessment, 92–93
        complications, 107–111
        delivering nutrition, methods of, 100–104
        electrolytes, 97–98
        micronutrients, 98–100
        monitoring, 106–107
        needs of patients, 95–97

O

Occupational lung disease, 221–255
    airway diseases (*see* Airway diseases,
        occupational)
    aluminum, 227–228
    animal confinement-related diseases, 244–245
    asbestos-related (*see* Asbestos-related
        disorders)

Occupational lung disease (cont.)
asthma, 239–240
beryllium, 227
bronchitis, 238–239
byssinosis, 245
cadmium, 227
CT of, high-resolution, 206–214
gases, chemical and toxic, 245
infections, 245
lung function tests in, 222–224
metals, 225–228
hard metal diseases, 226
methods, 221–225
radiography in, 221–222
in rural environment, 243–245
scientists and, 245–246
silica (see Silica)
society and, 245–246
welding, 225–226
Organic dust toxic syndrome: in rural
environment, 244
Oxygen supply: tissue, in carbon monoxide
poisoning, 290–291

P

Pacing: electrophrenic, of diaphragm in
ventilatory pump disorders, 73
Parainfluenza viruses, 124–125
Parasympathetic function: alteration in airway
hyperresponsiveness, 164–165
Parenteral nutrition in critical illness, 104–106
complications of, 108–111
Patients and ethics (see Ethics, patients)
Peak pressure: effect of flow and respiratory
rates on, 52
PEEP
auto, impact on inspiratory effort to trigger
assisted breath, 48
pressure-volume curves with, 56
with volume-cycled ventilation in ARDS,
57–58
Penicillamine: causing lung disease, 329–330
Perfusion circuit: of extracorporeal carbon
dioxide removal, 64
Pleural
disorders, benign, and asbestos, 230–231
effusions associated with drugs, 336
Pneumonia: chronic interstitial, CT of,
high-resolution, 196–200
Pneumonia, nosocomial, 1–28
antimicrobials in
definitive, 16–18

empiric, 14–15
empiric, listing of, 17
bacterial species in lung by different sampling
techniques, 7
brush cultures in, protected specimen, 9
brush specimens in, frequency of organisms
recovered from, 12
diagnosis, 5–10
etiologic agents, 10–13
mortality in trials, 20
pathogenesis, 2–5
pathogens
most frequently isolated, from lower
respiratory infections, 11
unusual, in immunocompromised hosts,
13
prevention, 18–21
therapy, 14–18
options with known etiology, 18
Pneumonitis
associated with drug-induced lung disease,
334
hypersensitivity, in rural environment,
243–244
Poisoning, carbon monoxide (see Carbon
monoxide poisoning)
Positive end-expiratory pressure (see PEEP)
Positive-pressure breath: volume-cycled, 47
Pressure-volume curves: with mechanical
ventilation, 56
Pulmonary
(See also Lung)
edema, drugs associated with, 335
medicine, ethics in, 29–41

R

Radiography: in lung disease, occupational,
221–222
Respiratory
central drive disorders, mechanical ventilation
in, 69–75
distress syndrome, adult (see ARDS)
failure, conversion from positive-pressure
mechanical ventilation in, 68
infections, lower, most frequently isolated
pathogens, 11
rates, effect on peak pressure, 52
syncytial virus, 123–124
viral infections (see Viral infections of
respiratory tract)
Rhinoviruses, 127–128
Rights of patients: recognition of, 35

S

Sarcoidosis
  advanced, upper lobes in, 203
  CT of, high-resolution, 200–201
  parenchymal changes in, 202
Scientists: and occupational lung disease,
    245–246
Silica, 234–238
  miner groups, 235
  case control studies, 235
  retrospective cohorts, 235
  relation of lung cancer to, 234–237
Silicosis, 235–238
  CT of, 212–213
Smoking: relation to allergy, 242
Society: and occupational lung disease,
    245–246

T

Technologic imperative: and intensive care unit,
    29–30
Theologic issues: in ethics, 30–31
Thoracic cage deformity: mechanical ventilation
    in, 69–75
Tomography, computed (*see* Computed
    tomography)
Toxic
  gases, occupational, 245
  organic dust toxic syndrome in rural
    environment, 244
T-piece: in ventilator dependence, 78
Trace elements: daily requirements, 99
Tracheal pressure: endotracheal tube resistance
    on, 80
Transplant: organ, and brain death, 35–36
Tube: endotracheal, resistance on airway and
    tracheal pressures, 80

V

Varicella-zoster virus, 128–129
V_{EI}, 52
Ventilation
  airway pressure-release, in ARDS, 62–63
  assist, proportional, in ventilator dependence,
    81–82
  extended expiratory time, in ARDS, 60–62
  extended inspiratory time (*see* inverse ratio
    below)
  inverse ratio
    airflow pressures with, 60
    airway pressures with, 60

alveolar pressures with, 60
  in ARDS, 60–62
mandatory, synchronized intermittent, in
    ventilator dependence, 80–81
mechanical, 43–90
  artificial airways, risks of, 45
  barotrauma with, 44–45
  cardiovascular compromise with, 66–69
  general considerations in, 44–46
  goals, 44
  hazards, 44–45
  hemodynamic consequences, 45
  in neuromuscular disease, 69–75
  positive-pressure, conversion from, in left
    ventricular dysfunction with respiratory
    failure, 68
  pressure-volume curves with, 56
  removal, 75–82
  removal, physiology, 75–77
  in respiratory central drive disorders,
    69–75
  in thoracic cage deformity, 69–75
  weaning, 75–82
minute, mandatory, in ventilator dependence,
    81
positive-pressure, by mouth or nose in
    ventilatory pump disorders, 73–75
pressure-controlled
  airflow pressures during, 59
  airway pressures during, 59
  alveolar pressures during, 59
  in ARDS, 58–60
pressure-support, in ventilator dependence,
    79–80
volume-cycled with PEEP in ARDS, 57–58
Ventilator(s)
  dependence, 77–82
  displacing abdominal contents in ventilatory
    pump disorders, 72–73
  guidelines in ARDS, 57
  negative-pressure, for ventilatory pump
    disorders, 71–72
Ventilatory
  pump disorders, ventilatory strategies for,
    71–75
  strategies
    for airflow obstruction, 48–54
    in ARDS, 55–66
    in asthma, 50–53
    in COPD, 53–54
    in hemodynamic disorders, 67–69
    in ventilator dependence, 77–82
    in ventilatory pump disorders, 71–75

Ventilatory (cont.)
support, general approach to, 45–46
Ventricle: left, dysfunction, conversion from positive-pressure mechanical ventilation in, 68
Vessels
compromise, and mechanical ventilation, 66–69
effects of carbon monoxide poisoning on, 291–292
Viral infections of respiratory tract, 119–141
adenoviruses, 125–126
coronaviruses, 128
cytomegalovirus, 130
herpes simplex viruses types 1 and 2, 129
influenza viruses, 119–123
measles virus, 130
nonrespiratory viruses, 128–130
parainfluenza viruses, 124–125
respiratory syncytial virus, 123–124
rhinoviruses, 127–128
varicella-zoster virus, 128–129
Vitamins: daily requirements, 99
Volume-pressure curves: with mechanical ventilation, 56

W

Weaning: physiology, 75–77
Welding: and occupational lung disease, 225–226

Z

Zoster-varicella virus, 128–129

Beclovent®   PRODUCT INFORMATION
(beclomethasone dipropionate, USP)
Inhalation Aerosol

For Oral Inhalation Only

DESCRIPTION: Beclomethasone dipropionate, USP, the active component of Beclovent® Inhalation Aerosol, is an anti-inflammatory steroid having the chemical name 9-chloro-11β,17,21-trihydroxy-16β-methylpregna-1,4-diene-3,20-dione 17,21-dipropionate and the following chemical structure:

Beclovent Inhalation Aerosol is a metered-dose aerosol unit containing a microcrystalline suspension of beclomethasone dipropionate-trichloromonofluoromethane clathrate in a mixture of propellants (trichloromonofluoromethane and dichlorodifluoromethane) with oleic acid. Each canister contains beclomethasone dipropionate-trichloromonofluoromethane clathrate having a molecular proportion of beclomethasone dipropionate to trichloromonofluoromethane between 3:1 and 3:2. Each actuation delivers from the mouthpiece a quantity of clathrate equivalent to 42 mcg of beclomethasone dipropionate, USP. The contents of one canister provide at least 200 oral inhalations.

CLINICAL PHARMACOLOGY: Beclomethasone 17,21-dipropionate is a diester of beclomethasone, a synthetic halogenated corticosteroid. Animal studies show that beclomethasone dipropionate has potent anti-inflammatory activity. When beclomethasone dipropionate was administered systemically to mice, the anti-inflammatory activity was accompanied by other features typical of glucocorticoid action, including thymic involution, liver glycogen deposition, and pituitary-adrenal suppression. However, after systemic administration of beclomethasone dipropionate to rats, the anti-inflammatory action was associated with little or no effect on other tests of glucocorticoid activity.

Beclomethasone dipropionate is sparingly soluble and is poorly mobilized from subcutaneous or intramuscular injection sites. However, systemic absorption occurs after all routes of administration. When given to animals in the form of an aerosolized suspension of the trichloromonofluoromethane clathrate, the drug is deposited in the mouth and nasal passages, the trachea and principal bronchi, and the lung; a considerable portion of the drug is also swallowed. Absorption occurs rapidly from all respiratory and gastrointestinal tissues, as indicated by the rapid clearance of radioactively labeled drug from local tissues and appearance of tracer in the circulation. There is no evidence of tissue storage of beclomethasone dipropionate or its metabolites. Lung slices can metabolize beclomethasone dipropionate rapidly to beclomethasone 17-monopropionate and more slowly to free beclomethasone (which has very weak anti-inflammatory activity). However, irrespective of the route of administration (injection, oral, or aerosol), the principal route of excretion of the drug and its metabolites is the feces. Less than 10% of the drug and its metabolites is excreted in the urine. In humans, 12%-15% of an orally administered dose of beclomethasone dipropionate was excreted in the urine as both conjugated and free metabolites of the drug.

The mechanisms responsible for the anti-inflammatory action of beclomethasone dipropionate are unknown. The precise mechanism of the aerosolized drug's action in the lung is also unknown.

INDICATIONS AND USAGE: Beclovent® Inhalation Aerosol is indicated only for patients who require chronic treatment with corticosteroids for control of the symptoms of bronchial asthma. Such patients would include those already receiving systemic

Beclovent® (beclomethasone dipropionate, USP)
Inhalation Aerosol

corticosteroids, and selected patients who are inadequately controlled on a nonsteroid regimen and in whom steroid therapy has been withheld because of concern over potential adverse effects.

Beclovent Inhalation Aerosol is NOT indicated:
1. For relief of asthma that can be controlled by bronchodilators and other nonsteroid medications.
2. In patients who require systemic corticosteroid treatment infrequently.
3. In the treatment of nonasthmatic bronchitis.

CONTRAINDICATIONS: Beclovent® Inhalation Aerosol is contraindicated in the primary treatment of status asthmaticus or other acute episodes of asthma where intensive measures are required.

Hypersensitivity to any of the ingredients of this preparation contraindicates its use.

WARNINGS:

Particular care is needed in patients who are transferred from systemically active corticosteroids to Beclovent® Inhalation Aerosol because deaths due to adrenal insufficiency have occurred in asthmatic patients during and after transfer from systemic corticosteroids to aerosol beclomethasone dipropionate. After withdrawal from systemic corticosteroids, a number of months are required for recovery of hypothalamic-pituitary-adrenal (HPA) function. During this period of HPA suppression, patients may exhibit signs and symptoms of adrenal insufficiency when exposed to trauma, surgery, or infections, particularly gastroenteritis. Although Beclovent Inhalation Aerosol may provide control of asthmatic symptoms during these episodes, it does NOT provide the systemic steroid that is necessary for coping with these emergencies.

During periods of stress or a severe asthmatic attack, patients who have been withdrawn from systemic corticosteroids should be instructed to resume systemic steroids (in large doses) immediately and to contact their physician for further instruction. These patients should also be instructed to carry a warning card indicating that they may need supplementary systemic steroids during periods of stress or a severe asthma attack. To assess the risk of adrenal insufficiency in emergency situations, routine tests of adrenal cortical function, including measurement of early morning resting cortisol levels, should be performed periodically in all patients. An early morning resting cortisol level may be accepted as normal only if it falls at or near the normal mean level.

Children who are on immunosuppressant drugs are more susceptible to infections than healthy children. Chickenpox and measles, for example, can have a more serious or even fatal course in children on immunosuppressant corticosteroids. In such children, or in adults who have not had these diseases, particular care should be taken to avoid exposure. If exposed, therapy with varicella zoster immune globulin (VZIG) or pooled intravenous immunoglobulin (IVIG), as appropriate, may be indicated. If chickenpox develops, treatment with antiviral agents may be considered.

Localized infections with *Candida albicans* or *Aspergillus niger* have occurred frequently in the mouth and pharynx and occasionally in the larynx. Positive cultures for oral *Candida* may be present in up to 75% of patients. Although the frequency of clinically apparent infection is considerably lower, these infections may require treatment with appropriate antifungal therapy or discontinuation of treatment with Beclovent Inhalation Aerosol.

Beclovent Inhalation Aerosol is not to be regarded as a bronchodilator and is not indicated for rapid relief of bronchospasm.

Patients should be instructed to contact their physician immediately when episodes of asthma that are not responsive to bronchodilators occur during the course of treatment with Beclovent Inhalation Aerosol. During such episodes, patients may require therapy with systemic corticosteroids.

Beclovent® (beclomethasone dipropionate, USP)
Inhalation Aerosol

There is no evidence that control of asthma can be achieved by the administration of Beclovent Inhalation Aerosol in amounts greater than the recommended doses.

Transfer of patients from systemic steroid therapy to Beclovent Inhalation Aerosol may unmask allergic conditions previously suppressed by the systemic steroid therapy, e.g., rhinitis, conjunctivitis, and eczema.

PRECAUTIONS: During withdrawal from oral steroids, some patients may experience symptoms of systemically active steroid withdrawal, e.g., joint and/or muscular pain, lassitude, and depression, despite maintenance or even improvement of respiratory function (see DOSAGE AND ADMINISTRATION).

In responsive patients, beclomethasone dipropionate may permit control of asthmatic symptoms without suppression of HPA function, as discussed below (see CLINICAL STUDIES). Since beclomethasone dipropionate is absorbed into the circulation and can be systemically active, the beneficial effects of Beclovent® Inhalation Aerosol in minimizing or preventing HPA dysfunction may be expected only when recommended dosages are not exceeded.

The long-term effects of beclomethasone dipropionate in human subjects are still unknown. In particular, the local effects of the agent on developmental or immunologic processes in the mouth, pharynx, trachea, and lung are unknown. There is also no information about the possible long-term systemic effects of the agent.

The potential effects of Beclovent Inhalation Aerosol on acute, recurrent, or chronic pulmonary infections, including active or quiescent tuberculosis, are not known. Similarly, the potential effects of long-term administration of the drug on lung or other tissues are unknown.

Pulmonary infiltrates with eosinophilia may occur in patients on Beclovent Inhalation Aerosol therapy. Although it is possible that in some patients this state may become manifest because of systemic steroid withdrawal when inhalational steroids are administered, a causative role for beclomethasone dipropionate and/or its vehicle cannot be ruled out.

Information for Patients: Patients who are on immunosuppressant doses of corticosteroids should be warned to avoid exposure to chickenpox or measles and, if exposed, to obtain medical advice.

Pregnancy: *Teratogenic Effects:* Glucocorticoids are known teratogens in rodent species and beclomethasone dipropionate is no exception.

Teratology studies were done in rats, mice, and rabbits treated with subcutaneous beclomethasone dipropionate. Beclomethasone dipropionate was found to produce fetal resorption, cleft palate, agnathia, microstomia, absence of tongue, delayed ossification, and partial agenesis of the thymus. Well-controlled trials relating to fetal risk in humans are not available. Glucocorticoids are secreted in human milk. It is not known whether beclomethasone dipropionate would be secreted in human milk, but it is safe to assume that it is likely. The use of beclomethasone dipropionate in pregnant women, nursing mothers, or women of childbearing potential requires that the possible benefits of the drug be weighed against the potential hazards to the mother, embryo, or fetus. Infants born of mothers who have received substantial doses of corticosteroids during pregnancy should be carefully observed for hypoadrenalism.

ADVERSE REACTIONS: Deaths due to adrenal insufficiency have occurred in asthmatic patients during and after transfer from systemic corticosteroids to aerosol beclomethasone dipropionate (see WARNINGS).

Suppression of HPA function (reduction of early morning plasma cortisol levels) has been reported in adult patients who received 1,600-mcg daily doses of Beclovent® Inhalation Aerosol for 1 month. A few patients on Beclovent Inhalation Aerosol have complained of hoarseness or dry mouth.

Rare cases of immediate and delayed hypersensitivity reactions, including urticaria, angioedema, rash, and bronchospasm, have been reported after the use of beclomethasone oral or intranasal inhalers.

DOSAGE AND ADMINISTRATION: Adults and Children 12 Years of Age and Older: The usual recommended dosage is two inhalations (84 mcg) given three or four times a day. Alternatively, four inhalations (168 mcg) given twice daily has been shown to be effective in some patients. In patients with severe asthma, it is advisable to start with 12-16 inhalations a day and adjust the dosage downward according to the response of the patient. The maximal daily intake should not exceed 20 inhalations, 840 mcg (0.84 mg), in adults.

Children 6-12 Years of Age: The usual recommended dosage is one or two inhalations (42-84 mcg) given three or four times a day according to the response of the patient. Alternatively, four inhalations (168 mcg) given twice daily has been shown to be effective in some patients. The maximal daily intake should not exceed 10 inhalations, 420 mcg (0.42 mg), in children 6-12 years of age. Insufficient clinical data exist with respect to administration of Beclovent® Inhalation Aerosol in children below the age of 6.

Rinsing the mouth after inhalation is advised.

Patients receiving bronchodilators by inhalation should be advised to use the bronchodilator before Beclovent Inhalation Aerosol in order to enhance penetration of beclomethasone dipropionate into the bronchial tree. After use of an aerosol bronchodilator, several minutes should elapse before use of the Beclovent Inhalation Aerosol to reduce the potential toxicity from the inhaled fluorocarbon propellants in the two aerosols.

Different considerations must be given to the following groups of patients in order to obtain the full therapeutic benefit of Beclovent Inhalation Aerosol.

Patients Not Receiving Systemic Steroids: The use of Beclovent Inhalation Aerosol is straightforward in patients who are inadequately controlled with nonsteroid medications but in whom systemic steroid therapy has been withheld because of concern over potential adverse reactions. In patients who respond to Beclovent Inhalation Aerosol, an improvement in pulmonary function is usually apparent within 1-4 weeks after the start of Beclovent Inhalation Aerosol.

Patients Receiving Systemic Steroids: In those patients dependent on systemic steroids, transfer to Beclovent Inhalation Aerosol and subsequent management may be more difficult because recovery from impaired adrenal function is usually slow. Such suppression has been known to last for up to 12 months. Clinical studies, however, have demonstrated that Beclovent Inhalation Aerosol may be effective in the management of these asthmatic patients and may permit replacement or significant reduction in the dosage of systemic corticosteroids.

The patient's asthma should be reasonably stable before treatment with Beclovent Inhalation Aerosol is started. Initially, the aerosol should be used concurrently with the patient's usual maintenance dose of systemic steroid. After approximately 1 week, gradual withdrawal of the systemic steroid is started by reducing the daily or alternate-daily dose. The next reduction is made after an interval of 1 or 2 weeks, depending on the response of the patient. Generally, these decrements should not exceed 2.5 mg of prednisone or its equivalent. A slow rate of withdrawal cannot be overemphasized. During withdrawal some patients may experience symptoms of systemically active steroid withdrawal, e.g., joint and/or muscular pain, lassitude, and depression, despite maintenance or even improvement of respiratory function. Such patients should be encouraged to continue with the inhaler but should be watched carefully for objective signs of adrenal insufficiency such as hypotension and weight loss. If evidence of adrenal insufficiency occurs, the systemic steroid dose should be boosted temporarily and thereafter further withdrawal should continue more slowly.

During periods of stress or a severe asthma attack, transfer patients will require supplementary treatment with systemic steroids. Exacerbations of asthma that occur during the course of treatment with Beclovent Inhalation Aerosol should be treated with a short course of systemic steroid that is gradually tapered as these symptoms subside. There is no evidence that control of asthma can be achieved by administration of Beclovent Inhalation Aerosol in amounts greater than the recommended doses.

Directions for Use: Illustrated Patient's Instructions for Use accompany each package of Beclovent Inhalation Aerosol.

CONTENTS UNDER PRESSURE. Do not puncture. Do not use or store near heat or open flame. Exposure to temperatures above 120°F may cause bursting. Never throw

Beclovent® (beclomethasone dipropionate, USP)
Inhalation Aerosol

container into fire or incinerator. Keep out of reach of children.

HOW SUPPLIED: Beclovent® Inhalation Aerosol is supplied in a 16.8-g canister containing 200 metered inhalations with oral adapter and patient's instructions (NDC 0173-0312-88). Also available is a 16.8-g refill canister only with patient's instructions (NDC 0173-0360-98).
Store between 2° and 30°C (36° and 86°F). As with most inhaled medications in aerosol canisters, the therapeutic effect of this medication may decrease when the canister is cold. Shake well before using.

ANIMAL PHARMACOLOGY AND TOXICOLOGY: Studies in a number of animal species, including rats, rabbits, and dogs, have shown no unusual toxicity during acute experiments. However, the effects of beclomethasone dipropionate in producing signs of glucocorticoid excess during chronic administration by various routes were dose related.

CLINICAL STUDIES: The effects of beclomethasone dipropionate on HPA function have been evaluated in adult volunteers. There was no suppression of early morning plasma cortisol concentrations when beclomethasone dipropionate was administered in a dose of 1,000 mcg per day for 1 month as an aerosol or for 3 days by intramuscular injection. However, partial suppression of plasma cortisol concentration was observed when beclomethasone dipropionate was administered in doses of 2,000 mcg per day either intramuscularly or by aerosol. Immediate suppression of plasma cortisol concentrations was observed after single doses of 4,000 mcg of beclomethasone dipropionate.
   In one study the effects of beclomethasone dipropionate on HPA function were examined in patients with asthma. There was no change in basal early morning plasma cortisol concentrations or in the cortisol responses to tetracosactrin (ACTH 1:24) stimulation after daily administration of 400, 800, or 1,200 mcg of beclomethasone dipropionate for 28 days. After daily administration of 1,600 mcg each day for 28 days, there was slight reduction in basal cortisol concentrations and a statistically significant ($p<.01$) reduction in plasma cortisol responses to tetracosactrin stimulation. The effects of a more prolonged period of beclomethasone dipropionate administration on HPA function have not been evaluated. However, a number of investigators have noted that when systemic corticosteroid therapy in asthmatic subjects can be replaced with recommended doses of beclomethasone dipropionate, there is gradual recovery of endogenous cortisol concentrations to the normal range. There is still no documented evidence of recovery from other adverse systemic corticosteroid-induced reactions during prolonged therapy of patients with beclomethasone dipropionate.
   Clinical experience has shown that some patients with bronchial asthma who require corticosteroid therapy for control of symptoms can be partially or completely withdrawn from systemic corticosteroids if therapy with beclomethasone dipropionate aerosol is substituted. Beclomethasone dipropionate aerosol is not effective for all patients with bronchial asthma or at all stages of the disease in a given patient.
   The early clinical experience has revealed several new problems that may be associated with the use of beclomethasone dipropionate by inhalation for treatment of patients with bronchial asthma.
   1. There is a risk of adrenal insufficiency when patients are transferred from systemic corticosteroids to aerosol beclomethasone dipropionate. Although the aerosol may provide adequate control of asthma during the transfer period, it does not provide the systemic steroid that is needed during acute stress situations. Deaths due to adrenal insufficiency have occurred in asthmatic patients during and after transfer from systemic corticosteroids to aerosol beclomethasone dipropionate (see WARNINGS).
   2. Transfer of patients from systemic steroid therapy to beclomethasone dipropionate aerosol may unmask allergic conditions that were previously controlled by the systemic steroid therapy, e.g., rhinitis, conjunctivitis, and eczema.
   3. Localized infections with *Candida albicans* or *Aspergillus niger* have occurred frequently in the mouth and

Beclovent® (beclomethasone dipropionate, USP)
Inhalation Aerosol

pharynx and occasionally in the larynx. It has been reported that up to 75% of the patients who receive prolonged treatment with beclomethasone dipropionate have positive oral cultures for *Candida albicans*. The incidence of clinically apparent infection is considerably lower but may require therapy with appropriate antifungal agents or discontinuation of treatment with beclomethasone dipropionate aerosol.
   The long-term effects of beclomethasone dipropionate in human subjects are still unknown. In particular, the local effects of the agent on developmental or immunologic processes in the mouth, pharynx, trachea, and lung are unknown. There is also no information about the possible long-term systemic effects of the agent. The possible relevance of the data in animal studies to results in human subjects cannot be evaluated.

January 1992

Allen & Hanburys®
DIVISION OF GLAXO INC.
Research Triangle Park, NC 27709

Ventolin® Inhalation Aerosol   PRODUCT INFORMATION
(albuterol, USP)
Bronchodilator Aerosol
For Oral Inhalation Only

Ventolin Rotacaps® for Inhalation
(albuterol sulfate, USP)
For Inhalation Only

Ventolin® Inhalation Solution, 0.5%*
(albuterol sulfate, USP)
*Potency expressed as albuterol.

Ventolin® Syrup
(albuterol sulfate)

Ventolin® Tablets
(albuterol sulfate, USP)

DESCRIPTION: The active component of **Ventolin® Inhalation Aerosol** is albuterol, USP, racemic (α^1-[(tert-butylamino)methyl]-4-hydroxy-m-xylene-α,α'—diol) and a relatively selective beta$_2$-adrenergic bronchodilator having the following chemical structure:

Albuterol is the official generic name in the United States. The World Health Organization recommended name for the drug is salbutamol. The molecular weight of albuterol is 239.3, and the empirical formula is $C_{13}H_{21}NO_3$. Albuterol is a white to off-white crystalline solid. It is soluble in ethanol, sparingly soluble in water, and very soluble in chloroform.

Ventolin Inhalation Aerosol is a metered-dose aerosol unit for oral inhalation. It contains a microcrystalline (95%≤10 μm) suspension of albuterol in propellants (trichloromonofluoromethane and dichlorodifluoromethane) with oleic acid. Each actuation delivers from the mouthpiece 90 mcg of albuterol. Each canister provides at least 200 inhalations.

The active component of **Ventolin Rotacaps® for Inhalation, Ventolin® Inhalation Solution, Ventolin® Syrup, and Ventolin® Tablets** is albuterol sulfate, the racemic form of albuterol and a relatively selective beta$_2$-adrenergic bronchodilator. It has the chemical name α^1-[(tert-butylamino)methyl]-4-hydroxy-m-xylene-α,α'-diol sulfate (2:1)(salt) and the following chemical structure:

Albuterol sulfate has a molecular weight of 576.7, and the empirical formula is $(C_{13}H_{21}NO_3)_2 \cdot H_2SO_4$. Albuterol sulfate is a white crystalline powder, soluble in water and slightly soluble in ethanol.

The World Health Organization recommended name for albuterol base is salbutamol.

Ventolin Rotacaps for Inhalation contain a dry powder presentation of albuterol sulfate intended for oral inhalation only. Each light blue and clear, hard gelatin capsule contains a mixture of 200 mcg of microfine (95%≤10 μm) albuterol (as the sulfate) with 25 mg of lactose. The contents of each capsule are inhaled using a specially designed plastic device for inhaling

Ventolin® (albuterol, USP) Inhalation Aerosol
Bronchodilator Aerosol For Oral Inhalation Only
Ventolin Rotacaps® (albuterol sulfate, USP) for Inhalation
For Inhalation Only
Ventolin® (albuterol sulfate, USP) Inhalation Solution, 0.5%* *Potency expressed as albuterol.
Ventolin® (albuterol sulfate) Syrup
Ventolin® (albuterol sulfate, USP) Tablets

powder called the Rotahaler®. When turned, this device opens the capsule and facilitates dispersion of the albuterol sulfate into the airstream created when the patient inhales through the mouthpiece. Ventolin Rotacaps for Inhalation are an alternative inhalation form of albuterol to the metered-dose pressurized inhaler.

Ventolin Inhalation Solution is in concentrated form. Dilute 0.5 mL of the solution with 2.5 mL of sterile normal saline solution before administration. Each milliliter of Ventolin Inhalation Solution contains 5 mg of albuterol (as 6 mg of albuterol sulfate) in an aqueous solution containing benzalkonium chloride; sulfuric acid is used to adjust the pH to between 3 and 5. Ventolin Inhalation Solution contains no sulfiting agents. Ventolin Inhalation Solution is a clear, colorless to light yellow solution.

Ventolin Syrup contains 2 mg of albuterol as 2.4 mg of albuterol sulfate in each teaspoonful (5 mL). Ventolin Syrup also contains the inactive ingredients citric acid, FD&C Yellow No. 6, hydroxypropyl methylcellulose, saccharin sodium, sodium benzoate, sodium citrate, artificial strawberry flavor, and purified water.

Each **Ventolin Tablet** contains 2 or 4 mg of albuterol as 2.4 or 4.8 mg, respectively, of albuterol sulfate. Each tablet also contains the inactive ingredients corn starch, lactose, and magnesium stearate.

CLINICAL PHARMACOLOGY: *In vitro* studies and *in vivo* pharmacologic studies have demonstrated that albuterol has a preferential effect on beta$_2$-adrenergic receptors compared with isoproterenol. While it is recognized that beta$_2$-adrenergic receptors are the predominant receptors in bronchial smooth muscle, recent data indicate that there is a population of beta$_2$-receptors in the human heart existing in a concentration between 10% and 50%. The precise function of these, however, is not yet established (see WARNINGS).

The pharmacologic effects of beta-adrenergic agonist drugs, including albuterol, are at least in part attributable to stimulation through beta-adrenergic receptors of intracellular adenyl cyclase, the enzyme that catalyzes the conversion of adenosine triphosphate (ATP) to cyclic-3',5'-adenosine monophosphate (cyclic AMP). Increased cyclic AMP levels are associated with relaxation of bronchial smooth muscle and inhibition of release of mediators of immediate hypersensitivity from cells, especially from mast cells.

Albuterol has been shown in most controlled clinical trials to have more effect on the respiratory tract, in the form of bronchial smooth muscle relaxation, than isoproterenol at comparable doses while producing fewer cardiovascular effects. Controlled clinical studies and other clinical experience have shown that inhaled albuterol, like other beta-adrenergic agonist drugs, can produce a significant cardiovascular effect in some patients, as measured by pulse rate, blood pressure, symptoms, and/or electrocardiographic changes.

Albuterol is longer acting than isoproterenol in most patients by any route of administration because it is not a substrate for the cellular uptake processes for catecholamines nor for catechol-O-methyl transferase.

Because of its gradual absorption from the bronchi, systemic levels of albuterol are low after inhalation of recommended doses. Studies undertaken with four subjects administered tritiated albuterol from a metered-dose aerosol inhaler resulted in maximum plasma concentrations occurring within 2-4 hours. Due to the sensitivity of the assay method, the metabolic rate and half-life of elimination of albuterol in plasma could not be determined. However, urinary excretion provided data indicating that albuterol has an elimination half-life of 3.8 hours. Approximately 72% of the inhaled dose is excreted within 24 hours in the urine, and consists of 28% as unchanged drug and 44% as metabolite.

Studies in asthmatic patients have shown that less than

Ventolin® (albuterol, USP) Inhalation Aerosol
Bronchodilator Aerosol For Oral Inhalation Only
Ventolin Rotacaps® (albuterol sulfate, USP) for Inhalation
For Inhalation Only
Ventolin® (albuterol sulfate, USP) Inhalation Solution,
0.5%* *Potency expressed as albuterol.
Ventolin® (albuterol sulfate) Syrup
Ventolin® (albuterol sulfate, USP) Tablets

Ventolin® (albuterol, USP) Inhalation Aerosol
Bronchodilator Aerosol For Oral Inhalation Only
Ventolin Rotacaps® (albuterol sulfate, USP) for Inhalation
For Inhalation Only
Ventolin® (albuterol sulfate, USP) Inhalation Solution,
0.5%* *Potency expressed as albuterol.
Ventolin® (albuterol sulfate) Syrup
Ventolin® (albuterol sulfate, USP) Tablets

20% of a single albuterol dose was absorbed following either intermittent positive-pressure breathing (IPPB) or nebulizer administration; the remaining amount was recovered from the nebulizer and apparatus and expired air. Most of the absorbed dose was recovered in the urine 24 hours after drug administration. Following a 3-mg dose of nebulized albuterol, the maximum albuterol plasma levels at 0.5 hours were 2.1 ng/mL (range, 1.4-3.2 ng/mL). There was a significant dose-related response in FEV_1 (forced expiratory volume in 1 second) and peak flow rate. It has been demonstrated that following oral administration of 4 mg of albuterol, the elimination half-life was 5-6 hours.

Albuterol is rapidly absorbed after oral administration of 10 mL of Ventolin® Syrup (4 mg of albuterol) and of 4-mg Ventolin® Tablets in normal volunteers. Maximum plasma concentrations of about 18 ng/mL of albuterol are achieved within 2 hours, and the drug is eliminated with a half-life of about 5 hours.

In other studies, the analysis of urine samples of patients given 8 mg of tritiated albuterol orally showed that 76% of the dose was excreted over 3 days, with the majority of the dose being excreted within the first 24 hours. Sixty percent of this radioactivity was shown to be the metabolite. Feces collected over this period contained 4% of the administered dose. Animal studies show that albuterol does not pass the blood-brain barrier.

Recent studies in laboratory animals (minipigs, rodents, and dogs) recorded the occurrence of cardiac arrhythmias and sudden death (with histologic evidence of myocardial necrosis) when beta-agonists and methylxanthines were administered concurrently. The significance of these findings when applied to humans is currently unknown.

The effects of rising doses of albuterol and isoproterenol aerosols were studied in volunteers and asthmatic patients. Results in normal volunteers indicated that albuterol is one half to one quarter as active as isoproterenol in producing increases in heart rate. In asthmatic patients similar cardiovascular differentiation between the two drugs was also seen.

In controlled clinical trials with Ventolin® Inhalation Aerosol involving adults with asthma, the onset of improvement in pulmonary function was within 15 minutes, as determined by both MMEF (maximum midexpiratory flow rate) and FEV_1. MMEF measurements also showed that near maximum improvement in pulmonary function generally occurs within 60-90 minutes following two inhalations of albuterol and that clinically significant improvement generally continues for 3-4 hours in most patients. Some patients showed a therapeutic response (defined as maintaining FEV_1 values 15% or more above baseline) that was still apparent at 6 hours. Continued effectiveness of albuterol was demonstrated over a 13-week period in these same trials.

In controlled clinical trials involving children 4-12 years of age, FEV_1 measurements showed that maximum improvement in pulmonary function occurs within 30-60 minutes. The onset of clinically significant (≥15%) improvement in FEV_1 was observed as soon as 5 minutes following 180 mcg of albuterol in 18 of 30 (60%) children in a controlled dose-ranging study. Clinically significant improvement in FEV_1 continued in the majority of patients for 2 hours and in 33%-47% for 4 hours among 56 patients receiving inhalation aerosol in one pediatric study. In a second study among 48 patients receiving inhalation aerosol, clinically significant improvement continued in the majority for up to 1 hour and in 23%-40% for 4 hours. In addition, at least 50% of the patients in both studies achieved an improvement in $FEF_{25\%-75\%}$ (forced expiratory flow rate between 25% and 75% of the forced vital capacity) of at least 20% for 2-5 hours. Continued effectiveness of albuterol was demonstrated over the 12-week study period.

In other clinical studies, two inhalations of albuterol taken approximately 15 minutes before exercise prevented exercise-induced bronchospasm, as demonstrated by the maintenance of FEV_1 within 80% of baseline values in the majority of patients. One of these studies also evaluated the duration of the prophylactic effect to repeated exercise challenges, which was evident at 4 hours in the majority of patients and at 6 hours in approximately one third of the patients.

In single, dose-range, crossover trials with Ventolin Rotacaps® for Inhalation in patients 12 years of age and older, the onset of improvement in pulmonary function was within 5 minutes, as determined by a 15% increase in FEV_1 following administration of either a 200- or 400-mcg dose. Maximum increases in FEV_1 occurred within 60 minutes following inhalation of either dose. The duration of effect (defined as an increase in FEV_1 of 15% or greater in a single-dose study) was 1-2 hours after the 200-mcg dose and 3-4 hours after the 400-mcg dose. In a single-dose study, an increase in $FEF_{25\%-75\%}$ of 20% or greater continued for 3-4 hours after the 200-mcg dose and for 3-6 hours following the 400-mcg dose. A therapeutic response continued for 4 hours in the majority of patients and for 6 hours in 38% of the patients following the 400-mcg dose. Twenty-two percent of the patients receiving 200-mcg dose had a duration of effect of 8 hours.

In 12-week, double-blind, comparative evaluations in patients 12 years of age and older of one 200-mcg Ventolin Rotacaps for Inhalation capsule versus two inhalations of Ventolin Inhalation Aerosol, the two dosage regimens were found to be equivalent. Based on a 15% or more increase in FEV_1 determinations, both provided a therapeutic response that persisted for 2 or 3 hours in 50% of 231 patients aged 12 years and older. Similar results were found in two controlled, 12-week clinical trials involving 204 children aged 4-11 years. Both formulations produced a therapeutic response (defined as maintenance of mean increase over baseline of at least 15% in FEV_1, or 20% in $FEF_{25\%-75\%}$). Therapeutic improvement of $FEF_{25\%-75\%}$ persisted for 3-5 hours in over 50% of the children throughout the study. Continued effectiveness and safety of Ventolin Rotacaps for Inhalation were demonstrated over the 12-week study periods in both adults and children.

In controlled clinical trials with Ventolin® Inhalation Solution, most patients exhibited an onset of improvement in pulmonary function within 5 minutes as determined by FEV_1. FEV_1 measurements also showed that the maximum average improvement in pulmonary function usually occurred at approximately 1 hour following inhalation of 2.5 mg of albuterol by compressor-nebulizer and remained close to peak for 2 hours. Clinically significant improvement in pulmonary function (defined as maintenance of a 15% or more increase in FEV_1 over baseline values) continued for 3-4 hours in most patients, with some patients continuing up to 6 hours. In repetitive dose studies, continued effectiveness was demonstrated throughout the 3-month period of treatment in some patients.

In controlled clinical trials with Ventolin Syrup and Ventolin Tablets in patients with asthma, the onset of improvement in pulmonary function, as measured by MMEF and FEV_1 and by MMEF, respectively, was within 30 minutes, with peak improvement occurring between 2 and 3 hours.

In a controlled clinical trial with Ventolin Syrup involving 55 children, clinically significant improvement (defined as maintenance of mean values over baseline of 15%-20% or more in the FEV_1 and MMEF, respectively) continued to be recorded up to 6 hours. No decrease in the effectiveness was reported in one uncontrolled study of 32 children who took Ventolin Syrup for a 3-month period.

In controlled clinical trials with Ventolin Tablets in which measurements were conducted for 6 hours, clinically significant improvement (defined as maintaining a 15% or more increase in

Ventolin® (albuterol, USP) Inhalation Aerosol
Bronchodilator Aerosol For Oral Inhalation Only
Ventolin Rotacaps® (albuterol sulfate, USP) for Inhalation
For Inhalation Only
Ventolin® (albuterol sulfate, USP) Inhalation Solution,
0.5%* *Potency expressed as albuterol.
Ventolin® (albuterol sulfate) Syrup
Ventolin® (albuterol sulfate, USP) Tablets

Ventolin® (albuterol, USP) Inhalation Aerosol
Bronchodilator Aerosol For Oral Inhalation Only
Ventolin Rotacaps® (albuterol sulfate, USP) for Inhalation
For Inhalation Only
Ventolin® (albuterol sulfate, USP) Inhalation Solution,
0.5%* *Potency expressed as albuterol.
Ventolin® (albuterol sulfate) Syrup
Ventolin® (albuterol sulfate, USP) Tablets

FEV_1 and a 20% or more increase in MMEF over baseline values) was observed in 60% of patients at 4 hours and in 40% at 6 hours. In other single-dose, controlled clinical trials, clinically significant improvement was observed in at least 40% of the patients at 8 hours. No decrease in the effectiveness of Ventolin Tablets has been reported in patients who received long-term treatment with the drug in uncontrolled studies for periods up to 6 months.

INDICATIONS AND USAGE: Ventolin® Inhalation Aerosol is indicated for the prevention and relief of bronchospasm in patients 4 years of age and older with reversible obstructive airway disease and for the prevention of exercise-induced bronchospasm in patients 12 years of age and older. Ventolin Inhalation Aerosol can be used with or without concomitant steroid therapy.

Ventolin Rotacaps® for Inhalation are indicated for the prevention and relief of bronchospasm in patients 4 years of age and older with reversible obstructive airway disease and for the prevention of exercise-induced bronchospasm in patients 12 years of age and older. This formulation is particularly useful in patients who are unable to properly use the pressurized aerosol form of albuterol or who prefer an alternative formulation. Ventolin Rotacaps for Inhalation can be used with or without concomitant steroid therapy.

Ventolin® Inhalation Solution is indicated for the relief of bronchospasm in patients with reversible obstructive airway disease and acute attacks of bronchospasm.

Ventolin® Syrup is indicated for the relief of bronchospasm in adults and children 2 years of age and older with reversible obstructive airway disease.

Ventolin® Tablets are indicated for the relief of bronchospasm in patients with reversible obstructive airway disease.

CONTRAINDICATIONS: The Ventolin® preparations are contraindicated in patients with a history of hypersensitivity to any of the components.

WARNINGS: As with other inhaled beta-adrenergic agonists, Ventolin® Inhalation Aerosol, Ventolin Rotacaps® for Inhalation, and Ventolin® Inhalation Solution can produce paradoxical bronchospasm that can be life-threatening. If it occurs, the preparation should be discontinued immediately and alternative therapy instituted.

Fatalities have been reported in association with excessive use of inhaled sympathomimetic drugs and with the home use of nebulizers. The exact cause of death is unknown, but cardiac arrest following the unexpected development of a severe acute asthmatic crisis and subsequent hypoxia is suspected. It is therefore essential that the physician instruct the patient in the need for further evaluation if his/her asthma becomes worse. In individual patients, any $beta_2$-adrenergic agonist, including albuterol inhalation solution, may have a clinically significant cardiac effect.

Immediate hypersensitivity reactions may occur after administration of albuterol, as demonstrated by rare cases of urticaria, angioedema, rash, bronchospasm, anaphylaxis, and oropharyngeal edema. Albuterol, like other beta-adrenergic agonists, can produce a significant cardiovascular effect in some patients, as measured by pulse rate, blood pressure, symptoms, and/or electrocardiographic changes.

The contents of Ventolin Inhalation Aerosol are under pressure. Do not puncture. Do not use or store near heat or open flame. Exposure to temperatures above 120°F may cause bursting. Never throw container into fire or incinerator. Keep out of reach of children.

PRECAUTIONS:
General: Although no effect on the cardiovascular system is usually seen after the administration of inhaled albuterol at recommended doses, cardiovascular and central nervous system effects seen with all sympathomimetic drugs can occur after use of inhaled albuterol and may require discontinuation of the drug. As with all sympathomimetic amines, albuterol should be used with caution in patients with cardiovascular disorders, especially coronary insufficiency, cardiac arrhythmias, and hypertension; in patients with convulsive disorders, hyperthyroidism, or diabetes mellitus; and in patients who are unusually responsive to sympathomimetic amines. Clinically significant changes in systolic and diastolic blood pressure have been seen in individual patients and could be expected to occur in some patients after use of any beta-adrenergic bronchodilator.

Large doses of intravenous albuterol have been reported to aggravate pre-existing diabetes mellitus and ketoacidosis. As with other beta-agonists, inhaled and intravenous albuterol may produce significant hypokalemia in some patients, possibly through intracellular shunting, which has the potential to produce adverse cardiovascular effects. The decrease is usually transient, not requiring supplementation.

Although there have been no reports concerning the use of Ventolin® Inhalation Aerosol or Ventolin Rotacaps® for Inhalation during labor and delivery, it has been reported that high doses of albuterol administered intravenously inhibit uterine contractions. Although this effect is extremely unlikely as a consequence of Ventolin Inhalation Aerosol or Ventolin Rotacaps for Inhalation use, it should be kept in mind.

Information for Patients: The action of Ventolin Inhalation Aerosol, Ventolin® Inhalation Solution, and Ventolin® Syrup may last up to 6 hours; the action of Ventolin Rotacaps for Inhalation may last for 6 hours or longer; and the action of Ventolin® Tablets may last for 8 hours or longer. Therefore, they should not be used more frequently than recommended. Do not increase the dose or frequency of medication without medical consultation. If the recommended dosage does not provide relief of symptoms or symptoms become worse, seek immediate medical attention.

While taking Ventolin Inhalation Aerosol or Ventolin Rotacaps for Inhalation, other inhaled drugs should not be used unless prescribed. While taking Ventolin Inhalation Solution, other antiasthma medicines should not be used unless prescribed.

In general, the technique for administering Ventolin Inhalation Aerosol to children is similar to that for adults, since children's smaller ventilatory exchange capacity automatically provides proportionally smaller aerosol intake. Children should use Ventolin Inhalation Aerosol and Ventolin Rotacaps for Inhalation under adult supervision, as instructed by the patient's physician.

See package inserts for Ventolin Inhalation Aerosol, Ventolin Rotacaps for Inhalation, and Ventolin Inhalation Solution for illustrated Patient's Instructions for Use.

Drug Interactions: Other sympathomimetic aerosol bronchodilators or epinephrine should not be used concomitantly with albuterol. If additional adrenergic drugs are to be administered by any route to patients using Ventolin Inhalation Aerosol or Ventolin Rotacaps for Inhalation, they should be used with caution to avoid deleterious cardiovascular effects.

In addition, the concomitant use of Ventolin Syrup or Ventolin Tablets and other oral sympathomimetic agents is not recommended since such combined use may lead to deleterious cardiovascular effects. This recommendation does not preclude the judicious use of an aerosol bronchodilator of the adrenergic stimulant type in patients receiving Ventolin Syrup or Ventolin Tablets. Such concomitant use, however, should be individualized and not given on a routine basis. If regular coadministration is required, then alternative therapy should be considered.

Albuterol should be administered with extreme caution to patients being treated with monoamine oxidase inhibitors or tricyclic antidepressants because the action of albuterol on the

Ventolin® (albuterol, USP) Inhalation Aerosol
Bronchodilator Aerosol For Oral Inhalation Only
Ventolin Rotacaps® (albuterol sulfate, USP) for Inhalation
For Inhalation Only
Ventolin® (albuterol sulfate, USP) Inhalation Solution,
0.5%* *Potency expressed as albuterol.
Ventolin® (albuterol sulfate) Syrup
Ventolin® (albuterol sulfate, USP) Tablets

vascular system may be potentiated.

Beta-receptor blocking agents and albuterol inhibit the effect of each other.

Carcinogenesis, Mutagenesis, Impairment of Fertility: Albuterol sulfate, like other agents in its class, caused a significant dose-related increase in the incidence of benign leiomyomas of the mesovarium in a 2-year study in the rat at doses corresponding to 93, 463, and 2,315 times, respectively, the maximum inhalational dose for a 50-kg human; to 42, 248, and 1,042 times, respectively, the maximum inhalational dose for a 50-kg human (Ventolin Rotacaps for Inhalation); to 10, 50, and 250 times, respectively, the maximum nebulization dose for a 50-kg human; to 2, 9, and 46 times the maximum human (child weighing 21 kg) oral dose (syrup); and to 3, 16, and 78 times, respectively, the maximum oral dose for a 50-kg human (tablets). In another study this effect was blocked by the coadministration of propranolol. The relevance of these findings to humans is not known. An 18-month study in mice (at doses corresponding to 10,417 times the human inhalational dose) and a lifetime study in hamsters (at doses corresponding to 1,042 times the human inhalational dose) revealed no evidence of tumorigenicity. Studies with albuterol revealed no evidence of mutagenesis. Reproduction studies in rats (at doses corresponding to 1,042 times the human inhalational dose) revealed no evidence of impaired fertility.

Pregnancy: Teratogenic Effects: Pregnancy Category C: Albuterol has been shown to be teratogenic in mice when given subcutaneously in doses corresponding to 14 times the human aerosol dose; to five times the maximum inhalational dose (Ventolin Rotacaps for Inhalation); to 0.2 times the maximum human (child weighing 21 kg) oral dose (syrup); to 0.4 times the maximum human oral dose (tablets); and when given in doses corresponding to the human nebulization dose. There are no adequate and well-controlled studies in pregnant women. Albuterol should be used during pregnancy only if the potential benefit justifies the potential risk to the fetus.

A reproduction study in CD-1 mice given albuterol subcutaneously (0.025, 0.25, and 2.5 mg/kg, corresponding to 1.15, 11.5, and 115 times, respectively, the maximum inhalational dose for a 50-kg human; to 0.52, 5.2, and 52 times, respectively, the maximum inhalational dose for a 50-kg human [Ventolin Rotacaps for Inhalation]; to 0.1, 1, and 12.5 times the maximum human nebulization dose; and to 0.04, 0.4, and 3.9 times, respectively, the maximum oral dose for a 50-kg human [tablets]) showed cleft palate formation in 5 of 111 (4.5%) fetuses at 0.25 mg/kg and in 10 of 108 (9.3%) fetuses at 2.5 mg/kg. None was observed at 0.025 mg/kg. Cleft palate also occurred in 22 of 72 (30.5%) fetuses treated with 2.5 mg/kg of isoproterenol (positive control). A reproduction study with oral albuterol in Stride Dutch rabbits revealed cranioschisis in 7 of 19 (37%) fetuses at 50 mg/kg, corresponding to 2,315 times the maximum inhalational dose for a 50 kg human; to 1,042 times the maximum inhalational dose for a 50-kg human (Ventolin Rotacaps for Inhalation); to 250 times the maximum human nebulization dose; to 46 times the maximum human (child weighing 21 kg) oral dose (syrup) of albuterol sulfate; and to 78 times the maximum oral dose for a 50-kg human (tablets).

Labor and Delivery: Oral albuterol has been shown to delay preterm labor in some reports. There are presently no well-controlled studies that demonstrate that it will stop preterm labor or prevent labor at term. Therefore, cautious use of Ventolin Rotacaps for Inhalation, Ventolin Inhalation Solution, Ventolin Syrup, and Ventolin Tablets is required in pregnant patients when given for relief of bronchospasm so as to avoid interference with uterine contractility. Use in such patients should be restricted to those patients in whom the benefits clearly outweigh the risks.

Nursing Mothers: It is not known whether albuterol is excreted in human milk. Because of the potential for tumorigenicity shown for albuterol in some animal studies, a decision should be made whether to discontinue nursing or to discontinue the drug,

Ventolin® (albuterol, USP) Inhalation Aerosol
Bronchodilator Aerosol For Oral Inhalation Only
Ventolin Rotacaps® (albuterol sulfate, USP) for Inhalation
For Inhalation Only
Ventolin® (albuterol sulfate, USP) Inhalation Solution,
0.5%* *Potency expressed as albuterol.
Ventolin® (albuterol sulfate) Syrup
Ventolin® (albuterol sulfate, USP) Tablets

taking into account the importance of the drug to the mother.

Pediatric Use: Safety and effectiveness have not been established in children below 12 years of age for Ventolin Inhalation Solution; in children below 6 years of age for Ventolin Tablets; in children below 4 years of age for Ventolin Inhalation Aerosol and Ventolin Rotacaps for Inhalation; and in children below 2 years of age for Ventolin Syrup.

ADVERSE REACTIONS: The adverse reactions to albuterol are similar in nature to reactions to other sympathomimetic agents, although the incidence of certain cardiovascular effects is lower with albuterol. Rare cases of urticaria, angioedema, rash, bronchospasm, hoarseness, and oropharyngeal edema have been reported after the use of inhaled albuterol. In addition to the reactions given below by specific dosage form, albuterol, like other sympathomimetic agents, can cause adverse reactions such as angina, vertigo, and CNS stimulation.

Ventolin® Inhalation Aerosol: A 13-week, double-blind study compared albuterol and isoproterenol aerosols in 147 asthmatic patients aged 12 years and older. The results of this study showed that the incidence of cardiovascular effects was: palpitations, fewer than 10 per 100 with albuterol and fewer than 15 per 100 with isoproterenol; tachycardia, 10 per 100 with both albuterol and isoproterenol; and increased blood pressure, fewer than 5 per 100 with both albuterol and isoproterenol. In the same study, both drugs caused tremor or nausea in fewer than 15 patients per 100, and dizziness or heartburn in fewer than 5 per 100 patients. Nervousness occurred in fewer than 10 per 100 patients receiving albuterol and in fewer than 15 per 100 patients receiving isoproterenol.

Twelve-week, double-blind studies involving the use of Ventolin Inhalation Aerosol 180 mcg q.i.d. by 104 asthmatic children aged 4-11 years showed the following side effects:

Central Nervous System: Headache, 3 of 104 patients (3%); nervousness, lightheadedness, agitation, nightmares, hyperactivity, and aggressive behavior, each in 1%.

Gastrointestinal: Nausea and/or vomiting, 6 of 104 (6%); stomachache, 3 of 104 (3%); diarrhea in 1%.

Oropharyngeal: Throat irritation, 6 of 104 (6%); discoloration of teeth in 1%.

Respiratory: Epistaxis, 3 of 104 (3%); coughing, 2 of 104 (2%).

Musculoskeletal: Tremor and muscle cramp, each in 1%.

Ventolin Rotacaps® for Inhalation: Results of clinical trials with Ventolin Rotacaps for Inhalation 200 mcg in 172 patients aged 12 years and older (adults) and 129 patients aged 4-12 years (children) showed the following side effects:

Central Nervous System: Adults: Headache, 4 of 172 patients (2%); nervousness, 2 of 172 (1%); dizziness, insomnia, lightheadedness, each in <1%. **Children:** Headache, 6 of 129 (5%); dizziness and hyperactivity, each in <1%.

Gastrointestinal: Adults: Burning in stomach in <1%. **Children:** Nausea and/or vomiting in 5 of 129 (4%), stomachache in 2 of 129 (2%), diarrhea in <1%.

Oropharyngeal: Adults: Throat irritation in 3 of 172 (2%); dry mouth and voice changes, each in <1%. **Children:** Throat irritation in 3 of 129 (2%), unusual taste in 2 of 129 (2%).

Respiratory: Adults: Cough in 8 of 172 (5%), bronchospasm in 2 of 172 (1%). **Children:** Cough and nasal congestion, each in 3 of 129 (2%); hoarseness and epistaxis, each in 2 of 129 (2%).

Musculoskeletal: Adults: Tremor in 2 of 172 (1%). **Children:** None reported.

Ventolin® Inhalation Solution: The results of clinical trials in 135 patients showed the following side effects that were considered probably or possibly drug related:

Central Nervous System: Tremors (20%), dizziness (7%), nervousness (4%), headache (3%), insomnia (1%).

Gastrointestinal: Nausea (4%), dyspepsia (1%).

Ear, Nose, and Throat: Pharyngitis (<1%), nasal

Ventolin® (albuterol, USP) Inhalation Aerosol
Bronchodilator Aerosol For Oral Inhalation Only
Ventolin Rotacaps® (albuterol sulfate, USP) for Inhalation
For Inhalation Only
Ventolin® (albuterol sulfate, USP) Inhalation Solution,
0.5%* *Potency expressed as albuterol.
Ventolin® (albuterol sulfate) Syrup
Ventolin® (albuterol sulfate, USP) Tablets

congestion (1%).
 Cardiovascular: Tachycardia (1%), hypertension (1%).
 Respiratory: Bronchospasm (8%), cough (4%), bronchitis (4%), wheezing (1%).
 No clinically relevant laboratory abnormalities related to Ventolin Inhalation Solution administration were determined in these studies.
 In comparing the adverse reactions reported for patients treated with Ventolin Inhalation Solution with those of patients treated with isoproterenol during clinical trials of 3 months, the following moderate to severe reactions, as judged by the investigators, were reported. This table does not include mild reactions.

**Percent Incidence of Moderate to
Severe Adverse Reactions**

Reaction	Albuterol n=65	Isoproterenol n=65
Central nervous system		
Tremors	10.7%	13.8%
Headache	3.1%	1.5%
Insomnia	3.1%	1.5%
Cardiovascular		
Hypertension	3.1%	3.1%
Arrhythmias	0%	3.0%
Palpitation*	0%	22.0%
Respiratory		
Bronchospasm†	15.4%	18.0%
Cough	3.1%	5.0%
Bronchitis	1.5%	5.0%
Wheezing	1.5%	1.5%
Sputum increase	1.5%	1.5%
Dyspnea	1.5%	1.5%
Gastrointestinal		
Nausea	3.1%	0%
Dyspepsia	1.5%	0%
Systemic		
Malaise	1.5%	0%

*The finding of no arrhythmias and no palpitations after albuterol administration in this clinical study should not be interpreted as indicating that these adverse effects cannot occur after the administration of inhaled albuterol.
†In most cases of bronchospasm, this term was generally used to describe exacerbations in the underlying pulmonary disease.

Ventolin® Syrup: The most frequent adverse reactions to Ventolin Syrup in adults and older children were tremor, 10 of 100 patients, and nervousness and shakiness, each in 9 of 100 patients. Other reported adverse reactions were headache, 4 of 100 patients; dizziness and increased appetite, each in 3 of 100 patients; hyperactivity and excitement, each in 2 of 100 patients; and tachycardia, epistaxis, and sleeplessness, each in 1 of 100 patients. The following adverse effects each occurred in fewer than 1 of 100 patients: muscle spasm, disturbed sleep, epigastric pain, cough, palpitations, stomachache, irritable behavior, dilated pupils, sweating, chest pain, and weakness.
 In young children 2-6 years of age, some adverse reactions were noted more frequently than in adults and older children. Excitement was noted in approximately 20% of patients and nervousness in 15%. Hyperkinesia occurred in 4% of patients, with insomnia, tachycardia, and gastrointestinal symptoms in 2% each. Anorexia, emotional lability, pallor, fatigue, and conjunctivitis were seen in 1%.

Ventolin® Tablets: The most frequent adverse reactions to Ventolin Tablets were nervousness and tremor, with each occurring in approximately 20 of 100 patients. Other reported reactions were headache, 7 of 100 patients; tachycardia and palpitations, 5 of 100 patients; muscle cramps, 3 of 100 patients; and insomnia, nausea, weakness, and dizziness, each in 2 of 100 patients. Drowsiness, flushing, restlessness, irritability, chest discomfort, and difficulty in micturition each occurred in fewer than 1 of 100 patients.
 The reactions to Ventolin Syrup and Ventolin Tablets are generally transient in nature, and it is usually not necessary to discontinue treatment. In selected cases, however, dosage may be reduced temporarily; after the reaction has subsided, dosage should be increased in small increments to the optimal dosage.

OVERDOSAGE: The expected symptoms with overdosage are those of excessive beta-stimulation and/or occurrence or exaggeration of any of the symptoms listed under ADVERSE REACTIONS, e.g., seizures, angina, hypertension or hypotension, tachycardia with rates up to 200 beats per minute, arrhythmias, nervousness, headache, tremor, dry mouth, palpitation, nausea, dizziness, fatigue, malaise, and insomnia. Hypokalemia may also occur.
 Treatment consists of discontinuation of albuterol together with appropriate symptomatic therapy.
 As with all sympathomimetic aerosol medications, cardiac arrest and even death may be associated with abuse of aerosol albuterol.
 The oral LD_{50} in male and female rats and mice was greater than 2,000 mg/kg. The inhalational LD_{50} could not be determined.
 Dialysis is not appropriate treatment for overdosage of Ventolin® Inhalation Aerosol, Ventolin Rotacaps® for Inhalation, or Ventolin® Syrup. The judicious use of a cardioselective beta-receptor blocker, such as metoprolol tartrate, is suggested, bearing in mind the danger of inducing an asthmatic attack. There is insufficient evidence to determine if dialysis is beneficial for overdosage of Ventolin® Inhalation Solution or Ventolin® Tablets.

DOSAGE AND ADMINISTRATION:
Ventolin® Inhalation Aerosol: For treatment of acute episodes of bronchospasm or prevention of asthmatic symptoms, the usual dosage for adults and children 4 years of age and older is two inhalations repeated every 4-6 hours; in some patients, one inhalation every 4 hours may be sufficient. More frequent administration or a larger number of inhalations are not recommended.
 The use of Ventolin Inhalation Aerosol can be continued as medically indicated to control recurring bouts of bronchospasm. During this time most patients gain optimal benefit from regular use of the inhaler. Safe usage for periods extending over several years has been documented.
 If a previously effective dosage regimen fails to provide the usual relief, medical advice should be sought immediately as this is often a sign of seriously worsening asthma that would require reassessment of therapy.
 Exercise-Induced Bronchospasm Prevention: The usual dosage for adults and children 12 years of age and older is two inhalations 15 minutes before exercise.
 For treatment, see above.
Ventolin Rotacaps® for Inhalation: The usual dosage for adults and children 4 years of age and older is the contents of one 200-mcg capsule inhaled every 4-6 hours using a Rotahaler® inhalation device. In some patients, the contents of two 200-mcg capsules inhaled every 4-6 hours may be required. Larger doses or more frequent administration are not recommended.
 The use of Ventolin Rotacaps for Inhalation can be continued as medically indicated to control recurring bouts of

Ventolin® (albuterol, USP) Inhalation Aerosol
Bronchodilator Aerosol For Oral Inhalation Only
Ventolin Rotacaps® (albuterol sulfate, USP) for Inhalation
For Inhalation Only
Ventolin® (albuterol sulfate, USP) Inhalation Solution,
0.5%* *Potency expressed as albuterol.
Ventolin® (albuterol sulfate) Syrup
Ventolin® (albuterol sulfate, USP) Tablets

Ventolin® (albuterol, USP) Inhalation Aerosol
Bronchodilator Aerosol For Oral Inhalation Only
Ventolin Rotacaps® (albuterol sulfate, USP) for Inhalation
For Inhalation Only
Ventolin® (albuterol sulfate, USP) Inhalation Solution,
0.5%* *Potency expressed as albuterol.
Ventolin® (albuterol sulfate) Syrup
Ventolin® (albuterol sulfate, USP) Tablets

bronchospasm. During this time most patients gain optimal benefit from regular use of the Ventolin Rotacaps for Inhalation formulation.

If a previously effective dosage regimen fails to provide the usual relief, medical advice should be sought immediately as this is often a sign of seriously worsening asthma that would require reassessment of therapy.

Exercise-Induced Bronchospasm Prevention: The usual dosage of Ventolin Rotacaps for Inhalation for adults and children 12 years of age and older is the contents of one 200-mcg capsule inhaled using a Rotahaler 15 minutes before exercise.

Ventolin® Inhalation Solution: The usual dosage for adults and children 12 years of age and older is 2.5 mg of albuterol administered three to four times daily by nebulization. More frequent administration or higher doses are not recommended. To administer 2.5 mg of albuterol, dilute 0.5 mL of the 0.5% inhalation solution with 2.5 mL of sterile normal saline solution. The flow rate is regulated to suit the particular nebulizer so that Ventolin Inhalation Solution will be delivered over approximately 5-15 minutes.

The use of Ventolin Inhalation Solution can be continued as medically indicated to control recurring bouts of bronchospasm. During this time most patients gain optimal benefit from regular use of the inhalation solution.

If a previously effective dosage regimen fails to provide the usual relief, medical advice should be sought immediately as this is often a sign of seriously worsening asthma that would require reassessment of therapy.

Ventolin® Syrup: The following dosages of Ventolin Syrup are expressed in terms of albuterol base.

Usual Dosage: The usual starting dosage for adults and children over age 14 is 2 mg (1 teaspoonful) or 4 mg (2 teaspoonfuls) three or four times a day.

The usual starting dosage for children 6-14 years of age is 2 mg (1 teaspoonful) three or four times a day.

For children 2-6 years of age, dosing should be initiated at 0.1 mg/kg of body weight three times a day. This starting dosage should not exceed 2 mg (1 teaspoonful) three times a day.

Dosage Adjustment: For adults and children over age 14, a dosage above 4 mg four times a day should be used *only* when the patient fails to respond. If a favorable response does not occur, the dosage may be cautiously increased stepwise, but not to exceed 8 mg four times a day.

For children 6-14 years of age who fail to respond to the initial starting dosage of 2 mg four times a day, the dosage may be cautiously increased stepwise, but not to exceed 24 mg per day (given in divided doses).

For children 2-6 years of age who do not respond satisfactorily to the initial dosage, the dosage may be increased stepwise to 0.2 mg/kg of body weight three times a day, but not to exceed a maximum of 4 mg (2 teaspoonfuls) given three times a day.

Elderly Patients and Those Sensitive to Beta-adrenergic Stimulators: The initial dosage should be restricted to 2 mg three or four times a day and individually adjusted thereafter.

Ventolin® Tablets: The following dosages of Ventolin Tablets are expressed in terms of albuterol base.

Usual Dosage: The usual starting dosage for adults and children 12 years of age and older is 2 or 4 mg three or four times a day.

The usual starting dosage for children 6-12 years of age is 2 mg three or four times a day.

Dosage Adjustment: For adults and children 12 years of age and older, a dosage above 4 mg four times a day should be used only when the patient fails to respond. If a favorable response does not occur with the 4-mg initial dosage, it should be cautiously increased stepwise up to a maximum of 8 mg four times a day as tolerated.

For children 6-12 years of age who fail to respond to the

initial starting dosage of 2 mg four times a day, the dosage may be cautiously increased stepwise, but not to exceed 24 mg per day (given in divided doses).

Elderly Patients and Those Sensitive to Beta-adrenergic Stimulators: An initial dosage of 2 mg three or four times a day is recommended for elderly patients and for those with a history of unusual sensitivity to beta-adrenergic stimulators. If adequate bronchodilatation is not obtained, dosage may be increased gradually to as much as 8 mg three or four times a day.

The total daily dose should not exceed 32 mg in adults and children 12 years of age and older.

HOW SUPPLIED: Ventolin® Inhalation Aerosol is supplied in 17-g canisters containing 200 metered inhalations in boxes of one. Each actuation delivers 90 mcg of albuterol from the mouthpiece. Each canister is supplied with an oral adapter and patient's instructions (NDC 0173-0321- 88). Also available, Ventolin Inhalation Aerosol Refill 17-g canister only with patient's instructions (NDC 0173-0321-98). **Store between 15° and 30°C (59° and 86°F). As with most inhaled medications in aerosol canisters, the therapeutic effect of this medication may decrease when the canister is cold. Shake well before using.**

Ventolin Rotacaps® for Inhalation, 200 mcg, are light blue and clear, with "VENTOLIN 200" printed on the blue cap and "GLAXO" printed on the clear body. Ventolin Rotacaps for Inhalation are supplied in a unit dose kit containing one unit dose pack of 96 capsules and one Rotahaler® inhalation device (NDC 0173-0389-81) and a hospital unit dose kit containing one unit dose pack of 24 capsules and one Rotahaler inhalation device (NDC 0173-0389-03). **Store between 2° and 30°C (36° and 86°F).**

Ventolin® Inhalation Solution, 0.5% is supplied in bottles of 20 mL (NDC 0173-0385-58) with accompanying calibrated dropper in boxes of one. **Store between 2° and 30°C (36° and 86°F).**

Ventolin® Syrup, a clear, orange-yellow liquid with a strawberry flavor, contains 2 mg of albuterol as the sulfate per 5 mL in bottles of 16 fluid ounces (one pint) (NDC 0173-0351-54). **Store between 2° and 30°C (36° and 86°F).**

Ventolin® Tablets, 2 mg of albuterol as the sulfate, are white, round, compressed tablets impressed with the product name (VENTOLIN) and the number 2 on one side and scored on the other with "GLAXO" impressed on each side of the score in bottles of 100 (NDC 0173-0341-43) and 500 (NDC 0173-0341-44).

Ventolin Tablets, 4 mg of albuterol as the sulfate, are white, round, compressed tablets impressed with the product name (VENTOLIN) and the number 4 on one side and scored on the other with "GLAXO" impressed on each side of the score in bottles of 100 (NDC 0173-0342-43) and 500 (NDC 0173- 0342-44).

Store between 2° and 30°C (36° and 86°F). Replace cap securely after each opening.

Allen & Hanburys®
DIVISION OF GLAXO INC.
Research Triangle Park, NC 27709

January 1992

Ventolin® Inhalation Aerosol/Ventolin Rotacaps® for Inhalation/Ventolin® Inhalation Solution/Ventolin® Tablets: Allen & Hanburys, Research Triangle Park, NC 27709

Ventolin® Syrup:
Manufactured for Allen & Hanburys, Research Triangle Park, NC 27709 by Schering Corporation, Kenilworth, NJ 07033